The Importance of Good Nutrition, Herbs and Phytochemicals

for Your Health, Good Looks and Longevity

Getty T. Ambau

Preface by John Pfeifer, M.D.

Foreword by Jessie Goodpasture, Ph.D.

Published by

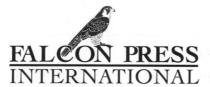

FALCON PRESS
INTERNATIONAL

P.O. Box 4113
Mountain View, CA 94040
Tele: 415-941-6691
E-mail: falconpress@slip.net

Printed and bound in the United States of America
Cover Art: by Fabrizio Camera Graphics
Cover Arrangement: by Fabrizio Camera Graphics/Getty T. Ambau
Illustrations: by Roy Minor Graphic Arts, Darrin Brunner and John Kimball
Typeset by Roy Minor of Roy Minor Graphic Arts

Library of Congress cat. card No. 93-086855
ISBN 1-884459-02-1

Important Note
The information contained in this book is meant to be used for educational purposes only. It is not meant to replace the advice or consultation of a trained professional.

ABOUT THE AUTHOR

Getty Ambau is a graduate of Yale University where he studied Molecular Biophysics and Biochemistry and Economics.

Before he started his own international distribution of health and nutritional products, he had worked as a research chemist in organic chemistry and in polymer and material sciences for several years.

A bestselling author on health and nutrition, he also holds a Master's degree in business and lives in Mountain View, California.

Dedication

This book is dedicated to my parents, who gave
me the freedom to go the distances in life.

Reader Comments

As a person interested in living a healthier, more abundant life, I have found this book to be an invaluable source and instructional tool. It is of tremendous value in understanding the way our body processes the food we eat, our body's nutritional needs and why our body needs supplements.

I appreciate that Getty has presented this detailed book in such a unique way. He has written the book to make it easy and interesting to read. He assumes the reader's intelligence while at the same time making it possible for the layman to understand complicated terms and processes. It is truly a remarkable book in many ways. I highly recommend this book to anyone who has an interest in proper nutrition ...

Dianne Radcliff
Los Gatos, California

The Importance of Good Nutrition, Herbs and Phytochemicals for Your Health, Good Looks, and Longevity presents a tremendous amount of information ... The wealth of information is written in understandable language for the lay person.

I have attended many seminars and classes on diet and nutrition, but none can compare with this comprehensive book, which gives in detail all areas of diet and good health, including all the latest information available....

Evalyne Shepherd
Bellingham, Washington

The Importance of Good Nutrition, Herbs and Phytochemicals for Your Health, Good Looks, and Longevity is an invaluable resource for my business. I find that when referring to certain sections, in order to prepare my product knowledge seminars, I keep reading on, unable to stop at the specific piece of information I need. The text is both enjoyable and understandable....

Nancy Cox-Konopelski
Santa Cruz, California

I wanted to let you know how much I am enjoying reading your book, *The Importance of Good Nutrition, Herbs and Phytochemicals for Your Health, Good Looks, and Longevity*. It is comprehensive and unusually "user friendly."

How nice to be able to refer to your book to answer a question and not only find the answer but also be able to understand the answer.

You can be sure that it will be a part of my reference library....

Enid Hey
Soquel, California

Contents

Preface

The 1990s herald a new era in health consciousness. The public has become focused on health, prevention of disease and longer life. At the same time, we are beginning to see that our crisis-oriented medical system (which is the best of its kind in the world) is a costly system and becomes more so each year. Analysis of results has suggested that crisis intervention is not the key to the management of disease. The medical care system is finally beginning to realize that prevention and nutrition may very well be the answer for many of the degenerative diseases of our society.

A simple study of current medical research and medical literature suggests that the key to survival lies in behavioral change. Cessation of smoking, the use of a high fiber, low fat diet, and regular exercise can make a difference of years of healthy active life. In the last few years, remarkable breakthroughs in nutrition have suggested that if we add to behavioral modification certain key nutritional supplements which target deficiencies in the human, we may extend life even further.

We live in a toxic society. We rarely experience clean air and pure water; the number of new toxins added to the environment multiplies each year. Thus the person of today is in a very different environment than the person of a hundred years ago. To counteract these toxins, we have now learned that antioxidant vitamins may well be vital to long-term health. At the same time, with the deficiencies in soil, we find that absorbable minerals must be added to the modern diet.

Thus, as we experience this shift from crisis orientation to prevention and nutrition, we are able to see that the person who modifies behavior and takes certain targeted supplements may very well live a more dynamic, healthy and longer life than those who ignore these factors.

This excellent book by Getty Ambau is a summary of current human needs and deals with specific nutritional topics that target and support those needs. It is an excellent and essential primer for all of those who are interested in the emerging awareness of prevention and nutrition.

John R. Pfeifer, M.D.
Adjunct Professor of Health Science, Oakland University;
Associate Clinical Professor of Surgery, Wayne University
School of Medicine

Foreword

Have you ever wondered what a free radical is, what makes a nutrient an essential nutrient, what an RDA is, what food labeling means or which foods really are good for you? These and hundreds of other questions about human nutrition are answered here by Getty Ambau. From lay beginners to health care professionals, this book acts as a teaching tool or reminder of the many faces of nutrition, and just how much can be achieved by paying attention to it.

Mr. Ambau provides a gentle beginning with topics such as nutritional allowances, units of measure and food labeling. He goes on to present in understandable terms all the components of nutrition including proteins, carbohydrates, and fats; vitamins and minerals; the food pyramid; and the all important fluid of life—water. Optimal health also depends on regular exercise, and Mr. Ambau presents an excellent chapter on what exercise really is and what forms it comes in.

Mr. Ambau steps beyond the basic components of nutrition, however, and presents state-of-the-art information on such exciting topics as amino acids and their development as "drugs of the future," agents which can do many things from fighting jet lag and curbing the appetite to treating arthritis and relieving pain.

This comprehensive book will be useful to anyone desiring to improve their health through consideration of what they allow past their lips and into their bodies. In today's world, our bodies are presented with substantial physical stresses every day, many of which can lead to ill health and some to serious ill health. These stresses range from environmental toxins to unhealthy foods, and to simply being alive another year. Fortunately, medical research has yielded much information in the recent past about how we can reduce the long term impact of these stresses on our bodies through good nutrition. It is not difficult to take advantage of this information, particularly with the availability of this book as a guide to what good nutrition is.

Treat your body with care and it will reward you. This book is an excellent beginning to helping you do so.

Jessie C. Goodpasture, Ph.D.,
Senior Clinical Program Director,
Institute of Immunology and Infectious
Diseases, Syntex Research

Acknowledgments

Most writing is a one-man show. But similar to a one-man show that can't successfully reach fruition without other production participants, writing a book like this one without the following people would not have been accomplished with any semblance of success. Therefore, I express my deep appreciation and acknowledgment to the following people.

I am grateful to Mrs. Marutha Menuhin whose exemplary lifelong commitment to healthy diet and nutrition inspired me to write this book. She died at almost 101 years of age and her remarkable wit, mental acumen and tremendous sense of humor never left her to the very end. She was also a very graceful and beautiful lady. I have no doubt that these and the aforementioned attributes were largely a result of good nutrition, good judgment, and the healthy life-style she led all her life.

I'd like to thank Dr. Jessie Goodpasture for taking time out from her busy work schedule to review this manuscript. Her comments and technical input have been invaluable. Many thanks to Al Fabrizio of Fabrizio Camera Graphics for doing an outstanding job in the design of the cover of this book and to Roy and Hinda Minor of Roy Minor Graphic Arts who spent countless hours crafting and typesetting the book and for being good friends. Also, thanks to Douglas Peck for excellent photography used on the cover of the book.

I'm thankful to Deborah Cady for editing the final manuscript and to Leila Hanson for proofing and editing the original draft of the manuscript and for being a good friend. Kudos to Darrin Brunner, John Kimball and Richard Waldron for their patience with my obsessive perfectionism. Thanks, too, for their computer wizardry with many of the illustrations in this book.

My last but not the least thanks go to Rosario Limas, Jerry Gora, Muffy Foster and Rosemary Mathson for their reviewing and proofing of the manuscript and for their support and encouragement.

"You are what you eat...

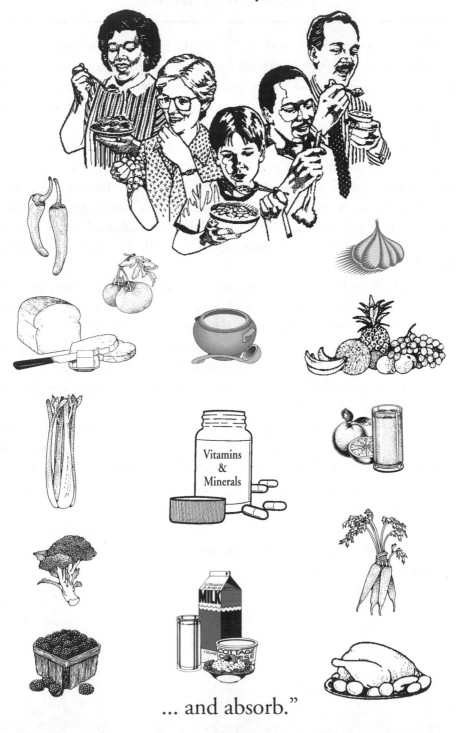

... and absorb."

Introduction

Nearly twenty-five hundred years ago, Hippocrates, the father of modern medicine, poignantly stated: *"Let thy food be thy medicine and thy medicine be thy food."* Unfortunately, this famous dictum has remained unheeded or unpracticed by man throughout history. Instead, over the centuries, man has sought plant extracts, witchcraft, or synthetic drugs to cure his ills and diseases.

The value of nutrients in foods as a way of preventing diseases or engendering good health and well-being has not always been acknowledged. Today, many of us see food merely as a device to fill an empty stomach or kill hunger. What's more, some of us also put many health-eroding, mind-altering and life-shortening substances in our bodies. Our ignorance stems largely from our lack of understanding of the impact foods or substances have on our health.

The information contained in this book is, therefore, intended to be used by anyone who wishes to learn about the basic components of nutrition and the roles these food components play in one's health and well-being.

Over the last few decades an increasing amount of research in nutrition and health care seems to indicate that if the body is kept free of the many health-eroding habits (such as excessive drinking, drugs, cigarettes) and is adequately nourished and exercised, it can properly maintain and protect itself from many harmful diseases. As mentioned above, however, the use of nutrition to build, enhance and protect the body from within seems to go contrary to our many established attitudes and practices towards it, i.e.,

- nutrition is an individual affair, and no corporation or government agency has control over what you may or may not eat. Most people, unless they have a major nutritional deficiency like scurvy (a lack of vitamin C) or beriberi (a shortage of thiamine), are lulled into believing that they are getting every thing they need from their normal diet.

- alarmingly, the problem of subclinical or marginal deficiency is rampant in this country. According to one government survey, one-third of Americans were found to be low in iron and vitamins A and C, while one-half were found to be low in B6, calcium and magnesium. Only 3% of the people surveyed were free of any deficiencies.[1] The problem with marginal and subclinical deficiencies is that they don't express themselves until later in life. When they do, they usually manifest themselves as cancer, diabetes, heart disease, etc.[2]

- the medical profession itself doesn't seem to take nutrition seriously, and nutrition is rarely taught at medical schools. For example, a survey that covered 45 of the 127 medical schools in this country found that only about one-fourth of them required even one course in nutrition.[3] According to one report, the average medical student in this country receives 2.5 hours worth of education in nutrition in his or her four years of medical school.[4] Moreover, because the nutrition field has never been a glamorous or high paying profession, not many students go into it as a career.

- since vitamins and minerals can't be patented as chemicals or drugs are, pharmaceutical companies have never found nutritional products commercially appealing. These companies would rather push their patent-protected products than treat specific ailments, although those ailments themselves may have resulted from bad diet or malnutrition.

There is an increasing amount of evidence that a good nutrition program alone can shield you from many sicknesses—from a head cold to cancer and heart disease. According to one expert "not only is nutrition an excellent tool for preventing disease, but it can also heal and improve certain conditions. Instead of using drugs and surgery to remove the *symptoms*, nutrients can often clear up the problem itself."[5] Pharmacists and doctors, however, would rather have you take drugs than suggest nutritional remedies.

- the nation's nutritional standard—the RDA—against which the nutritional values of foods are measured, has constantly been attacked by many medical and nutritional experts. Even the advocates themselves have had disagreement as to what the RDAs are supposed to do for us—whether they are to be used to protect us from slipping into nutritional deficiencies or to buffer us from the onset of diseases. This difference of opinion by the top experts who write the golden rules of our nutritional standard does little to inspire the general public's confidence in the RDAs and nutrition as a whole.

To whom, then, do you turn for your nutritional guidance? You. You become your own nutritionist, your own doctor when it comes to the food you eat. This doesn't entail your having to go to school and learning every technical detail about nutrition. It is simply knowing enough to avoid the substances known to be bad and making those that are believed to be beneficial your allies in helping you fend off diseases and slow the process of aging. This is particularly so, since several studies have shown that a well-balanced nutrition program is one of the most important methods of engendering good health, good appearance and longevity.

It's the author's best hope that the information contained in this book will assist you in becoming your own best nutritionist and that you, like many others, will not be a casualty of diseases and early death.

PART I
Nutritional Allowances and Food Labeling Reforms

Table 1.1 Recommended Dietary Allowance[1]

Category Age (years) or Condition	Weight[2] (kg)	(lb)	Height[2] (cm)	(in)	Protein (g)	Fat-Soluble Vitamins Vit. A (µg RE)	Vit. D (µg)	Vit. E (µg αTE)	Vit. K (µg)	Water-Soluble Vitamins Vit. C (mg)	Thiamin (mg)	Riboflavin (mg)	Niacin (mg)	Vit. B6 (mg)	Folate (mg)	Vit. B12 (µg)	Minerals Calcium (mg)	Phosphorus (mg)	Magnesium (mg)	Iron (mg)	Zinc (mg)	Iodine (mg)	Selenium (mg)
Infants 0.0-0.5	6	13	60	24	13	375	7.5	3	5	30	0.3	0.4	5	0.3	25	0.3	400	300	40	6	5	40	10
0.5-1.0	9	20	71	28	14	375	10	4	10	35	0.4	0.5	6	0.6	35	0.5	600	500	60	10	5	50	15
Children 1-3	13	29	90	35	16	400	10	6	15	40	0.7	0.8	9	1.0	50	0.7	800	800	80	10	10	70	20
4-6	20	44	112	44	24	500	10	7	20	45	0.9	1.1	12	1.1	75	1.0	800	800	120	10	10	90	20
7-10	28	62	132	52	28	700	10	7	30	45	1.0	1.2	13	1.4	100	1.4	800	800	170	10	10	120	30
Males 11-14	45	99	157	62	45	1000	10	10	45	50	1.3	1.5	17	1.7	150	2.0	1200	1200	270	12	15	150	40
15-18	66	145	176	69	59	1000	10	10	65	60	1.5	1.8	20	2.0	200	2.0	1200	1200	400	12	15	150	50
19-24	72	160	177	70	58	1000	10	10	70	60	1.5	1.7	19	2.0	200	2.0	1200	1200	350	10	15	150	70
25-50	79	174	176	70	63	1000	5	10	80	60	1.5	1.7	19	2.0	200	2.0	800	800	350	10	15	150	70
51 +	77	170	173	68	63	1000	5	10	80	60	1.2	1.4	15	2.0	200	2.0	800	800	350	10	15	150	70
Females 11-14	46	101	157	62	46	800	10	8	45	50	1.1	1.3	15	1.4	150	2.0	1200	1200	280	15	12	150	45
15-18	55	120	163	64	44	800	10	8	55	60	1.1	1.3	15	1.5	180	2.0	1200	1200	300	15	12	150	50
19-24	58	128	164	65	46	800	10	8	60	60	1.1	1.3	15	1.6	180	2.0	1200	1200	280	15	12	150	50
25-50	63	138	163	64	50	800	5	8	65	60	1.1	1.3	15	1.6	180	2.0	800	800	280	15	12	150	55
51 +	65	143	160	63	50	800	5	8	65	60	1.0	1.2	13	1.6	180	2.0	800	800	280	10	12	150	55
Pregnant					60	800	10	10	65	70	1.5	1.6	17	2.2	400	2.2	1200	1200	320	30	15	175	65
Lactating 1st 6 mos					65	1300	10	12	65	95	1.6	1.8	20	2.1	280	2.6	1200	1200	355	15	19	200	75
2nd 6 mos					62	1200	10	11	65	90	1.6	1.7	20	2.1	260	2.6	1200	1200	340	15	16	200	75
USRDA					45-65*	1000	10	22	—	60	1.5	1.7	20	2.0	400	2.6	1000	1000	400	18	15	150	—

* Based on protein quality: 45 grams of protein comes from eggs, fish, milk, or poultry; 65 grams if it doesn't.

1. The RDAs are given as average daily intakes over time. They are figured assuming individual variations among most normal persons that live under normal environmental stresses. They also assume that diets come from major food groups: i.e., grains, vegetables, and fruits, meats, and dairy products.

2. There new RDAs are based on actual median weights and heights rather than on ideal estimates.

Pitfalls: Aside from what has been discussed in the text, these RDAs have two major pitfalls:

a. The oldest group represented is 55+. There is no specific category for the elderly or for menopausal or postmenopausal women, as there is for pregnant or lactating women.

b. The figures in this table are only for "healthy" individuals. There are many people who don't fall into these categories and whose nutritional needs are considerably higher than what is given in this table.

CHAPTER 1
Nutritional Allowances

The Recommended Dietary Allowance (RDA)*

Nowadays, it's almost impossible to read food labels without observing a reference to the USRDA or RDA. It is important that you understand what it is supposed to mean so that when you see ingredient lists that are many times the RDAs in some supplements, for example, you won't worry about overdosing yourself. As a guardian of your health, you need to become an astute observer and learner of all the nutritional information you find around you.

During World War II, the U.S. government delegated the Food and Nutrition Board of the National Academy of Sciences to devise nutritional guidelines that could be used uniformly for all the armed forces. These guidelines were called the Recommended Dietary Allowances (RDAs). After the war, the applications of the RDAs were expanded to include use by hospitals, boarding schools and nursing care facilities.

These initial standards were set to establish the minimal amounts of nutrients necessary to avert any diseases arising from nutritional deficiencies. These diseases might be rickets, arising from vitamin D shortage, or scurvy, from a lack of vitamin C. The RDAs are now aptly defined as "the levels of intake of essential nutrients that, on the basis of scientific knowledge, are judged by the Food and Nutrition Board to be adequate to meet the known nutrient needs of practically all healthy people."[1]

This definition (and the RDA values in Table 1.1) may have some relevance as a guideline for the population at large, but to the individual, they have very little significance. Bear in mind that these figures are only statistical averages based on median heights and weights of certain groups of "healthy" people. Depending on your life situation, you as an individual may have nutrition needs that vary significantly from what is given in the RDA table. According to current findings, even those people who are healthy may have nutritional needs many times greater than the RDAs.[2]

In addition, some individuals' nutritional requirements are far greater than what

---

* Now called Reference Daily Intake (RDI).

one finds in the RDA tables. These individuals include the sick, the elderly, people under emotional and physical stress, athletes and other physically active people such as laborers or construction workers. The RDAs also don't account for the genetic, metabolic and physiological differences of people.[3] These inherent variations can lead to differential absorption of nutrients from the digestive tract.

Furthermore, the RDAs don't account for pollution[*] in the air and water and the various food additives the average American consumes daily. They don't account for cigarette smokers,[†] other drug users or people who drink excessive alcohol. Drugs, including nicotine and alcohol, often either interfere with the absorption of nutrients from the intestinal tract or increase the amount required by the body.

In short, to quote one expert, "The variations in requirements reported by the scientists are too great to presume that any committee could determine the needs of a diverse population and thus the RDAs bear little or no relation to nutritional reality."[4] This is also to say that the RDAs, which are supposed to be our reference point for "normal" health, are not necessarily the rule to follow for "optimal" health.

Because of the above limitations, the best thing you as an individual can do, besides eating a balanced diet, is to include quality supplements as part of your overall health program. Vitamins, minerals, amino acids and essential fatty acids, beyond controlling deficiency-related diseases, have also been found to be health promoting and disease preventing.[4]

For example, a ten-year study by a group of researchers at UCLA revealed that intake of vitamin C in excess of the National Research Council (RCA) recommended amount can increase the life expectancy of men by six years. (The current RDA for vitamin C is 60 mg.) This study had followed 11,000 adult Americans for over a decade, and it was found that those men who supplemented their diet with 300 to 400 milligrams of vitamin C had a 42% lower overall death rate and a 45% lower death rate from heart diseases than those who used the RDA or lower amounts of the vitamin.[5]

In this study the results with the women were not as dramatic. Compared to those that consumed lower amounts of the vitamin, women had a 10% reduction in

---

[*] City dwellers, for example, experience a higher level of air pollution than those who live in the country or small towns.

[†] With the last revision, the RDA of vitamin C for smokers was increased to 100 mgs/day. This quantity is not really sufficient when you realize that one cigarette can wipe out from 25–100 mgs of vitamin C. The current RDA for nonsmokers is 60 mgs/day.

overall death rate and a 25% reduction in deaths from heart-related conditions. These recent findings are good illustrations of how the RDAs are inadequate for overall good health and longevity.

Similarly, in a recently released study, high doses of vitamin E were shown to lower the risk of heart disease significantly. This study included 87,000 female nurses (ages 34 to 59 years of age) and 40,000 male health professionals (ages 40 to 75) and covered a period of four to eight years. It was found that those who supplemented their diet with high doses of vitamin E (at least 10 times the RDA, the amount found in regular foods) had a 40% reduction in heart diseases.[6]

Although the researchers who did the study caution that this should not lead people to start taking massive doses of the vitamin,* this preliminary finding is another good indicator of the inadequacy of the RDA values of the nutrients we consume.

Nowadays, like many other things that affect the U.S. Population, RDAs have become political and economic issues for certain interest groups. Do you remember the outcry the meat and dairy industries made in 1991 when the U.S. Department of Agriculture (USDA) proposed to re-configure the four food groups?

Because fibers and grains have, for some time, been known to be more healthy than meat and dairy products, in 1991 the USDA proposed to re-configure the existing food groups pyramid. Fibers and grains would have been assigned to the bottom of the pyramid—thus making them the foundation of the nutritional hierarchy. These were followed by fruits and vegetables, which were to be followed by dairy products (such as cheese and milk) and eggs, fish, meats, nuts and beans. The top was going to be allotted for sweets, oils and fats. The lobbyists for the meat and dairy industry protested so loudly and clearly that the USDA withheld publication of the new Food Guide Pyramid until August 1992. (The Food Guide Pyramid is shown on page 344.)

Besides the disagreement or conflict that often rages in the Food & Nutrition Board of the National Academy of Sciences as to the true meaning of the RDAs, recipients of certain food programs (such as schools, nursing homes or hospitals), food manufacturers and others influence the decisions board members make on the RDAs. For example, in 1985, one of the changes considered (strictly for economic reasons) was lowering the RDA for vitamins A and C. Government agencies that are responsible for certain food

---

*Because the results may not be conclusive and that we don't know what the long-range effect would be from the consumption of high amounts.

programs base their funding on RDA requirements. By lowering the amounts of vitamins A and C, they could use cheaper food sources or reduce the quantities of the same
foods. This created a major uproar not only from the recipients of the food programs
but also from other groups, such as food supplement manufacturers.

Because of these and a few other reasons, the tenth edition of the RDA was not
released until 1989—four years past its scheduled publication! When it was finally
released, the following changes had been incorporated: the adolescent's RDA for
calcium was increased to 1,200 mg up to age 24 (instead of 18), since human bone
mass is believed to increase up to age 25. For the first time, values for vitamin K and
selenium were included. On the other hand, the RDAs for folate, iron, magnesium
and vitamins B6 and B12 were reduced.

The U.S. Recommended Daily Allowance (USRDA)

As you can see in Table 1.1, there are many different sets of RDAs—varying from
those for infants to those for pregnant and lactating women. For nutritional information on food products such as cereals and vitamin and mineral supplements, the different RDA values are rather confusing. To simplify this problem and create uniformity for
food labeling purposes, the Food and Drug Administration (FDA) established the
USRDA. (See bottom section of Table 1.1 for the USRDAs.)

According to the USRDA, calories plus ten nutrients must be included on food
labels. These nutrients are protein, carbohydrates, fats, vitamin A, vitamin C, thiamin,
riboflavin, niacin, calcium and iron. The FDA was able to circumvent the obvious
problem by taking the highest value of the 1968 RDAs for each nutrient and by using a
percentile as a reference point. RDA figures for people over four years of age (excluding
pregnant and lactating women) were chosen. The USRDA for vitamin E, for example,
is 22 micrograms. If you see a food label that says 35% of USRDA, it means that this
food product contains 7.7 micrograms of the nutrient.

Although there were no changes made to the USRDA when the tenth edition
of the RDA was released in 1989, beginning with 1993, new nutritional information began to appear on food labels. Most of the manufacturers were given until
May 1994 to comply with many of the new labeling requirements. These changes
reflected the new regulations passed since 1990. The USRDA name was changed to
RDI (Reference Daily Intake).[5] (Read "Food Labeling Reforms" on page 9 for more
information on this subject.)

Units and Measurements Used in Food Labeling

Part of being an astute protector of your health is understanding or knowing about units and measurements you find on food labels. Unless you know what they mean, some of them can be quite confusing. For example, some of the vitamins are measured in milligrams or micrograms, while others are in international units (IUs).

To better understand what they all mean, remember that all the fat-soluble vitamins (vitamins A, E, D and K) are commonly expressed in international units and all the water-soluble vitamins and minerals are given in metric weight units— milligrams and micrograms. Although you rarely see it on regular food labels, vitamin A is sometimes expressed in retinol equivalent (RE) in the literature.

As you probably know, there are two forms of vitamin A. These are retinol,[*] which comes from animal sources, and beta carotene[†] which you find largely in plant products. By using the biological activity (BA) of retinol as a reference point, the BA's of other vitamin A's can be evaluated. Thus, when an RE is used, it's intended to show the amount (in weight) of a provitamin present in a food source that is equivalent to retinol.

Thus, 1 RE is equal to 1 microgram (mcg, or μg) of retinol or 6 mcg of beta carotene. One IU of vitamin A is equal to 0.3 mcg of retinol, which is to say that 3.33 IU is equal to 1 RE. Through a somewhat complicated computation, however, it turns out that retinol equivalents (REs) are actually equal to one-fifth of international units (IUs.) Hence, for example, from Table 1.1 you see that the vitamin A RDA for females between the ages of 11 and 51 is given as 800 RE. This number is equal to 4,000 IUs. For your own practical applications, all you need to remember is that IUs are 5 times the REs.

Table 1.2 illustrates some common units of measurement.

---

[*] The most common sources of retinol are cod liver oil, halibut, shark and tuna.

[†] Beta carotene is a member of the carotenoid provitamins.

Table 1.2 Units of Measurement

Going from large to small units of measure

Unit	Abbreviation	Conversion value
1 kilogram	kg	1000 gram
1 gram	g	1000 milligram
1 milligram	mg	1000 micrograms
1 gram	g	1,000,000 micrograms

Going from small to large metric units of measure

Unit	Abbreviation	Conversion value
1 milligram	mg	1/1000 gram
1 microgram	mcg (µg)	1/1000 milligram
1 gram	g	1/1000 kilogram
1 microgram	mcg (µg)	1/1,000,000 gram

Going from English to metric units of measure

Unit	Abbreviation	Conversion value
1 ounce	oz	28.35 grams
16 ounces (1 pound)	oz, Ib	453.6 grams

Units of fluid measure

Unit	Abbreviation	Conversion value
1 liter	1	1000 milliliter (or cc*)
1 milliliter	ml	1000 microliter (mcl or µl)

Units of fluid measure

1 teaspoon	tsp	4 cc (or fluid gram)
1 tablespoon	tbsp	15 cc (or 1/2 fluid ounce)
1/2 pint	pt	240 cc (or 8 fluid ounces)

Units of energy measure**

Unit	Abbreviation	Conversion value
1 kilocalorie	kcal	1000 calories

* cubic centimeters

** The energy units of measure that you see on food labels or those we use to describe a person's daily caloric intake are not exactly what they appear to be. The energy values we use in these instances are really kilocalories, not calories. Somehow, by convention "kilo calories" and "calories" have come to mean the same thing. For example, if you see on a food label 100 calories for an ingredient, it actually means 100 kilocalories (100,000 calories). The former figure is a shortcut representation of kilocalories.

Food Labeling Reforms

For a long time, most companies voluntarily provided information about the nutritional content of their packaged foods. The exception has been companies that manufactured fortified foods or those that made nutritional claims. This option and the absence of full regulation by the FDA meant that companies could put just about anything they wished on their food labels.

Some of the confusing labels involved terminologies. For instance, words like "low," "diet" and "reduced" on food labels were meant to describe the calorie content of foods. Other words such as "free," "low" and "reduced" were to give information about the sodium level in foods. For years, many manufacturers have used these terms indiscriminately.

Then there was the "cholesterol-free" statement we used to see on just about every food label, so it seemed. Cholesterol comes only from animal sources, but references to cholesterol had continuously appeared on foods that had nothing to do with cholesterol.

The FDA finally said "enough is enough" to all these confusing and often deceptive practices used by food and beverage manufacturers. Effective May 1994, all food and supplement manufacturing companies had to comply with many of the sweeping changes introduced by the agency.[5] These changes were made because, according to FDA commissioner Dr. David Kessler, the FDA wanted to: "...clear up confusion;...help us make healthy choices; and... encourage product innovation, so that companies are more interested in tinkering with the food in the package, not the words on the label."[6]

As you can see below, the proposed rulings are more comprehensive and far-reaching than just keeping a few overzealous companies honest. The new rulings are also intended to standardize and incorporate some of the recent advances in nutritional science into an everyday practical use so that we, the consumers, will be able to make wiser decisions on the foods we buy. [7]

For quite some time, for example, there has been a strong link between cholesterol, saturated fats and sodium and some degenerative or chronic diseases. Now, with the new rulings, standardized values have been appearing on food labels for these and other similarly worrisome food substances. Hence, as consumers, we are now able to compare the cholesterol, saturated fat or sodium amounts in the foods we buy against the given reference values and make wise decisions.[8]

The format and nutritional content of packaged foods have also become explicit enough so that we won't have to guess, for example, what the manufacturer really means when he says "low-fat" or "cholesterol-free." Thus, according to the FDA, the emphasis now is "on nutrients that will have a significant impact on the health of today's consumers,"[9] not simply hype and promotion.

Here are some of the FDA's rulings that took effect starting May 1994:[10]

1. All food and supplement manufacturers, save for a few exceptions,* are mandatorily required to give nutritional information on all packaged and manufactured foods. In the past, only those that manufactured fortified or processed foods were required to do this, and even then, only about 60% of such foods have had the required information on their labels. These required listings were serving size, servings per container, the number of calories, sodium and the ten required nutrients mentioned on page 2.

    Food labels that appeared beginning May 1994 have been more informative and comprehensive. Included in these labels are total calories, calories derived from fat, total fat, saturated fat, cholesterol, total carbohydrates, complex carbohydrates, sugars, dietary fiber, protein, sodium, vitamins A and C and calcium and iron.** Three nutrients—thiamin, riboflavin and niacin—which used to appear under the old food label are no longer mandatory listings. It's thought that since these nutrients are widely available in many foods, their inclusion on food labels would be optional.

    Because of the many diseases associated with fat, however, all those hidden fats that you had unknowingly been consuming are now "glistening" right before your eyes. It is hoped that this explicit information will enable you to go along with your sensibilities and not with the whim of your palate. Fat is given in grams or as a percentage of the new nutritional standard, the Daily Reference Values, DRVs or simply DVs.

    With the new ruling, DVs are meant to be used as reference values for foods that previously did not have standard values but in recent years have been recognized as important determinants of health. These are fats, cholesterol, carbohydrates, dietary fiber, sodium and potassium. The RDIs, as was mentioned

---

* Exempted will be most spices and miniature packages, restaurant foods and foods produced by small businesses whose food sales amount to no more than $50,000 a year with total sales of no more than $500,000 a year.

** These and other facts on these pages are based on a new FDA publication called FDA Backgrounder.

earlier, have replaced the USRDAs. But unlike the USRDAs, which were based on the 1968 highest RDA values for protein, vitamins and minerals, the RDIs are based on the 1989 RDA average values. (See the reasoning below.)

2. Those terms such as "free," "reduced" and "low" that have commonly been used to designate the calorie and sodium contents in foods are now used for other nutrients as well. These and other relevant terms have been clearly defined, and consumers as well as food manufacturers should know what each stands for. For instance, "calorie-free" is used for all those foods that have fewer than 5 calories per serving. Similarly, "sugar-free" is used for foods that contain less than 0.5 gram per serving.

   "Low-fat" applies only if the food has 3 or fewer grams of fat per serving and per 100 grams of food. "Cholesterol-free" means the food contains less than 2 milligrams of cholesterol per serving and 2 or fewer grams of saturated fat per serving. Relative terms such as "less," "reduced" and "light" are used only when referenced to other foods or values. For instance, "light" may be used if a given food contains less than one-third the calories of a comparable food. "Less" means that the nutrient content of a given food is reduced by at least 25%.

3. For the first time, food labels are allowed to make health claims based on known relationships between certain foods and health benefits or risks. Ten such relationships have been under consideration, and now four of them have been allowed to appear on food labels: fats and cardiovascular diseases, sodium and hypertension, fat and cancer, and calcium and osteoporosis. Food manufacturers have been able to make these claims since May 1993. Other relationships, such as those between fiber and heart disease and between fiber and cancer, are still under consideration.

4. Starting May 1994, the FDA has required ingredients listings on all foods, including those that were exempted in the past, such as mayonnaise, ketchup and macaroni. The agency's aim is to get all food manufacturers to give complete nutritional information to the public without an exception. In the new proposal, manufacturers are also required to list the names of all additives: coloring agents, flavor enhancers, preservatives and other ingredients. In doing so, those who may be allergic or have some religious or cultural dietary requirements would be informed about these ingredients.

   All the food ingredients, including any sweeteners, have to be listed and be given in a descending order of proportion by weight. Likewise, fruit and vegetable juice products that contain different juices have to identify the juices and

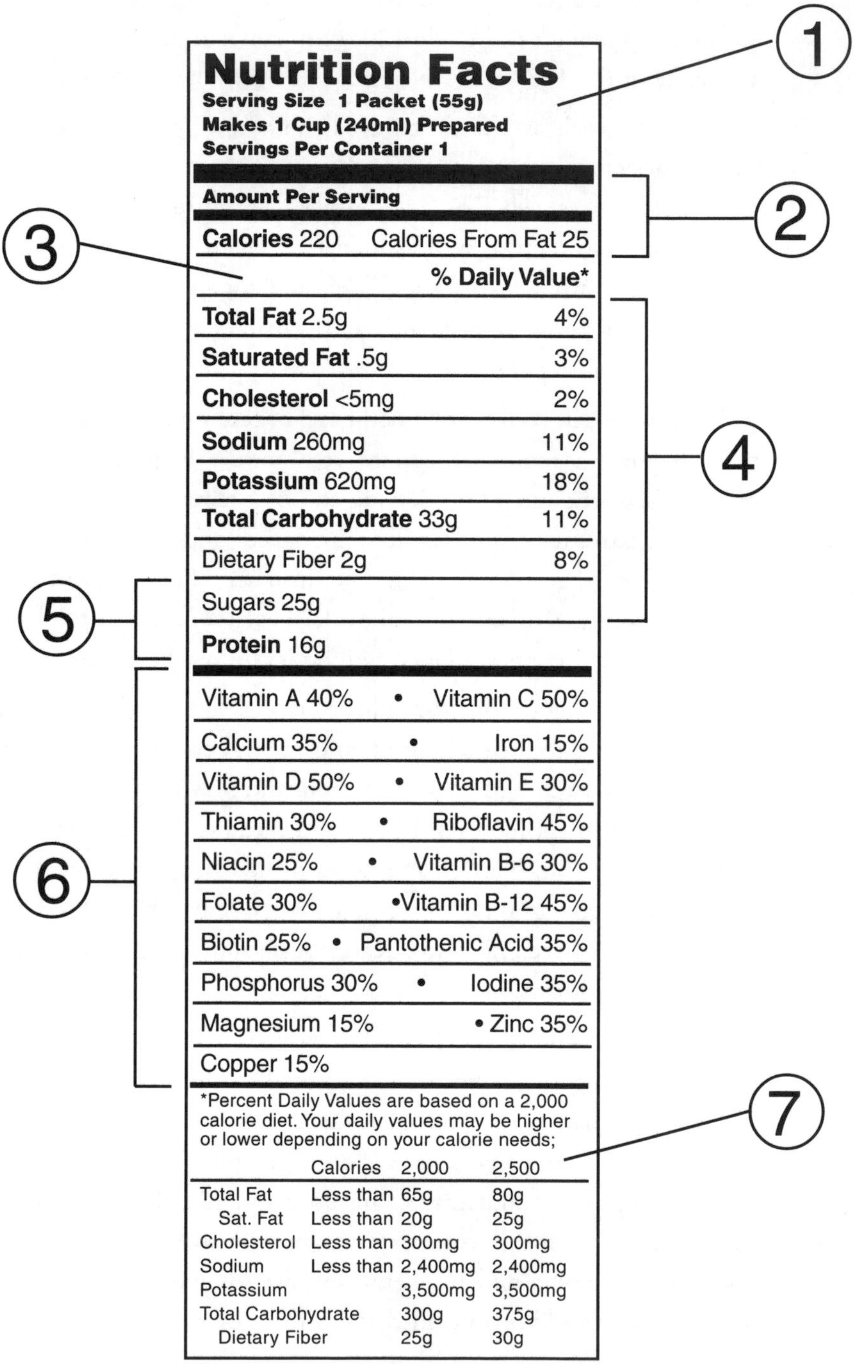

Nutrition Facts
Serving Size 1 Packet (55g)
Makes 1 Cup (240ml) Prepared
Servings Per Container 1

Amount Per Serving

Calories 220   Calories From Fat 25

% **Daily Value***

Total Fat 2.5g	4%
Saturated Fat .5g	3%
Cholesterol <5mg	2%
Sodium 260mg	11%
Potassium 620mg	18%
Total Carbohydrate 33g	11%
Dietary Fiber 2g	8%
Sugars 25g	
Protein 16g	

Vitamin A 40%	•	Vitamin C 50%
Calcium 35%	•	Iron 15%
Vitamin D 50%	•	Vitamin E 30%
Thiamin 30%	•	Riboflavin 45%
Niacin 25%	•	Vitamin B-6 30%
Folate 30%	•Vitamin B-12 45%	
Biotin 25% • Pantothenic Acid 35%		
Phosphorus 30%	•	Iodine 35%
Magnesium 15%	• Zinc 35%	
Copper 15%		

*Percent Daily Values are based on a 2,000 calorie diet. Your daily values may be higher or lower depending on your calorie needs;

		Calories	2,000	2,500
Total Fat	Less than	65g	80g
Sat. Fat	Less than	20g	25g
Cholesterol	Less than	300mg	300mg
Sodium	Less than	2,400mg	2,400mg
Potassium		3,500mg	3,500mg
Total Carbohydrate		300g	375g
Dietary Fiber		25g	30g

Figure 1.1 An Illustration of Food Labeling

the relative amounts of each juice given as percentages. Grocery stores are now also required to give nutritional information on raw fruit, raw vegetables and raw fish.

5. Finally, effective May 1994, vitamin and mineral supplement labels have been given as percentages of the RDIs—Reference Daily Intakes. The RDIs, as mentioned before, now represent adjusted average values of the 1989 RDA figures for proteins, vitamins and minerals, different from USRDAs, which had long used the 1968 highest RDA values.

   Although the RDIs for vitamins and minerals are now going to be 14% less than those given by USRDA, the FDA feels that the average approach would give the public a more unified "measuring stick" to compare "the contents of all labeled nutrients among different foods." Since fats, cholesterol and fibers are also included, to take the highest value of the RDA for these new nutrients would be self-defeating. The goal is to minimize our intake of fats and cholesterol, not to maximize it.

Food Labeling—An Illustration

The food label you see on your tomato soup can or breakfast cereal box is not something that is put together at the whim of the individual manufacturer. From the specific nutritional information to the layout of the label and the prominence and conspicuousness of the information given, labels have to follow certain standards and guidelines. These requirements are illustrated in Figure 1.1. Let's look closely at each section of the panel.

As you can see, the label titled "Nutrition Facts" contains several categories. For ease of reference, I have assigned numbers to each of these categories.

1. Serving size and serving per container, presented in both household measures and metric units, give the amount of food of the particular product. This information is particularly important when observed in the context of the nutritional breakdown that appears in numbers 2 and 3. Because a high intake of fat, cholesterol and sodium is associated with health risks, the serving size and servings per container can help you decide how much of the given food you may want to consume and still keep the amounts of the aforementioned substances within the recommended values, discussed in number 7.

2. If you are concerned about your weight, you may want to watch your daily intake of calories. High amounts of fat calories are particularly bad not only

because they are easily converted into body fat but also because they have been associated with the onset of certain degenerative diseases. Authorities have recommended that our fat calories not exceed 30%* of our total daily calories.

3. % Daily Value (DV) is the reference standard for different food components you consume every day. The last section of Figure 1.1 lists the DVs for total fat, saturated fat, cholesterol, etc. Your goal should be to get at least 100% DV of the healthful foods such as carbohydrates, fiber, vitamins and minerals, and less than 100% DV of foods that have been linked to health risks. You may need to take significantly higher (than the RDI) amounts of the antioxidants vitamins and some of the B-complex vitamins.

4. This section gives the various components of food calories as well as sodium, sugar and fiber. For the reasons given in number 1, keep some of these foods within the recommended DVs. For example, the Daily Value for saturated fat is less than 10% of total calories, and for cholesterol it is to be less than 300 mgs.

   The percentages that appear in this section were computed against the Daily Values given at the bottom of the panel. For instance, a total is given as 2.5 grams of fat. Dividing this figure by 65 grams, the daily amount of fat recommended in a 2,000-calorie diet is 4%—the amount of fat contributed by this food toward your Daily Value.

5. Although excessive consumption of sugar can negatively affect your health, there is no DV for this nutrient. Health authorities have not set a limit for sugar primarily because sugar comes in many different forms and from many different sources: table sugar, honey, milk and fruits and vegetables like carrots, beets and sweet potatoes. Similarly, protein has not had a DV because a conclusive study has not been done as to its health risk when taken in excessive amounts.

6. Companies can also give the vitamin and mineral content of their products. The percentages for these nutrients are computed from the RDIs (formerly RDAs), values that are normally found in a table like the table on page 2. In general, the higher the percentages for these foods, the better the food values.

7. You usually see this portion of the panel mainly on larger packages. For the first time, you can now compare your daily intake of total fat, cholesterol, etc. against the standardized figures that appear in this section of the label. As you can see, all those items that present a health risk are given as maximums, while those

---

* Some experts suggest the our daily fat caloric intake should be less than 20%.

that contribute to health such as fiber and carbohydrates are shown as minimums. You adjust your intake of these foods according to your daily caloric intake, which, as shown, can be either 2,000 calories or 2,500 calories.* Let's see how you figure Percent Daily Values for total fat and saturated fat from recommended total calories.

For a 2,000-calorie diet, the suggested DV for total fat is 65 grams. We know that there are 9 calories per gram of fat. When we multiply 65 grams by 9 calories per gram, we obtain 585 calories. As a percentage of total calories, this figure translates to 29% (585 divided by 2,000), which is less than the 30% suggested value. Saturated fat is given as 20 grams, which contains 180 calories. As a percentage of total calories, this is 9%, which again is less than the suggested 10% calories for saturated fat.

In summary, for the first time, you have food serving sizes that are consistent for all products. And now you also have reference values for total fat, saturated fat, cholesterol, sodium, total carbohydrates and fiber on food labels. For the first time you have information that can help you make healthy food choices whether you are sitting in a restaurant or shopping for groceries. It would be helpful for you to study the food label above, memorize the key information and use it every time you have the opportunity to make healthy food choices.

---

* The 2,000 calories are recommended for less active men, teenage girls and most women. The 2,500 calories may be consumed by many men, teenage boys and very active women.

PART II
Nutrition and Longevity

Malnutrition Examples

Subclinical
(harder to detect)

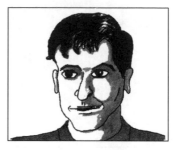

Marginal
(sometimes observable)

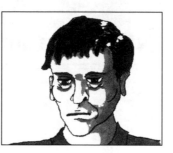

Obesity
(observable)

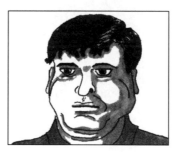

Figure 2.1 Malnutrition Examples
These three faces embody the subtle but health-eroding forms of malnutrition that are often found in the U.S. and other industrial nations. In the subclinical case, a nutritional deficiency is hard to detect unless one takes the nutrient-analysis exam described in Appendix I and illustrated in Appendix J. Marginal deficiency symptoms, on the other hand, may be experienced occasionally, as when you feel depressed, irritable or fatigued for no apparent reason. The bottom face is the counterpart of the malnutrition that is frequently found in Third World countries. Here in the U.S., for example, some people suffer from eating too much of the wrong food, while in the Third World people starve from lack of sufficient food.

CHAPTER 2
Optimal Nutrition

Current Health Issues in the United States

Increasingly people are living longer today. This is particularly so when you realize that two-thirds of the people who have ever lived past 65 years of age are alive today.[1] This piece of information is astounding in another way. A little over a hundred years ago, people did not expect to live past 40 years of age. Now, because of the eradication of many of the epidemic diseases (such as tuberculosis and smallpox), average life expectancy is nearly double what it was a hundred years ago. Today the average person can expect to live to roughly 76 years of age.

The future of human life is even more impressive. According to experts on aging, not only will there be a greater number of people living past 100 years, but some may even live as long as 120 years, the current maximum biological age for humans.[2,3] Nonetheless, to a large extent, how you care for yourself is what will determine how many years you can expect to live.[4,5] See Figure 2.2 on page 20 for past, present and future survival curves.

Nowadays, venereal diseases, influenza and tuberculosis are not the main killers in the United States and other industrialized societies. Instead, the main killers are cancer, cardiovascular diseases, diabetes and other degenerative diseases. These diseases as a group, which were relatively unknown in the early part of this century, account for 9 out of 10 deaths in the United States.[6,7]

Just to give you some statistics, cancer, the number two cause of death in this country, kills 1 in 3 people today. This is, a dramatic increase from 1 in 25 people in the early 1900s and 1 in 8 in the 1950s. Since 1962 alone, the cancer death rate has risen by 25%. Deaths from cardiovascular diseases (heart attacks, stroke and other circulatory complications) are equally astounding. These diseases have risen from 1 in 9 in the 1920s to 1 in 2 currently, making them as a group the number one cause of death in this country.[8]

Yet what's interesting about these statistics is that many of these diseases are caused by factors that may be preventable. Most of the cardiovascular diseases, for example, are caused by fatty deposits or are due to a sedimentation of cholesterol-bound calcium along the arterial walls.[9] When these fats collect in the arteries, they block the flow of blood, and this can lead to heart attack. Calcium and cholesterol deposits, on the other hand, cause the blood vessels to become rigid and brittle. This condition can result in breakage or rupture of the blood vessels as well as stroke

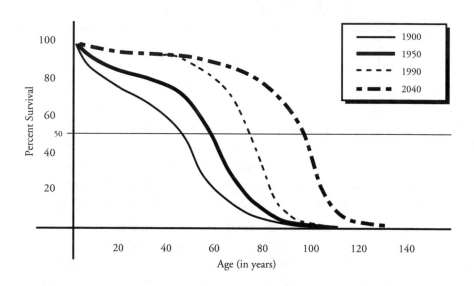

These Life Expectancy Curves show past, present and future U.S. population life span profiles. Average life expectancies at a 50% survival rate are shown below:

1900	44 years
1950	60 years
1990	76 years
2040	89 years*

> * The National Institute on Aging projects that by the year 2040, the life expectancy for men will be 86 and for women will be 91.5; the average of these two numbers is roughly 89 years.

Dr. Ken Dychtwald, in his book *The Age Wave*, says that if we somehow could eliminate heart diseases, stroke and cancer, the average life expectancy would rise by 18 years. That means if we minimize the incidence of these preventable diseases, we could expect to live to an average of 94 years, instead of the present 76 years.

We hope the nutritional information you find in this book and your own precautions will help you reach these new life expectancies.

Figure 2.2 Survival Curves for the U.S. Population

if the blood vessels are in the brain. Both these problems could be a result of the food you eat.

The other nutrition-related circulatory disorder is one that comes from electrolyte imbalance. Both the heart muscles and nerves need certain minerals like sodium, calcium, potassium, and magnesium for their normal functioning. Severe shortage of these minerals can lead to spasms and even sudden death.[10,11,12]

The best solution to any of these health hazards is to avoid or minimize the consumption of foods that are rich in saturated fats and cholesterol. Foods that are rich in saturated fats, such as red meat, whole milk and coconut and palm oils, can be some of the major culprits. Lowering stress level and exercising regularly can also help you clear up some of these circulatory problems.

Current Nutrition Status

Given the present health problems, Americans are far from getting what would be considered optimal nutrition for good health, vigor and well-being.[13] Malnutrition or some form of nutritional deficiency is common in this country.[14] However, the kind of malnutrition that exists in the United States and most industrialized nations today is not your classical type where children's stomachs become bloated and people end up with protruding bones and emaciated faces.[15,16]

More often, the malnutrition that exists in Western countries is of the subtle, undetectable type, referred to (see Figure 2.1 on page 18) as *subclinical.* In this type of nutritional deficiency you may have nourished yourself just enough to meet all your body's minimum requirements but not sufficiently enough to give you that extra zest in life.

Subclinical malnutrition is not observable because for all practical reasons you feel OK. The problem with this form of malnutrition, as with the other two discussed below, is that in the long run, your health will be seriously compromised. Like subterranean termites that slowly eat away at the wooden foundation of your home and finally bring the house tumbling down, a subclinical type of malnutrition could do the same to your body. Often, like those hidden termites, you would not notice that something is amiss until it's too late. Particularly predisposed to this type of nutritional deficiency are pregnant women, infants, teenagers and the elderly.[17]

Marginal deficiency (also shown in Figure 2.1) is another type of malnutrition. With this, your body might be low in one or more nutrients, but you go on living without any outright sign of sickness, except perhaps for slight behavioral changes you might be experiencing from time to time.[18]

People who have the third kind of malnutrition, *obesity,* can have the marginal or subclinical type in addition to being overweight. The problem with obese people is not that they get enough nutrients, but more often that they get too much of the wrong food. For example, if you gorge on fat-laden meals similar to those you find in fast-food outlets and some restaurants, drink too much beer and eat too many processed foods, you will be malnourished. The fat, alcohol and sugars in these foods have no nutritional value for your body. They merely make you fat.

In addition, over time, fat begins to clog the arterial walls, alcohol starts to erode the health of your liver and brain cells and sugar undermines the proper function of the pancreas. You now become a strong candidate for cardiovascular diseases, diseases of the liver, diabetes and premature death.

Ironically, in the United States the above nutrition problems are not necessarily a condition of the poor, the homeless or a particular class or race of people. Several government surveys have shown that they are problems that affects people of all socioeconomic classes.[19] According to one expert, "Everyone who has in the past eaten processed sugar, white flour, or canned food has some deficiency disease, the extent of the disease depending on the percentage of such deficient foods in the diet."[20] That means practically everybody.

The chart below and Figure 2.3 show what could happen to the body as a result of chronic malnutrition. As you can see in these illustrations, nutritional deficiency

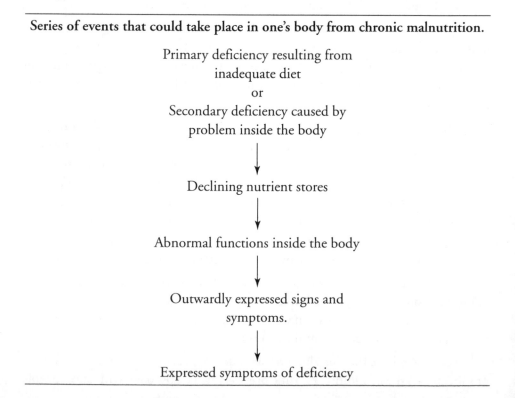

Series of events that could take place in one's body from chronic malnutrition.

Primary deficiency resulting from
inadequate diet
or
Secondary deficiency caused by
problem inside the body

↓

Declining nutrient stores

↓

Abnormal functions inside the body

↓

Outwardly expressed signs and
symptoms.

↓

Expressed symptoms of deficiency

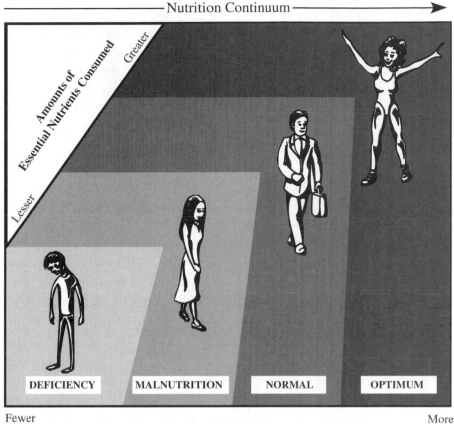

Figure 2.3 Nutrition Continuum

This nutrition continuum illustrates the four possible levels of nutrition and serves as a model that accommodates individual differences and nutritional need variabilities among humans.

can come about as a result of either inadequate diet or from the body's inability to process the food properly due physiological or metabolic disorders. In either case, when this happens, nutrient stores in the body begin to decline. This problem leads first to abnormal function of tissues and organs then to an outwardly expressed symptoms or diseases such as scaly or coarse skin, cracking or ridging nails and thin and weak hair or scurvy, pellagra or rickets. To determine the causes of these symptoms or diseases, a health care professional first assesses a person's diet and medical history. These assessments are followed by a series of laboratory tests and physical examinations and measurements.

Causes of Malnutrition

Besides having a problem with processed foods, Americans have had a great love affair with dairy and meat products. These foods are rich in saturated fats and protein, which may contribute to cardiovascular diseases, obesity and a number of other problems. Milk, for example, could interfere with proper absorption of foods, and in infants, it could cause diarrhea and iron deficiency anemia. Furthermore, the high protein content in milk, could, among other things, lead to the depletion of a number of vitamins and minerals from the body, including potassium, calcium, magnesium and B vitamins.

More often than not, the food you eat is naturally nutritionally sparse.[21] Because of overfarming, the agricultural lands of this country have long been depleted of their minerals, and the fertilizers used today have no more than three or four nutrients in them.[22,23,24] A high concentration of these few nutrients may help plants to grow big and attractive, but these plants are far from being nutritionally balanced and complete. This is so when you realize that plants need as many as 16 essential nutrients to grow well. As you can see in Table 20.1 on page 240, there is a great variation in the nutritional content of vegetables grown in the United States.

The other major problem of malnutrition is simply a practical one. In these days of working couples and single men, single women and single parents, people don't seem to have the time, the desire, the discipline or the knowhow to prepare well-balanced meals. These folks often opt for TV dinners, fast food or restaurant meals. The food from these sources either is not nutritious or has too much of the wrong things, such as fat, white bread, excess sugar, additives and a number of other unhealthy substances.

Whatever the causes or the reasons—subclinical, marginal or obesity—malnutrition will definitely shorten the path to your grave. If you are serious about your health and quality of life, you need to take important steps right now! Since nutrition is the basis of it all, one of the first things you can do is to eat a well-balanced meal every day. As a margin of safety you also may want to take supplements: vitamins, minerals, amino acids and other nutrients. Your goal is not to have just normal nutrition but rather optimal nutrition.

Optimal Nutrition—Your Answer to Health and Longevity

As we mentioned earlier, current estimations put the maximum human biological age in the 115- to 120-year range. Among many factors that influence your chance of reaching this range, nutrition ranks on top. To illustrate this point, we'll call that nutrition level that may help us reduce the gap between our current life expectancy of 76 years and the biological limit, the "optimal" nutrition.

However, because of the biological, physiological and gender variations among people as well as their age, stress level, physical conditions or type of work they do, people's nutritional needs will vary accordingly. This variability creates a problem for us to come up with a single nutritional or optimal standard.

Moreover, researchers have so far shown that we need at least 45 to 50 essential nutrients—nutrients that our bodies are not capable of producing. These include two essential fatty acids, eight essential amino acids, fifteen vitamins, twenty minerals and another five that are not conclusively known to be essential. Researchers have also shown that quantities higher than current RDA values of these nutrients can help us deal with many health-related issues, some of which are described below.

One, since your body depends on the food you eat for practically everything it does, the greater availability of the above nutrients in the tissues, the more effectively and vigorously it accomplishes its tasks or activities. For example, with optimal nutrition, your immune system can marshal its forces (immune cells) quickly and efficiently to defend your body in times of invasion by foreign elements like virus, bacteria or parasites. It can equally quickly suppress or destroy potential dangers (such as the growth of cancer) from within the body.

Two, if you are one of those people with special circumstances—e.g., have a stressful life-style, live or work in a polluted environment, are pregnant, are elderly or have a certain genetic defect—your need for nutrients may consequently be higher than most people's. Similarly, if you have surgery, are undergoing drug treatment or are having therapy, your need for nutrients may also be higher than most people's.

Three, certain nutrients when taken in higher doses do things that normal RDA amounts may not do for you.[25] For example, when vitamin A (as beta carotene) is taken in higher quantities, it protects the body from the destructive side effects of chemotherapy.[26] Higher-than-RDA amounts of vitamin E improve circulation. In women with premenstrual syndrome, vitamin E also may help reduce breast tenderness.[27] Similarly, higher amounts of vitamin C and zinc speed up recovery from wounds and infections.[28]

According to recent reports, greater amounts of vitamin C (300 to 400 mgs per day) can prolong the life of men by six years. The current RDA for vitamin C is 60 mgs. Similarly, higher-than-RDA amounts of Vitamin E were found to reduce the risk of heart disease.[29,30]

Thus, to accommodate nutrient needs and quantity variabilities, we have to treat nutrition as a continuum. This means that in Figure 2.2 the two variables can be adequately represented. In this graph, office workers, physically active or sick people, as well as others with special nutritional needs, will also have their places. Let's see exactly what this graph tells us.

The horizontal axis represents the number of essential daily nutrient intakes. The vertical axis represents the amount of those intakes. The results of combining these two axes describe the nutritional conditions that we have labeled *deficiency, malnutrition, normal* and *optimum*. The figures in the chart represent each one of these conditions, or the z-axis of coordinate geometry.

Thus, as we go from left to right on the continuum, we are moving from nutritionally low foods (such as white bread, candy, pastries and soda pop) to those that are nutritionally dense* and balanced (such as liver and fish), which may bring you closer and closer to optimal health. How far along and how wide you are in the "optimal" range will depend on your own individual needs. If you are a person who is concerned about your looks and well-being or the appearance of your hair and skin, you want to be as far along the continuum and as high up on it as your individual needs dictate.

If you are a growing person, elderly, sick, athletic or physically or emotionally stressed, you need nutrients and nutrient levels that can adequately help you meet these conditions. Are you a smoker, heavy drinker or other drug user? If so, your nutritional needs will be equally high and further to the right and higher up on the continuum. In this manner, as you provide your body with all the good nutrients it needs, all the organs (heart, lungs, liver, brain, etc.) should function to their maximum efficiency and capacity.[†]

Good nutrition, simply speaking, means eating a well-balanced diet—rich in vitamins, minerals, proteins, fibers, essential fatty acids and carbohydrates. Such a combination of nutrients and in higher concentrations may bring peace and order to your body. In the end you may feel a heightened sense of well-being, contentment and happiness.

How to Achieve Your Own Optimal Levels

The first thing you should do is find out where you are nutritionally on the chart. You can do this by asking your physician to do a series of tests that evaluate your overall health as well as your nutritional status. Depending on your particular situation, you can have done all of the following items or just the part on nutrition. It would be advisable, however, to undergo comprehensive exams for the first time. In the future, you can use these first exams as references to gauge how your health and nutritional profiles have changed.

Tests your physician can do or have done for you:

---

[*] Nutrient density is defined as the amounts of proteins, carbohydrates, vitamins and minerals contained in 100 kilocalories of any food. The health value (or desirability) of the food depends on the density of the nutrient per kilocalorie. This means, the greater the density, the more valuable (or desirable) the food. White bread has few nutrients, and therefore it is the least valuable.

[†] This assumes, of course, that you have no genetic abnormality or other complications in your body.

1. General Physical Exam—This evaluates your body's overall physical/mechanical operations, such as tendon reflexes, the function of your heart and lungs, joint mobility, muscle tone and strength, and assesses the condition of your ears, eyes and mouth.

2. Specific Clinical Exams—These are equally varied and range from blood sugar levels to blood cell counts, urinalysis, cholesterol (both HDL and LDL) and triglyceride (fat) levels, to blood chemistries, electrocardiograms and others.

3. Specific Nutritional Exams

    a. Comprehensive Digestive Stool Analysis—This test helps determine how well your digestive system operates. Stool analysis is particularly important as you get older. Some of the problems older people have are the improper digestion and utilization of foods. Thus, this test looks for over 20 different components of the stool—bacterial, yeast and undigested food levels, unexpected organisms, chemicals and other components.

    b. Vitamin Analysis—This test determines specific vitamin profiles as well as the blood level of all the known essential vitamins. This analysis can ascertain both the subclinical and the marginal or clinical conditions of vitamin deficiency. Vitamins are critical to life. Since many of the life-sustaining processes depend on vitamins, anytime you are low in even one vitamin, important metabolic functions can be jeopardized. This, in turn, will undermine your health and your body's ability to fight infections and diseases.

        SpectraCell Laboratories in Houston, Texas, has perhaps the best techniques for analyzing the nutrient status of the body. By using methods called Essential Metabolics Analysis (EMA™) and Spectrox, it assesses the nutritional status of the body by directly examining the nutrient function of lymphocytes or white blood cells. While EMA is used to examine individual nutrient status of the cells, Spectrox is used to assess the functional antioxidant level of the cells. Reportedly, the two methods are superior to urine, serum or hair analysis—methods that have long been used to assess the nutritional status of an individual—because, among other things, deficiency levels not detected by traditional methods can be picked up by the two methods. See page 403 for sample runs of the test.

    c. Nutrient and Toxic Mineral Levels and Mineral Ratios—Minerals are the other class of nutrients in which many people could be deficient. Samples for these tests can be hair, urine or blood. The results of tests on hair samples are often better correlated with tissue stores of minerals than the results for either blood or urine.

As you can see by the sample on page 402 of Appendix J, all the mineral levels contained in the specimen are listed as parts per million (PPM) and are compared to standard numerical ranges. Nonnumerical terms such as high and low are also used to compare results against the references. Hence, if you are eating well-balanced meals and have no digestion or absorption problems, your test results should fall within the reference ranges, preferably on the high end. Otherwise, you might be deficient or borderline deficient. This can mean you either are outright malnourished or have subclinical/marginal deficiencies.

Mineral ratios are also important. All the minerals in your body should be in tolerable ranges in relation to each other. For example, the ideal ratio of calcium to phosphorus is 1:1 and of calcium to magnesium is 2:1. Too much deviation from these ratios often leads to the improper utilization of one of the minerals. This test can also determine levels in the body of toxic minerals such as cadmium, lead, nickel, mercury and arsenic. Knowing the amounts of each will help you in taking remedial and preventive measures against these dangerous minerals.

4.   Allergy and Tissue Toxicity Tests—Although these two tests are lumped together in one category, they are actually two separate tests. Food allergy tests assess your body's sensitivity to various foods. This can help you be watchful of food-related allergies and minimize any potential problems.

The toxicity tests, on the other hand, try to ascertain your body's level of exposure to various industrial, agricultural, household and other toxic chemicals. These can be PCBs, formaldehyde, PBBs, asbestos, gasoline, herbicides, pesticides (such as DDT, EDB, DBCP), a number of organophosphates and others. Many of these chemicals are known to be carcinogens, and they often collect in the fatty tissues of the body.

Considering the air and water pollution levels we have in this country, chemical toxicity tests may be important, particularly if you know you have been exposed to these chemicals in the past or are working in a heavily polluted environment.

When you look at the above list of tests, you will probably ask yourself, "Who in the world would bother to do all these, let alone be able to afford them?" It's true that most people don't even get an annual physical exam let alone such elaborate and, in some instances, esoteric tests.

First, you must realize that any corrective measures you take now regarding nutritional deficiencies could save you a lot of money in the future. The costs of many of these tests vary depending upon whether you use your hair, urine or blood and the type of nutrient levels you want analyzed. The tests could range from roughly $45 for hair-mineral analysis to $170 for amino-acid urine analysis. For more information on these and other tests, call the respective test laboratories listed in Appendix K on page 411 or the clinics in your area.

Second, since preventive medicine through proper nutrition is gaining popularity, such tests as the above are perhaps the beginning of more to come. Modern medicine has long focused on curing the symptoms instead of preventing the causes. You might want to take any warranting corrective steps now.

The financial and human cost of degenerative diseases (cancer, diabetes, arthritis, circulatory disease, etc.) prevalent today have been astronomical. In the past few decades, millions have died, and billions of dollars have been expended trying to cure or find answers to these diseases. Unless we as individuals take preventive measures early on, diseases, such as the above and many others, will continue to cost more. Some of the preventive steps you can take include eating foods that are rich in vitamins, minerals and amino acids and supplementing your diet with quality products. Along with these, you should have annual physical exams and nutritional analyses. The costs of these preventative steps are significantly less, compared to what it could cost you later, in terms of medical expenses (both insurance and hospital), lost wages, quality of life and your longevity.

In short, what all the above exercises of prudence can do for you is optimize your health and level of well-being. Your body has many of the attributes of a mechanical system. It needs proper and periodic maintenance if you want it to last and function at optimal efficiency.

From the list of tests above, you can choose one that fits your particular needs. If you have long abused your body by drinking, smoking and eating indiscriminately , or have worked in a stressful and polluted environment, you might want to do all, or almost all, of the tests in the above list. On the other hand, if you have always taken care of yourself, have never smoked, have eaten and drunk wisely or have lived and worked in a clean environment, you might want to take specific nutritional exams* (#3 on page 27). This actually would be a good starting point

---

* These tests are also important for people who are going to go into surgery. It's reported that nearly 50% of preoperative patients are malnourished. Knowing the importance of nutrition, both in your body's ability to go through the operation and for rapid recovery afterwards, it would be useful to find out how well equipped you are nutritionally before you go into surgery. This rest would also be crucial for pregnant women, infants, teenagers and the elderly.

because whatever you have done to your body, nutritionally or otherwise, will be picked up by the tests in this category.

Once you have done all these, your goal should be to take all the necessary nutrients to protect yourself from many of the health hazards mentioned earlier. For example, vitamins A, C, E and the mineral selenium and a number of amino acids have a neutralizing or purging effect on a number of toxins and pollutants that might have collected in your body.

The Role Top Quality Supplements Can Play in Optimizing Your Health, Happiness and Longevity

Considering what we face every day or the life-styles we lead, we have little chance of reaching the optimal level in the nutrition continuum from our everyday ordinary diet. Besides facing environmentally related challenges (such as pollution, irradiation and the sun) we have to deal with stresses, poor eating habits and consumption of excessive alcohol, coffee and cigarettes. These last three substances not only interfere with the absorption of nutrients from your intestinal tract but also deplete your tissue nutrient reserve. As a result, most of us fall somewhere in the middle—malnourished to normal—area of the continuum.

If you personally wish to close the gap or move farther to the right on the graph, you may need, among other things, to include quality supplements as part of your daily meals. Top-quality supplements, besides filling your nutritional chasm, are easy to prepare. In all these areas.

Let's see how quality nutritional supplements can help you move further to the right on the nutrition continuum on page 23. One of the problems encountered with the food you consume every day is that you don't exactly know the quantities of nutrients you get with each meal. Unfortunately there is no device that can help you measure the amount of protein, vitamins and minerals contained in the foods you eat every day.

Instead, when you can, you try to mix vegetables with meats, carbohydrates and fruit in your meal and hope that you get all the nutrients you need. This is nothing short of casting your oats in the wind and praying that they grow healthy and strong.

As was mentioned earlier, not only is there naturally a great variation in nutrients among foods, but a greater percentage of the nutrients that already exist in certain foods are stripped out during processing and canning. For instance, processing wheat could remove 99% of chromium, 86% of vitamin E, 50% of the pantothenic acid (vitamin B5), 72% of vitamin B6 and nearly 100% of the zinc contained in the original grain.[31] According to research findings, only "two percent of the flour consumed in America is whole wheat."[32] Canning and freezing equally destroy or remove many of the nutrients in foods.

Then there is the problem with absorption. Minerals and vitamins found in natural foods such as vegetables and grains are not completely absorbed. In some cases you would be lucky to have even a 10% absorption rate. Some companies chelate (wrap) minerals in amino acids or other organic compounds to significantly increase the absorption of these nutrients. Chelation can increase, in some cases, by as much as 90%, absorption of these nutrients.

As you get older, not only does your metabolism go down, but you also have problems with digestion and absorption. This means that to obtain the amount of nutrients you used to get when you were younger, you may need to consume larger portions at every meal. The problem with this is that at the expense of increasing your nutrient absorption, you will end up gaining unwanted pounds. Since less and less of the food you eat is metabolized (used up) as you get older, any excess amount of it is converted and stored as fat. Obviously, this is not an optimal situation.

Our discussion of the various nutrients and total or optimal health cannot be complete without including water, exercise and mental discipline. Considering the type of pollution that exists today, drinking clean water is of paramount importance to your health. Water is the medium in which all biochemical processes take place in your body. Thus, it's important that it be free from any antagonistic chemicals or pollutants that would hinder or disrupt these important processes.

Regular exercise is equally important for your health. When you engage in physical activities such as aerobic exercise, you help your body burn excess calories, improve circulation and purge any accumulated waste. Exercise also heightens your sense of well being and euphoria. An integral part of physical exercise is mental exercise. This may involve meditation, yoga, praying or some other form of mental discipline that can help integrate your physical and spiritual self.

PART III
Aging

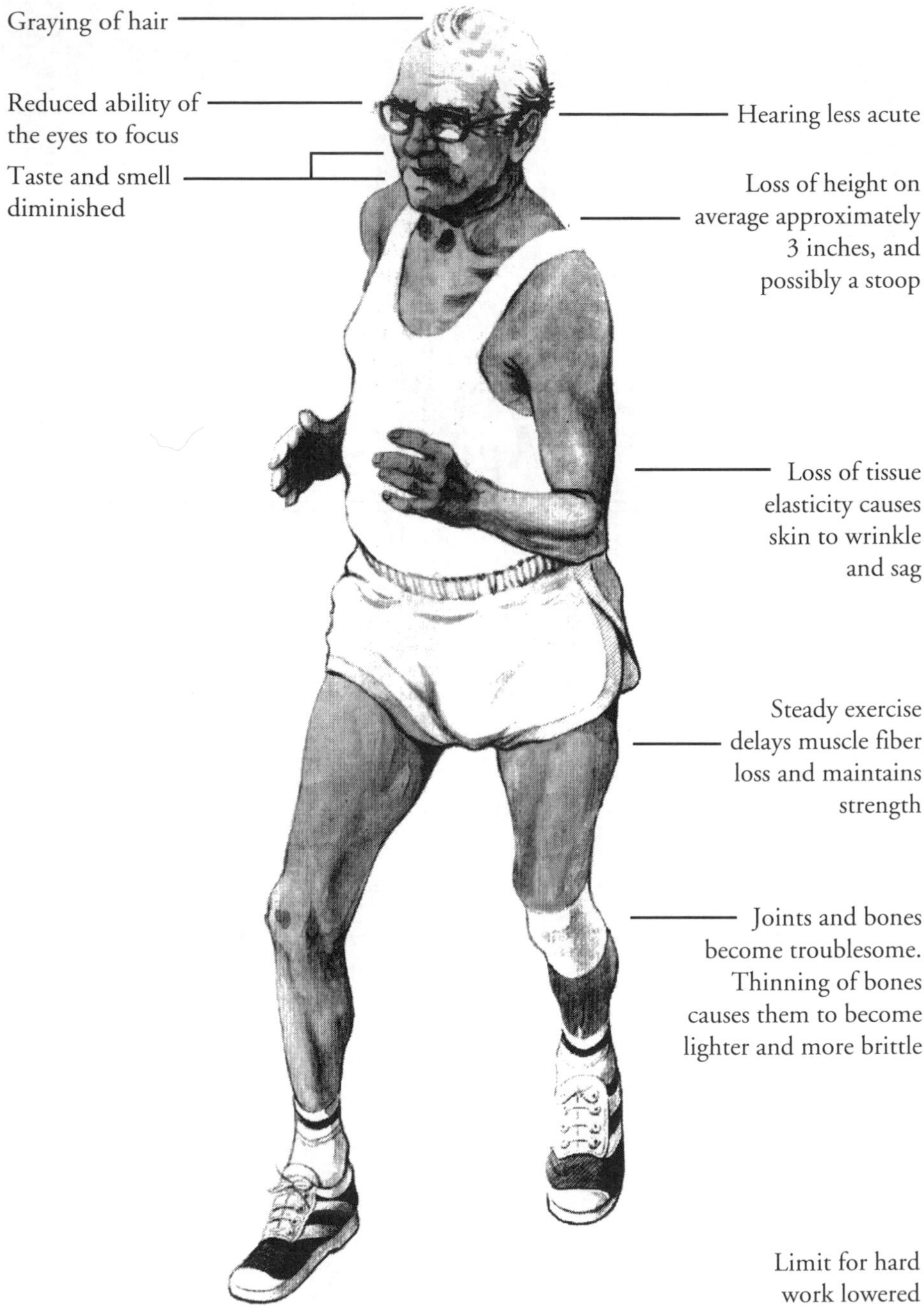

Graying of hair

Reduced ability of the eyes to focus

Taste and smell diminished

Hearing less acute

Loss of height on average approximately 3 inches, and possibly a stoop

Loss of tissue elasticity causes skin to wrinkle and sag

Steady exercise delays muscle fiber loss and maintains strength

Joints and bones become troublesome. Thinning of bones causes them to become lighter and more brittle

Limit for hard work lowered

Figure 3.1 Typical Example of Aging
From *The Human Body*, © Marshall Editions, 1992.

CHAPTER 3
Aging

A major concern to many nowadays is the issue of aging. Several of the health problems that come later in life relate as much to our biological aging as to the absence of good nutrition. In this century, medicine has greatly contributed to preventing diseases and sustaining life, but why we age and die is still a mystery to scientists.

The following few pages attempt to explain some of the current interpretations of aging studies and the nutritional remedies that may control or slow down the process of aging.

What Is Aging?

One theory of aging is that it is a result of a series of cellular "accidents" that take place within our body over time. As an illustration, imagine each cell in your body as a factory that houses thousands of truck drivers, foremen, janitors, assembly workers, security officers and administrators, as well as hundreds of raw materials. When you have this many individuals involved in one place, you'll occasionally have accidents and errors happening. Accidents can be those involving workers themselves or accidents on the manufacturing or assembly line with equipment and material. Some of these accidents can be big enough to require outside intervention, whereas others may be small and can be remedied by the people from within. In either case, the key is to minimize the number of accidents. Otherwise, if errors and accidents are allowed to continue, the morale of the people, as well as the long-term survival of the business itself, is severely compromised.

In your body at a microscopic level, your cells are subjected to the same "rules" or phenomena. In these tiny factories, there are thousands of substances: enzymes, hormones, glucose molecules, proteins, vitamins, minerals and others, each having its own function, or role, to play in your cells. Like the example above, the individual molecules within the cells can experience accidents. Examples of these are the loss of an electron (free radical formation) or a fragmentation or destruction of the molecules. This may arise from the molecules bumping into each other during construction or assembly of a new molecule (like a protein or some other substance).

There are also substances or situations that initiate accidents. In a chemist's

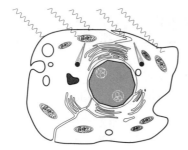

1. Radiant energy penetrating cell membrane
   initiates lipid peroxidation, releasing
   free radicals

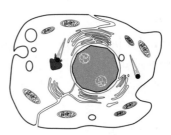

2. A free radical collides with a lysosome,
   puncturing its membrane and allowing
   the release of hydrolytic enzymes.

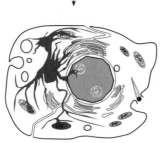

3. The hydrolysate spreads through the cell,
   destroying cellular components. Another free
   radical ruptures the cell membrane.

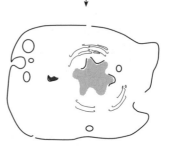

4. The end product of lipid peroxidation:
   a ruptured cell membrane, a distorted nucleus,
   and of the lysosome, only a "clinker" remains.
   The host has become one cell older.

Source: *Nutrition Today* magazine, Baltimore, MD: Williams and Wilkins, December, 1967

Figure 3.2 Free Radicals and the Life of a Cell

jargon, these are called free radical initiators, and they include radiation, heavy metals, such as mercury, cadmium and lead, and certain chemicals. Any situation that generates free radicals in the body can damage the cell membrane as well as other molecules in the cell. This problem can undermine the structural integrity and even the survival of the cell.

The illustrations in Figure 3.2, on page 36, show how your cells degenerate over time as a result of free radical attacks. In diagram 1, exposure to radiation leads to a chemical reaction, which makes free radicals from lipids or other organic compounds in the cell. The radicals created cause the membranes inside and surrounding the cell to rupture, and the cell begins to lose its function (diagrams 2 and 3). Finally, diagram 4 shows a cell that has lost everything it possessed except for a useless and disfigured nucleus.

Interestingly, these accidents start right after conception and continue on through the rest of our lives. How we control, or minimize, their occurrence will affect our health and longevity.

At another level of thinking and as a corollary to the above scenario, aging may be a result of entropy (or disorder) as it's explained by the Second Law of Thermodynamics. This law states that if things are left to their own devices, they tend to move toward maximum disorder (or entropy). Applying this theory to the contents of the cell, this means that the greater the disorder, the greater the chance for error.

Thus, although we may not have control over certain laws of nature concerning the aging process, it has been shown from both animal and some human studies that we can slow down the rate at which the body atrophies. We can do this, as it will be explained at various points in this book, by fortifying our cells and their contents with the right nutrients. The right nutrients can help improve the quality of our lives by shielding us from many of the degenerative diseases that come with age.

Bodily Changes That Take Place with Age

The diagrams used to describe the life of a single cell on page 36 are microcosmic illustrations of what happens to your total body as you age. With time, your organs and tissues atrophy, and they become less efficient in their functions. For instance, with aging, the skin loses its elasticity and color; the muscles shrink and the bones become thin and brittle—making them susceptible to breakage or fracture. The hair grays and thins out, and metabolic rate slows down. A drop in metabolism causes one to gain weight, which, consequently, makes one vulnerable to heart or other diseases by overstressing the organs.

Other changes in organs and tissues occur with aging. The eyes begin to weaken, and taste, smell and hearing are reduced. The pulmonary (lungs), circulatory, digestive and nervous systems also show a gradual decrease in their functions. Figure 3.1, on page 34 and the list below show you additional changes that take place with age.

If we ascribe 100% capacity for our various organs' functions at 20 years of age, the changes that take place for the average person by the time we are in our 70s or older are as follows:

Table 3.1 Changes in Body Functions

Bodily Parts Functions	Functional Percentage Changes
Brain Weight	85
Basal Metabolic Rate*	80
Cardiac Output (rest)	65
Lung Efficiency	55
Liver Weight	63
Liver Bloodflow	50
Kidney Mass	65
Nerve Impulse Transmission	85
Respiratory Capacity of Lungs	55
Kidney Filtration Rate	50
Body Water Content	85
Manual Dexterity and Strength	55

*Refers to the minimum amount of energy needed to maintain vital processes—e.g., breathing, digestion, circulation.

Several studies in gerontology now show that disease and debility are not necessarily a result of old age. Bad nutrition, bad habits like smoking, drinking and substance abuse and lack of exercise are major factors contributing to diseases and the decline in the body's function. Improving your life-style and eating habits can slow down, or even reverse, the aging process.

To give you an example, in one biological aging study,[1] a 39-year-old individual who smoked and consumed alcohol, fast foods, sweets, coffee and soft drinks regularly and was overweight showed a dramatic reversal, or slowing of the aging process after he changed his habits.

This study, a series of tests—which included testing the functional capacity of the cardiovascular system, the immune system, blood chemistry, vision and hearing, the pulmonary system and others—showed this 39-year-old subject to have the biological age of a 61-year-old man. He was evidently a primary target for any of the degenerative diseases (cancer, heart diseases, emphysema, etc.), as well as early death.

This life-threatening situation worried this subject so much that he made a dramatic change in his life-style. He stopped smoking and drinking, switched to a strictly vegetarian diet and began running on a regular basis, achieving the stamina of a marathon athlete. After three years of this regimen, a similar test was done on him. The result was astounding. His body had changed from its chronological age of 42 to the biological age of a 17-year-old.

Some of the Popular Theories on Aging

As stated above, the medical and scientific community still doesn't know exactly what causes aging. It is generally believed that aging represents the cumulative damage done to the body's tissues over the years, either by the environment or by a preprogrammed genetic process that takes place over the course of a human life. The National Institute on Aging has proposed the following theories as some of the causes of aging.

Cross-linking—Random interlocking between protein molecules in the human cells, which leads to loss of flexibility in the tissues. The collagen fibers in your skin, tendons and cartilage, for example, harden as you age. This causes the skin to wrinkle or sag and the tendons and cartilage to stiffen.

Wear and Tear—Consider the body as a mechanical system that over the course of time degrades and weakens, until it finally comes to a halt. Just as with a machine, any maintenance you give your body grants you an extension of life, not immortality.

A corollary to this theory is the notion that says the more you "use" your body, the faster it ages. In other words, if you eat too much or too often, your body works harder to process the food, and the harder it works, the faster it wears out.[2]

This postulation, although it has yet to be proven with humans, actually has been shown to be true with mice. In an experiment, one group of mice was given more to eat, while the control group was given normal amounts. Interestingly, the ones that were fed more than normal died at a faster rate than the control group.[3]

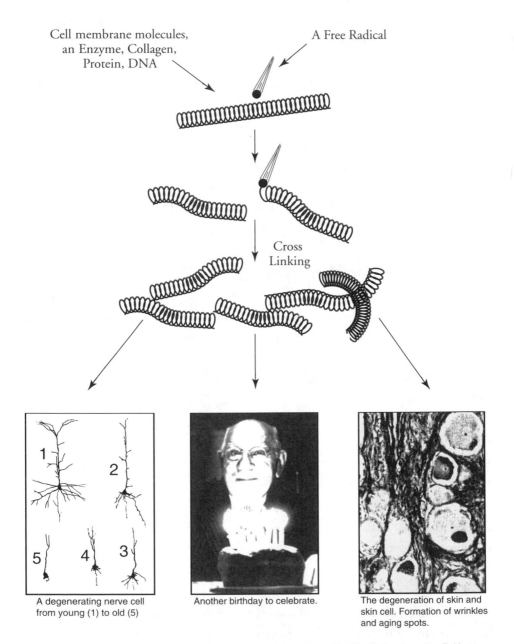

Figure 3.4 Free Radicals and the Aging Process

Somatic Mutation—This theory proposes that the genetic material (DNA) becomes exhausted as it goes through replications over time and begins to introduce spontaneous changes within itself.

Programmed Senescence—Aging and death, according to this theory, are proposed to be pre-programmed events in our genetic material that are inescapable. Certain hormones in our bodies, it's believed, control the onset of these events.

Free Radicals—The free radical theory of aging relates to the gradual atrophying of the body and mind that is due to the "rusting" effect of substances known as free radicals. Free radicals are generated during a normal metabolic process or are imported from outside via the foods we eat. Of all the theories, this one has been the most widely accepted as a probable cause of aging. Unlike the others, with this one we can have some level of control, because certain nutrients, called antioxidants, have been found to slow down the activities of free radicals in certain experiments. The following chapters address the chemical and molecular interpretation of free radicals.

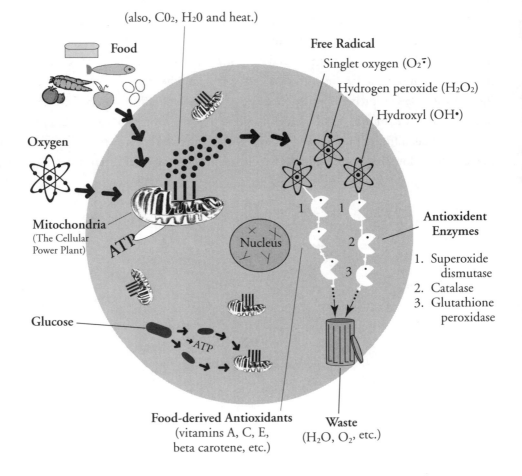

(also, CO_2, H_2O and heat.)

Food

Free Radical

Singlet oxygen (O_2^-)

Hydrogen peroxide (H_2O_2)

Hydroxyl ($OH\cdot$)

Oxygen

Mitochondria
(The Cellular
Power Plant)

ATP

Nucleus

**Antioxident
Enzymes**

1. Superoxide
   dismutase
2. Catalase
3. Glutathione
   peroxidase

Glucose

ATP

Food-derived Antioxidants
(vitamins A, C, E,
beta carotene, etc.)

Waste
(H_2O, O_2, etc.)

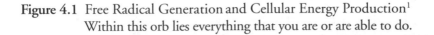

Figure 4.1 Free Radical Generation and Cellular Energy Production[1]
Within this orb lies everything that you are or are able to do.

CHAPTER 4
Free Radicals and Antioxidants

Free Radicals

Atoms are the basic building blocks of any substance. When atoms combine, they form stable molecules, like oxygen in our atmosphere (two oxygen atoms combined as one molecule) or water (two hydrogen atoms and one oxygen atom). When certain molecules combine, they form long chain substances (or polymers) like proteins, fats and carbohydrates—just to name a few.

Atoms or molecules are bonded together by electrons. In organic compounds, the most frequent number of electrons shared between atoms is two. These bonds are not permanent. Depending on the presence of other forces (temperature, radiation and chemical agents), these bonds can break and separate from each other, leading to an uneven number of electrons in each molecule or atom. As shown in Figure 3.2 on page 36, the same situation can result when a molecule is stripped off one of its outer electrons. In either case, the resulting molecule or atom is referred to as a free radical. In the body, free radicals are generated during the normal course of metabolism, or they may be induced by environmental factors, such as radiation and pollution.

Free radicals are unstable substances that cause havoc in the area in which they roam or with the things they encounter. A free radical's ultimate goal is to find another atom or molecule with which to pair up or from which to steal an electron to become stable again. When this happens, however, new free radicals are formed that go around attacking more molecules to generate still more free radicals. Such a chain reaction could produce millions of free radicals. If this reaction goes unchecked, it can lead to major complications in the body.

Cell membranes are damaged. Collagen and elastin proteins cross-link, allowing wrinkles or lines to form in the skin. Fats become rancid. Contacts between nerve cells are severed, and the DNA malfunctions. The cumulative effect is physical and mental aging, as well as the onset of various degenerative diseases like cancer, stroke, arthritis, arteriosclerosis, diabetes and senility.[1]

Figure 3.4, on page 40, illustrates what happens in the nervous system and the skin as you age and when you let free radicals run amok. Like moths that shred your wool clothes to pieces or termites that gnaw away the inner workings of your

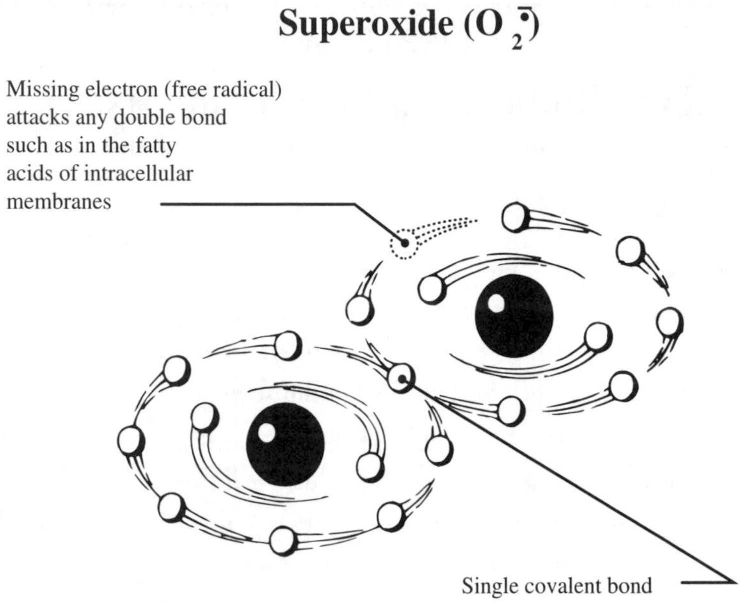

Superoxide (O$_2$$^{\cdot -}$)

Missing electron (free radical)
attacks any double bond
such as in the fatty
acids of intracellular
membranes

Single covalent bond

This superoxide radical is one of the by products of metabolic processes and is known to be highly reactive. In a normal situation the oxygen molecule has a two-electron covalent bond. In a superoxide free radical, as above, the molecule is held together by a single covalent bond.

Source: B. Halstead, *The Scientific Basis of EDTA Chelation Therapy*.
Colton, California: Golden Quill Publishers, 1979 p. 53
Artist: R.H. Knabenbauer

Figure 4.2 An Illustration of a Free Radical

house, uncontrolled free radicals can do the same to the delicate tissues of your body. The aftermath of free radical damage is poignantly illustrated by a degenerating nerve cell (on the left), heavily damaged skin tissue (on the right) and an aging gentleman, who tacitly accepts the effects of these molecular sharks as he sits down to celebrate his birthday.

Sources of Free Radicals

Inside the body, free radicals can be generated from normal metabolic processes and by white blood cells, which use them as a weapon to kill disease-causing foreign elements in the body. They can also be generated by oxidation of unsaturated fats, such as those found in the brain and other parts of the body.[2]

Some of the environmental sources of free radicals are x-rays, ultraviolet light, chemical toxins in the air and water (such as lead, cadmium, mercury, copper and even iron) and nuclear radiation.[3]

Cigarette smoking and dietary fats and oils—particularly those oils processed by the heat extraction method—are other common sources of free radicals. Barbecued and fried foods, such as those you buy at fast-food outlets, are also a great source of free radicals. The combination of high-temperature heated oils (used to prepare these foods) and oxygen is the ideal condition for the generation of enormous numbers of free radicals. The high temperature at the burning tips of cigarettes and the tar that results are also major sources of free radicals.[4]

A single puff of cigarette smoke, for example, can contain up to 100 trillion free radicals, never mind the 3000 plus different aromatic compounds some of which are known carcinogens, it contains.[5]

Perhaps the greatest source of free radicals is the oxygen we consume every day. It's reported that for every 25 molecules of oxygen we inhale, 1 free radical is produced. Considering that we consume trillions of oxygen molecules, with a single gulp of air, you can imagine how many free radicals can be generated every time you breathe in air.

In the mitochondria, during food metabolism, oxygen is reduced to water and carbon dioxide through an addition of electrons one at a time. Hence addition of one electron to a food-derived molecule generates the superoxide free radical (shown in Figure 4.2) two electrons, the hydrogen peroxide free radical, and four electrons, water molecules. In the presence of energy such as UV light, x-ray, iron and copper the hydrogen peroxide converts to the hydroxyl free radical which is the most noxious of the radicals formed in the body.[6] (Hydrogen peroxide and hydroxyl free radicals are shown in Figure 4.1 on page 42)

It is important to note that free radical generation takes place throughout a person's lifetime but increases with age. Particularly vulnerable are brain cells and white blood cells because they are rich in unsaturated fats. A destruction of large numbers of white blood cells can lead to the weakening of your immune system. This is one of the reasons why you become more susceptible to diseases and infections as you get older.

Antioxidants

Luckily, we are not entirely without defense against these freaks of nature—free radicals. Through our body's manufacture of its own antioxidant enzymes and by the food we eat, we can help shield our tissues and organs from free radical damage. The two most powerful antioxidant enzymes are superoxide dismutase (SOD), glutathione peroxidase and catalase. These enzymes are manufactured by the body to promote good health. (See Figure 4.1 for an illustration of these enzymes.)

Superoxide dismutase specifically works to help fight oxygen free radicals. Our body burns the food we eat by using oxygen through a process called metabolism. During this process, many oxygen free radicals are produced, the most common one being the superoxide free radical (see Figure 4.2). The SOD helps neutralize this free radical before it attacks tissues and begins a chain reaction.

What is interesting is that there are two types of SOD—one that exists inside the mitochondria of the cell, the other outside but within the cell. The one inside the mitochondria has manganese as its component, and the one outside has zinc and copper in its structure. It has been shown that a small deficiency in any of these elements greatly affects the SOD activity in our body, thus speeding up our cellular attack by free radicals and our biological aging.[7] The minerals zinc, copper and manganese aid the body to manufacture its own SOD. Similarly, catalase is an antioxidant enzyme that is formed with and activated by iron. In collaboration with the other enzymes, it helps nuetralize free radicals generated in the cell. Its function is primarily to neutralize the hydrogen peroxides.

The other antioxidant enzyme, glutathione peroxidase, is a very versatile molecule involved in a variety of activities in the body. This enzyme promotes the effectiveness of vitamin C and vitamin E and enhances the immune system. Glutathione peroxidase can also help neutralize the unhealthy effects of heavy metals such as cadmium, mercury, lead and aluminum. It saves cells from oxidation. Both white and red blood cells depend on this enzyme for their proper functioning. The power behind glutathione peroxidase comes from the mineral selenium, which is one of the major components of the enzyme. The importance of selenium in human health is discussed in pages 50-52 and 181-184.

Food-Derived Antioxidants

There are many well-documented antioxidants obtained from the food you eat. Some of the prominent ones are vitamins A, C and E, beta carotene, minerals such as selenium, copper, zinc, manganese and iron, glutathione and the amino acids cysteine, methionine and lysine. Recently a new class of compounds called phytochemicals has been added to the list. You find these mainly in green, red and yellow vegetables as well as in herbs. Each one of these nutrients has many benefits to our health besides its role as an antioxidant. Let's look at each one separately.

Beta Carotene—Precursor of Vitamin A

"Eat your carrots. They can help you see better at night." Perhaps you heard your mother chirp this when you were little. And from that time on you have associated the absence of carrots in your diet with night blindness. You try to include a few sticks of these tuberous vegetables whenever you get a chance.

Perhaps you now know that carrots are good for you because they contain a substance known as beta carotene. It is beta carotene that converts to vitamin A in the body and helps the *visual purple*—the pigment in the retina that enables your eyes to quickly adapt when you go from light to darkness.

For a long time, scientists had associated vitamin A with night vision. Vitamin A is now known, however, to have many different functions and benefits for the human body. One of these functions is fighting free radicals. In the body the two most common free radicals are those that form from oxygen molecules and polyunsaturated fatty acids (PUFAs). PUFAs are an integral part of the cell membrane, body fat and some of the food you eat. Beta carotene is known to be an excellent scavenger of the PUFA-generated and singlet oxygen free radicals. Singlet oxygen free radical is one of the most damaging of the oxygen radicals in the body.

In test experiments, vitamin A was also found to inhibit chemically induced cells from becoming cancerous. This, in itself, is very important because our body is constantly exposed to all kinds of chemical carcinogens found in foods as additives, e.g., preservatives, coloring and flavoring agents and texturizers. Vitamin A can also help fight the cancerous effect of drugs, cigarettes, radiation, water and air pollutants.

Vitamin C

Unlike vitamins A and E (the fat-soluble antioxidants), vitamin C has the distinct advantage of being water soluble. Since nearly two-thirds of our body is water, it means this vitamin can go just about anywhere in the body. As an antioxidant, Vitamin C can travel freely in the bloodstream and aid the cells and tissues from the effects of free radicals.

Vitamin C, in effect, acts as your body's sacrificial lamb. A vitamin C molecule gives up one of its electrons to a free radical substance, and in so doing, self-destructs. This battle between vitamin C and free radicals takes place thousands, if not millions, of times a second (depending on the number of free radicals present in your body and the vitamin C level in your bloodstream).

Free radicals, besides contributing to your aging process, are responsible for a variety of cancers. Vitamin C, by neutralizing these marauding chemical species and by boosting your immune forces (antibodies, white blood cells, lymphocytes), protects your body from bacterial and viral infections as well as from cancerous growth. In addition, vitamin C is known to block the formation of nitrosamines—cancer-initiating compounds formed from proteins and nitrites (such as sodium nitrite), which are used as food preservatives.

Vitamin E

Vitamin E is the other food-based antioxidant that has important functions in the body. As one of the few fat-soluble vitamins, vitamin E's primary function is to protect fat molecules from free radical attack. These include the triglycerides and cholesterol in the circulatory blood and the polyunsaturated fats (PUFs) found in the cell membranes and the brain cells.

As said earlier, free radicals are generated during a normal metabolic process or are imported from outside via the water and foods we consume. These ravaging chemical species attack everything they encounter, but they have an affinity for the fundamental building units of your tissues and organs: the cells. A significant portion of the membrane that covers the cells and the sheath that coats nerve axons is made from proteins and substances known as polyunsaturated fatty acids (PUFAs).

As mentioned above, PUFAs are highly vulnerable to a free radical attack. Vitamin E is one of the few fat-soluble vitamins and lodges itself in the membranes of the cells and neutralizes the free radicals before they harm the membrane substances. In doing so, this vitamin averts the onset of many diseases and premature aging.

This effect of vitamin E has been shown in several experiments. Researchers in one study showed the protective level of vitamin E by giving a group of people 600 I.U. of the vitamin for ten days and then subjecting their red blood cells to oxygen and light. When they compared these results with that of the control group (those who had not received vitamin E), the red blood cells from the group who were supplemented with vitamin E oxidized by only 8% while those of the control group

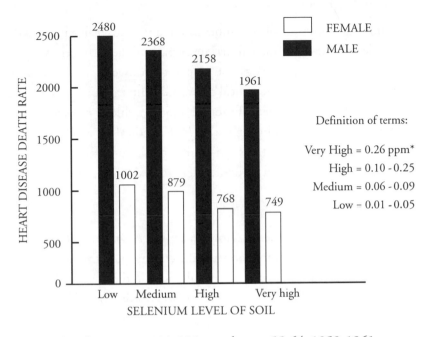

Death rates per 100,000 people, age 55-64, 1959-1961.

Source: Ambau drawing based on the average of data for coronary,
hypertensive, cardiovascular, renal and cerebrovascular diseases.
Data by R. Shamberger, May 11-13, 1976, *Proceedings of the
Symposium on Selenium-Tellurium in the Environment,* University of
Notre Dame, p. 256.
*ppm - parts per million used to define blood selenium level.

Figure 4.3 U.S. heart disease death rates and selenium

were completely destroyed.[8]

In another experiment, rats supplemented with vitamin E had a greater resistance to the damaging effects of lead poison than those that weren't given the vitamin.[3] Vitamin E in collaboration with vitamin C has also been shown to counter the cancerous effects of several food additives (such as sodium nitrite) that lead to the formation of nitrosamines—well-known carcinogens. Nitrogen dioxide, a common pollutant and by-product of automobile exhaust, is also known to be damaging to the lungs. There is evidence to show that vitamins C and E help prevent this problem, too.

The Mineral Antioxidants

The antioxidant property of the minerals copper, zinc, manganese, iron and selenium has largely to do to their function as part of the enzymes systems discussed earlier. Copper, zinc and manganese are part of the two superoxide dismutases that neutralize the superoxide free radical produced from the consumption of oxygen. Iron and selenium, as partners of catalase and glutathione peroxidase, respectively, help in destroying the hydrogen peroxide free radicals as well as free radicals generated from the breakdown of fats. Of course, these minerals have many other functions and benefits to the body besides their antioxidant properties.

Selenium

Selenium has many great benefits to your health. As an antioxidant, selenium can function by itself or in conjunction with the enzyme glutathione peroxidase, a powerful enzyme that plays many important functions in the body, including fighting free radicals, boosting the immune system, cancer prevention and detoxification of heavy metals (such as cadmium, mercury, lead, arsenic) from the body. The mineral selenium is an integral part of this enzyme. Each molecule of the enzyme cradles four atoms of selenium. Many of the metabolic free radical fragments, such as hydrogen peroxides, and those generated from the breakdown of fats are neutralized with the help of this enzyme.

Selenium, together with vitamin E, has also been shown to fight the onset of two major killers: heart disease and cancer, so much so that the incidence of these diseases and the level of selenium in the soil have been correlated. In the areas of the country where there is a low level of selenium in the soil, there are more deaths from cancer and heart disease.[9] (See Figure 14.2, on page 184 for the geographical distribution of selenium in the U.S.)

This amazing mineral has many other benefits. The prevalence of cancer, for example, is equally consistent with the level and geographical distribution of selenium around the world. According to studies from many different countries, the use of selenium in the diet helps minimize the incidence of several types of cancer, including breast, uterine, lung, pancreatic, rectal, mouth, prostate, lymph gland, liver, thyroid, colonic and ovarian cancer. Selenium was found to be equally effective against cancer of the bladder, skin, cervix, esophagus, intestine, pharynx and kidneys.[10,11]

Interestingly, even those who have already succumbed to cancer seem to realize improved survival time, fewer malignancies or metastases and less recurrence of

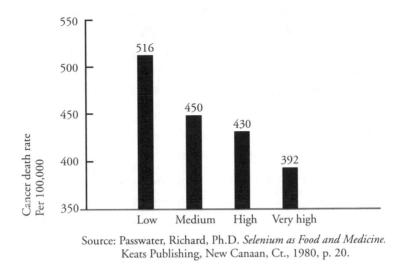

Source: Passwater, Richard, Ph.D. *Selenium as Food and Medicine.*
Keats Publishing, New Canaan, Ct., 1980, p. 20.

Figure 4.4 Cancer and heart disease death rates and selenium

lesions when they received sufficient selenium. A study in which mice were infected with a virus that induces mammary cancer showed a reduction by eightfold in the occurrence of the tumor with a selenium-containing diet. This is a dramatic improvement considering that these mice ordinarily develop tumors in a purported 95% to 100% of the time when infected with the same virus.[12]

Because of the close similarity to the way breast cancer develops in humans, the scientist who did the above study feels that the incidence of breast cancer in this country would be reduced significantly if women took 250 to 350 micrograms of selenium supplements daily.[13]

Selenium is also very important for the proper functioning of the sex organs. The production of sperm cells, as well as their strength and motility, is aided by the level of selenium in these organs. More than half of the body's selenium is found in the testicles and seminal ducts. This means that every time men have sex, they lose a fair amount of it. To maintain an adequate body level of this mineral, they have to keep replenishing it.

In other areas, selenium has been found to be beneficial in the efficient production of energy, in relieving arthritis and in reducing the incidence of cataracts. All these, incidentally, have something to do with selenium's ability to fight free radicals.

Selenium is, indeed, a remarkable mineral. The bar graphs in Figures 4.1 and 4.2 (depicting the relationships between different levels of selenium in the soil and the incidence of heart disease and cancer) are good illustrations of what adequate amounts of this mineral in our diet can do in promoting good health.

Cysteine, Glutathione, Methionine and Lysine

In addition to vitamins and the mineral selenium, there is a group of amino acids that are well-known antioxidants. Glutathione is a small peptide molecule consisting of glutamic acid, cysteine and glycine.

Glutathione helps in the synthesis of the enzyme glutathione peroxidase. This enzyme, as was discussed earlier, has many protective benefits in your body. Glutathione, in collaboration with selenium, helps fight free radicals, guards against cirrhosis of the liver, boosts the protective power of vitamins E and C, assists in removing toxic metals from the system and helps in the production and fortification of immune cells.

Cysteine and methionine are the two sulfur-containing amino acids that are known to be good antioxidants. These amino acids, besides functioning as building components for the regeneration of tissues, are great at mopping up accumulated toxins, such as metabolic by-products, tobacco and alcohol derivatives and heavy metals, such as mercury, lead and cadmium, from the body.

All these are deleterious to the body's organs and tissues. Lysine is known to help boost the immune system by encouraging the production of antibodies. In addition, a daily dose of 1,000 mgs of lysine was shown to reduce herpes breakout in those who carry the virus.

Herbal Antioxidants

Over the past few years, plant-derived substances called phytochemicals or phytonutrients have been toted, after vitamins, as the next group of substances that may have many beneficial properties in our health. These compounds, which are extracted from the green, red, blue, black and yellow of vegetables and fruits, are not exactly nutrients (at least so far as we know), in the sense that they don't get involved in energy production or in repairing and building of tissues, but they apparently have many influences in the health and wellness of our bodies. One of these influences is in serving as antioxidants. The other is by interacting or interfering with certain enzymes and substances in our tissues in ways that enhance and maintain the health and well-being of our bodies.

Some of these compounds are sulforaphane (from broccoli), lycopene (from tomatoes), lutein (from alfalfa), allylic sulfides (from garlic), genistein (from soybeans) and capsaicin (from red peppers). There are many other compounds found in different herbs and spices that have been shown to have beneficial properties in our bodies. (Read Chapters 15, 17 and 18 for more information on phytochemicals and herbal antioxidants).

A Team of Antioxidants for Maximum Health

If you notice, in a well-formulated supplement, all antioxidant vitamins, minerals and phytonutrients appear together. There are reasons for this:

1. All the antioxidants do not necessarily have the same function; that is to say, certain antioxidants are more effective than others in neutralizing certain types of free radicals. For example, beta carotene and selenium (as part of the enzyme glutathione peroxidase) are more powerful neutralizers of the singlet oxygen free radicals. This means, for instance, that during a strenuous physical exertion, like exercise or physical labor, you tend to use up a higher volume of oxygen, which consequently increases the metabolic activities of your cells and the production of the singlet oxygen free radicals. Taking the recommended amounts of these nutrients prior to your physical activity will thus minimize the damage these radicals can cause.

    Vitamin E and selenium, on the other hand, are great suppressors of fat peroxidation. Fat peroxidation (the rupturing of fat molecules leading to the formation of free radicals) can be initiated by a number of agents, including radiation, toxic metals and chemicals, singlet oxygen free radicals and a number of other substances. Tissues that are highly vulnerable to some of these agents are the lungs, the digestive tract and the liver.

    As you must know, the lungs and the digestive tract are the primary contacts of everything that enters the body, including the various chemicals and pollutants that come along with food, water and air. The liver, besides serving as main distribution center, is the place where many of the body's toxins accumulate. Consequently, these three organs take the brunt of many of the effects posed by substances that come in from outside as well as by those generated from within the body. The vitamins E and C and the mineral selenium are known to be excellent protectors of these tissues.[14]

    The phytoantioxidants also have their own special functions in the body. Some of them activate enzymes that are intimately involved in the health and proper function of the cell. Hence, for instance, while sulforaphane induces the synthesis of enzymes that are closely involved with the proper function of the cells, others like coumaric acid and cholorogenic acid help remove unfriendly substances from them.[15,16] There are also phytoantioxidants involved in the health of certain tissues of the body. For example, the anthocyanosides (in bilberry) help with the health of the retina, and leucoanthocyanin (in grape seed extract) is important for the well being of the blood capillaries.[17]   Likewise, the flavonoid molecules found in ginkgo biloba are important for the health and proper function of the brain and circulatory system.[18,19]

2.   When antioxidants are present together, besides enhancing your tissues, they protect one another and other nutrients from the effects of the free radicals. For instance, vitamin A protects vitamin C, which, in turn, protects vitamins A and E and some of the B complex vitamins from free radicals or other oxidative process. Vitamin E, similarly, can serve as a "bodyguard" for vitamins C, D and F* and the B complex vitamins.[20]

As you can see, you should have not only high concentrations of the antioxidants in your tissues but also all of them together so that each one will adequately complete its specific job without getting destroyed before it reaches its destination—usually the cells. As an illustration, think of military airplanes that are on a bombing mission. Unless these planes are adequately shielded from enemy air fire by escorting aircraft, they may never reach their target.

Inside your body, at a microcosmic level, a raging battle goes on between the free radicals and antioxidants. As in the real world, who wins this battle depends on the number and strength of the forces involved.

---

* Essential fatty acids like omega-3 and omega-6 fatty acids.

CHAPTER 5
Your Skin, Hair and Nails:
Where the First Aging Signs Begin

Much of the apparent change that takes place in your body, whether as a result of malnutrition, free radical or environmental damage, is first registered on your skin and to some degree in your hair and nails. As you age, your skin begins to show hairline creases and wrinkles and becomes dry, coarse and scaly. Similarly, the hair begins to gray, recede from your forehead and fall out in greater numbers. Although not as obviously, your nails also go through their own degeneration.

Besides the various antioxidants we talked about in the previous chapter, there are other specific nutrients (vitamins, minerals and amino acids) that can help you minimize the deterioration of the aforementioned body parts. Many of these nutrients are discussed in the appropriate chapters in the rest of the book. Your awareness and the inclusion of these nutrients in your daily meals can greatly help you delay the aging process, as well as improve the health, vitality and appearance of your skin, hair and nails. To practice necessary maintenance and correct any nutritional inequities, you should know exactly what the above bodily features are and how they function.

The Skin

The skin is your body's thermostat, an effective communication medium, a repository of waste, a protector and a tightly woven, thick mesh that holds everything about you together. The skin can be your provenance of pleasure (as when you have beautiful skin) or a source of anguish and pain (as when you have a bad complexion). Your skin is your body's largest organ, measuring some 15 to 25 square feet and weighing 8 to 10 pounds. The skin is home for billions of cells, thousands of hair follicles, oil and sweat glands, and is the outermost destination of nerve fibers and blood vessels.

As a thermostat, the skin maintains your body temperature at 98.6 degrees Fahrenheit by opening its pores when the air around you is hot and closing them when it is cold. Indirectly, the skin also maintains this constancy of temperature by signaling to you to cover up when it's cold or to take your clothes off when it's too warm.   It is your body's greatest communicator. The tickling morning sun on your back, the soft touch of a hand and the presence of a potentially dangerous disease from deep within your body are all first registered and expressed on the skin. In other ways, your skin reflects your feelings and emotions. A beading forehead, the pale, taut look when you're under stress and feeling anxiety and the radiance you emit when you are happy are all conveyed through your skin.

The skin is your first line of defense against many pollutants, bacteria and viruses that impinge upon you every day. The skin also produces many biochemicals and enzymes that help neutralize and detoxify many substances that either are metabolic by-products or manage to enter the inner layers of the skin.

Your skin produces vitamin D, which helps facilitate the absorption of calcium and phosphorus from your intestinal tract. Calcium and phosphorus are important for the development of strong bones and teeth.

Finally, your skin often can give many of your secrets away. How you have treated your body physically (as in excessive sun exposure), chemically (as in cigarette smoking, excessive drinking and drug abuse) and nutritionally (as in eating the wrong foods or a lack of sufficient food) is mirrored in your skin. No matter how you feel about your age or your looks, if there have been nutritional deficiencies or you have advanced in age, somehow your skin seems to give away these confidential matters.

The Structure of Skin and Nutrition

The skin is divided into three main layers. The topmost layer is the epidermis, which consists of an outer dead layer (keratin) and three other consecutive layers below. The epidermis measures about one twenty-fifth of an inch. Below it is the dermis, which houses blood vessels, oil and sweat glands and hair follicles. The collagen and elastin fibers, which give skin its form, strength and elasticity, are embedded in the dermis. At the bottom of the dermis is the subcutaneous (fatty) tissue that helps cushion the skin layers, the bones and vital organs.

The epidermal layer contains three important cells. Keratinocytes synthesize the protein keratin, which eventually becomes your hair, nails and the thin topmost dead tissue of your skin. This layer constantly sheds off—the entire skin being replaced about every two weeks. Melanocytes produce the pigment melanin, which gives color to your hair and skin. Melanin, which protects the skin from the damaging, cancer-causing effects of the sun, is produced in copious amounts when your skin is exposed to strong sun. This is your natural sunscreen. Then you have the Langerhans, whose main function is to protect the body from any bacterial, chemical or other substances that may cross to the dermal layer of the skin.

The well-being and the proper functioning of all these cells is very important for the health and appearance of the skin. New cells are continuously being born, rise to the top as they mature and finally die and flake off. The point is to have this process continue by giving the body the right foods from within and by properly treating the skin with cleansing and exfoliating.

The nutritional aspect of skin care is just as important as, if not more important than, the topical treatment. The quality and the appearance of your skin, hair and nails depend on the health and well-being of the respective cells born every day. These, in turn, will depend on the quality and diversity of the nutrients you eat.

A poor and unbalanced diet can lead to a number of skin conditions. For example, vitamin A deficiency can lead to dry and rough skin. Shortages of vitamin B2 and B6 can cause cracks and inflammation in the soft tissues of the mouth and nose. A deficiency of niacin can result in pellagra, a disease that often manifests itself as a scaly, dry and ugly-looking skin. A deficiency of iron can lead to wrinkles and dryness in the skin and loss of luster and form to your nails. With severe iron deficiency, nails can become concave or flat.

The strength and vitality of the network of blood vessels and skin tissues are also very important for the skin to function and mend itself properly. Capillaries in the skin are a network of tiny vessels that bring food and water to the cells. The structural integrity and proper functioning of these tissues are greatly aided by the presence of an adequate level of vitamin C in the body. Easy bruises or cuts in the skin can often be attributed to a vitamin C deficiency in the diet. The weakness of these minuscule blood vessels contributes to the inefficient distribution of nutrients and water to the skin.

The Hair

Hair is one of the most important parts of your personal appearance. We, as a nation, spend billions of dollars every year on hair and hair products. Most of the money is spent on topically used products. Although such items as shampoos and conditioners are great for cleansing the hair and temporarily fixing any damage, the most fundamental contributor to your hair's appearance (good or bad) is nutrition.

Hair, after all, is dead. But contradictory as it may sound, it is also one of the fastest growing tissues in your body. Like your skin, it is made from the food you eat, nearly all of it being protein. The quality and the completeness of your diet are what will determine the quality, strength and appearance of your hair. The specific hair-building nutrients you take have more influence on how your hair grows, looks and feels than any treatment you apply to it from outside.

Like the dead layer of your skin, hair starts its journey from deep within the skin and comes out through a pit, referred to as a follicle. The aggregate of cells at the bottom of the follicles that give rise to hair are called papillae. The papilla is supplied with blood vessels, which bring nutrients and water to it. As these cells mature, they produce keratin, the pigmented or nonpigmented product we refer to as hair. The keratin in your hair is very similar to the keratin in the top layer of your skin.

Unlike the keratin in your skin, which flakes off periodically, the hair in your scalp can stay with you for up to three years before it falls out and gets replaced with a new growth. During the hair's growing period, the oil glands, found alongside each follicle, keep the hair lubricated and moisturized to minimize breakage and hair loss. However, there are a number of circumstances whereby hair loss, either temporary or permanent, can come about.

The permanent type of hair loss, like balding or a receding hairline, can be caused by heredity, aging and hormonal changes. Nonetheless, there are also a number of circumstances that can cause temporary and, in some cases, permanent hair loss. These range from an unbalanced diet, stress, bad circulation and sudden weight loss to radiation exposure, hormonal imbalances, poor scalp hygiene and the use of medications such as antibiotics and cortisone.

During pregnancy and after the discontinuance of birth control pills, women often experience some level of temporary hair loss. It is important to remember that the average adult loses 50 to 100 strands of hair a day. It should be a cause of concern if the loss is considerably higher than that. However, it is also possible to reduce this loss to half or less by deeply cleansing and treating the hair with quality hair products.

Nails

These vestigial claws have very important mechanical and structural functions. From picking up a pin to buttoning your shirt, nails serve important daily functions. Because the tips of the fingers are made from a soft and fleshy tissue, nails give these tips form and strength.

Like hair and the top layer of your skin, nails are composed of the protein keratin, and their hardness is typically characteristic of their high sulfur content. Like hair, nails are born from a clump of cells (matrix) deep within the skin or the cuticle. Since nails are also dead tissue, there is nothing you can do to improve their appearance once they are formed (other than, of course, coating them with varnishes, enamels or lacquers to add artistic appeal to them).

The appearance of your nails is greatly influenced by your nutrition and the general condition of your health. Nails can often have pits, ridges, cracks, grooves or discolorations. All these can come about from nutritional deficiencies, poor circulation, sudden changes in diet (like fad diets) and sometimes severe physical and emotional stress. Exposure to harsh cleaning chemicals and the presence of fungi, psoriasis, eczema and other skin conditions, which can affect the keratin-producing cells (the matrix), can lead to malformed nails.

Under emotionally stressful conditions, as, for instance, when you have surgery, the body channels nutrients to take care of those specific internal needs. In these situations, the maintenance of beautiful nails, hair or skin is of less importance. Thus, any physical changes that appear on your nails can be attributed to these stressful conditions and a multitude of other factors.

You can effectively deal with the above problems, as well as enhance the appearance of your nails, by taking the right nutrients. These include vitamins A, Bl, B2, B5, B6 and B12, biotin, niacin, folic acid, inositol, the minerals potassium, iron, iodine, zinc, manganese, magnesium and calcium and amino acids (particularly those that contain sulfur, such as methionine, cysteine and taurine). The essential oils, such as omega-3 and omega-6, are also important.

These ingredients are involved in the metabolism of the food you eat and in the building and repair of your skin, hair and nails. The specific vitamins and minerals in your diet create the proper conditions for the proteins, carbohydrates and essential fatty acids you eat to work more efficiently.

Although it is not observable to you, your body wears and tears continuously—some parts (like the kidneys, heart, lungs, liver and blood cells) at a faster rate than others (muscles and bones). To retard the process of aging and the onset of diseases, you may want to assist your body by giving it the proper nutrients to rebuild and repair itself. As was mentioned regarding skin, the generation and growth of hair and nail tissues are continuous processes. These processes will take place smoothly and efficiently only if you provide your hair and nail tissues with the necessary proteins, carbohydrates, vitamins and minerals.

For more information, read the appropriate sections on each of these nutrients. For supplements, go to your health food store and find a product that is specifically designed for these body parts and use it as part of your diet. You may also ask around for an independent distributor in your area who sells vitamin and mineral supplements.

PART IV
Understanding the Food You Eat

CHAPTER 6
Macronutrients, Micronutrients and Fibers

Macronutrients

Every day, we perform the most basic of activities—activities that our very existence depends on. We breathe, drink and eat. Yet, most of us pay little attention to the quality or quantity of the food we eat, the water we drink or the air we breathe and what ultimately happens to them in our body. It seems that this negligence is largely the reason why we have so many health problems in this country and why we cannot attain optimal health and maximum longevity. Let's look at our daily nutrient intakes closely.

The basic raw materials we depend on for our survival are oxygen, water, carbohydrates, proteins and certain fats.

Oxygen

Oxygen is your body's fundamental life sustainer. Unlike water deprivation, which can kill you in five days, or food deprivation, which can kill you in five weeks, you can die within minutes without oxygen. For the cells in your body to function continuously, they need a steady supply of it. Oxygen combines with glucose in the cells to provide you with the energy you need to perform the most basic functions, as well as major physical tasks.

Oxygen enters the body after it's picked up from your lungs by hemoglobin—a protein molecule found in the red blood cells. Many of the metabolic processes—the conversion of foods into tissues and energy, or the breakdown of substances in the cells—depend on the availability of oxygen.

Water

After oxygen, water is the next most important substance in your body. It serves as an integral part of your tissues and as a medium in which nutrients and many biochemical components are conveyed from one part of the body to another. It also serves as the medium in which many biological reactions—the conversion of the food you eat into energy and bulk—take place. Water helps to remove toxins and acids that collect in your tissues during the normal metabolic process or during physical exertion like exercise.

Carbohydrates

There are two main dietary sources of energy for the body: carbohydrates and fats. Starch and sugar are perhaps the most common and frequently consumed carbohydrates used for this purpose. Carbohydrates are divided into three major classes.

1. *Monosaccharides* are the simplest type of carbohydrates. They include glucose, galactose and fructose.

2. *Disaccharides* consist of two linked saccharide molecules. They are sucrose (table sugar), lactose (milk sugar), honey and maltose.

3. *Polysaccharides* are made up of long chains of saccharide molecules.

Except for lactose (milk sugar) and ribose (animal nucleic acid sugar), all carbohydrates are synthesized by plants. Cereals, vegetables and fruits are the main sources of sugar, starch and cellulose. These food groups also contain a fair amount of vitamins, minerals and proteins. When these foods are consumed in their natural forms (unrefined), you get the maximum nutrients. Refined carbohydrates, like sugar and white flour, are devoid of many important nutrients.

During digestion, carbohydrates are broken down to simple sugars, such as glucose, galactose and fructose. The liver converts these sugars into glucose for utilization as fuel by the body. Unlike other foods, fats and proteins, for example, carbohydrates are the most efficient source of your daily energy needs.

Glucose is the preferred fuel in the digestive system. It fuels the body's processes and functions without creating too much waste. Any excess amount of glucose is converted into glycogen and stored in the liver or muscles for future need. When these storage sites are overloaded with glycogen, the body converts and saves glucose as fat.

Proteins

Proteins are long chain substances built from small units of molecules called amino acids. There are 20 commonly known amino acids in all living things. The hundreds of different proteins found in the human body are built from various combinations of most of these amino acids. The liver synthesizes nearly half of the amino acids that our bodies need. The other half—so-called *essential amino acids*— must be obtained from dietary sources. These are arginine, histidine, isoleucine,

leucine, lysine, methionine, phenylalanine, threonine, tryptophan and valine.

Proteins serve two major purposes in the body. Structurally, they serve as your body's building blocks and scaffolding. Practically of all the muscles, organs, glands, ligaments, nails, hair and some of the body fluids are composed of proteins. The health and structural integrity of all these body parts depend on the quality and variety of the amino acids and other nutrients you supply your body.

Functionally, proteins serve as enzymes and hormones and as an integral part of genes and the immune system. Of all the functional proteins, enzymes are the most prevalent (over 20,000 known) and the most important because nearly every process in the body depends on them. Enzymes are catalysts. They assist in bodily chemical reactions without being consumed themselves.

The most important of these processes is the digestion of food. Every step of the way—from the mouth to the stomach and small intestine to its final destination in cells, the food we eat is broken down with the assistance of enzymes. Once in the cell—some of it is used for energy, some of it for repair of tissue or growth and the remainder is converted into a form that can be stored and reused later. These steps, too, are accomplished with the help of enzymes.

In short, you could say enzymes are the construction workers that build muscle tissues, nerve cells, glands, bones, hair, nails and many other body parts. The number and quality of the workers available to do all these tasks depend on the variety and quality of the raw material you give your body. This requires you to consume quality proteins, carbohydrates, vitamins and minerals regularly. See Chapter 32 for more information on the function of enzymes.

Micronutrients (Vitamins and Minerals)

Perhaps the most astounding thing about the several million biochemical reactions that take place every second in our bodies is not that they happen at all, but that they happen in such orderly and sequential fashion with thousands of synchronous participants most of which have no similarities or relationships with one another. In this regard, you might draw the analogy of a symphony orchestra of a thousand instruments coming together to create the music of life—you or everything that has to do with the organic you.

Just as symphonic music doesn't exist until it is brought to life by the conductor and performers, you won't "exist" until all the right kinds and numbers of nutrients have come together in the right amounts and at the right place and time. These include not only the macronutrients (carbohydrates, proteins and oxygen) discussed above, but also the star performers—vitamins and minerals (also known as micro-nutrients because the body needs them in small amounts).

Vitamins are organic compounds that act as cofactors (or partners) or regula-tors of various metabolic processes. As co-workers of enzymes, vitamins enable the various chemical reactions in your body to take place quickly and smoothly. But unlike enzymes, which are synthesized in the body, vitamins must be obtained from outside. Plants, with a few exceptions, are the main sources for practically all the vitamins your body needs. There are over 13 different vitamins. They are generally divided into two groups according to their solubility, which defines their function and duration in the body.

Vitamins A, D, E and K are fat soluble, and they stay in the body longer. All the others—vitamin C and the B-complex group are water soluble. The water-soluble vitamins are eliminated from the body regularly through urine and, in some cases, also through the feces. The longest this group of vitamins stays in the body is four days. This means you need to consume these nutrients more frequently than the ones that are fat soluble. Moreover, vitamins are not evenly distributed in plants—some plants have more than others. For this reason, supplements that have a good mix of these important nutrients can be an asset to your health.

Minerals, on the other hand, are not compounds or chemicals like vitamins, but are atoms (elements that cannot be further broken down or formed from other components). Like vitamins, minerals serve as cofactors during metabolic processes. They also serve as structural components in the body—like calcium and phospho-rous in the bones and teeth, iron in the hemoglobin of the red cells and magnesium and copper in the free-radical-fighting enzyme superoxide dismutase (SOD).

The minerals used for biological processes are generally divided into macro (bulk) minerals, such as calcium, magnesium, sodium, potassium and phosphorus, and micro (trace) minerals, such as zinc, iron, copper, manganese, chromium, sele-nium and iodine.

Since the body doesn't make minerals, they, too, have to be provided through the food or supplements you take. If your body doesn't get all the minerals and vitamins it needs, it suffers. Some of the symptoms may be subtle; others may mani-fest as outright sickness.

Just as a symphonic performance would lose its vitality and harmony if the key instruments or performers were absent, so would your body if you didn't give it all the vitamins and minerals it needs to carry out its daily functions. The food you eat would not be used efficiently. Critical enzymes or hormones will not be synthesized in proper amounts, and your body will lose its ability to defend itself from diseases and infections. (See Chapters 12-14 for details on these crucial nutrients.)

Fibers

Fibers are indigestible substances that have no nutritive significance whatsoever. Because of this, for a long time fibers have been some of the least understood and most unsung heroes of the nutrition world. Only recently, scientists have come to recognize the importance of these inert, stringy substances in our diet. As you can see below, fibers do play a crucial role in our health.

Fibers come from many different sources, and depending on their origin, they have different functions and classifications. The so-called water-soluble fibers include the ones in apples, squash, potatoes and all the citrus fruits. These are the pectin family. The gums, which are in oat bran, lentils, guar gum, peas and beans, are also water soluble. These and pectin are great at absorbing fats, cholesterol and bile acids (involved in fat processing) in our stomach and intestinal tract. Because these fibers expand as they absorb water, they can quickly give you a sense of fullness. For those who want to lose or control weight, fibrous foods can help suppress the temptation to overindulge.

The insoluble fibers are also divided into two major groups. The lignins are in green beans, broccoli stalks, celery, popcorn hulls, eggplant and cereals. The cellulose and hemicellulose consist of beans, brussels sprouts, wheat flour and carrots. The insoluble fibers function as vacuum cleaners in your intestinal tract. They suck up toxic chemicals, fats, cholesterol and heavy metals, such as cadmium, lead, mercury and aluminum. Because of their fibrous consistency, these substances move relatively fast through the alimentary canal, which, as explained below, is a great benefit to your health.

The advantages of these fibers' short transit time in the gastrointestinal tract and their toxin-gathering ability can be explained by the difference in the health of those people who consume a lot of fiber and those who don't. For example, in those countries, such as the U.S., in which people consume a significant amount of processed foods (and too little fiber), the incidence of cancer, obesity and heart disease is very common. By contrast, in those countries, such as Japan and many African countries, in which the people eat fiber-rich foods, the aforementioned health hazards are much less common.

The Importance of Fibers for Your Health

Constipation When one thinks of fibers one often associates their benefit with minimizing constipation—abnormally difficult and irregular bowel movements. Because of the highly refined and processed foods people consume in this country, constipation is a frequent problem—particularly among older adults. This, in itself, is not a life-threatening situation. As food stays longer in the intestinal tract, however, it could lead to potential health hazards. These include cancer of the colon, hiatus hernia, diverticulosis (the ballooning of intestinal membrane due to hard feces accumulation), appendicitis, hemorrhoids, irritable bowel syndrome and other maladies.

To give you an idea of the prevalence and significance of some of these health problems, colon and rectal cancers, for example, are the second (after lung cancer) most common cancers in the U.S. Each year there are over 60,000 deaths from these two cancers. Scientists attribute these mortalities to the fat- and protein-rich and low-fiber foods people consume in this country. In one study, for instance, people who had low-fiber diets had four times the incidence of colon cancer as those who ate fiber-rich foods. Similarly, diverticulosis is a common health problem among the older generation. According to one report, 30% of Americans over 60 years old suffer from diverticulosis—a condition that can lead to internal bleeding, pain and distress.[1] Irritable bowel syndrome, which can lead to diarrhea, flatulence, cramps and spasms, is also a frequent problem among millions of Americans.

Heart Disease Fiber can play a very important role in keeping your circulatory system trouble-free. Since nearly all heart disease is caused by an excessive presence of artery-clogging fat in the bloodstream, a high-fiber diet serves as a purging device to your cardiovascular system. Fiber does this by absorbing fat and cholesterol from your stomach and small intestine and eliminating them along with other waste before it has a chance to get absorbed by the bloodstream.

The fibers that are highly effective in absorbing fat are the pectin and the gum family mentioned above. In a Stanford University study, when patients were given a concentrated level of guar gum with their meals, they showed a reduced level of the LDL cholesterol while at the same time showing an increase in their HDL level (the good cholesterol).[2] Similar results were also shown with locust bean gum, oat bran and pectin (from apples, pears and potatoes).[3]

Blood Pressure Fiber is also known to minimize high blood pressure (hypertension). Normal blood pressure is created when the heart pumps blood through the arteries. The accumulation of cholesterol and fats in the arterial walls can, however, impede the blood flow, thus forcing the heart to pump harder. The constriction of blood vessels due to hardening of the arteries can lead to a similar situation.

In addition to these culprits, hypertension can result from smoking cigarettes and excessive consumption of stimulants like coffee or tea, drug use and high sodium intake. One of the best and most natural ways to deal with this problem is to include a fair amount of fiber in your diet. By absorbing fat and cholesterol in the digestive tract, fiber can reduce the occurrence of high blood pressure. Hypertension is sometimes age-related. For this and the above reasons, it is important that you increase your fiber intake as you get older.

Environmental Pollution Through the food and water we consume, our bodies are constantly exposed to toxins and some of the cancer-causing agents like food additives and heavy metals, such as cadmium, mercury and lead. When you have a high amount of fiber in your diet, these toxins and pollutants will have a smaller chance of getting into the bloodstream. They will be sucked up and carried out of your digestive tract.[4]

Blood Sugar The consumption of sweets and processed foods can cause havoc in one's body. Since these foods are easily digestible, they are absorbed into the bloodstream quickly. This leads to an elevated blood sugar level, which triggers the secretion of a large amount of insulin to help burn off the excess sugar. As a result, a person could experience unpleasant mood swings—including depression, irritability, etc.

When your food is rich in fiber, however, you experience fewer problems. The fiber, by trapping the sweets longer and releasing them gradually, can provide a more even sugar level in the blood. For some diabetics, this can be a realistic and welcome alternative to insulin injection or the use of antidiabetic drugs. In addition to their cholesterol-lowering effect, gaur gum, xanthan gum, oat bran, pectin and locust bean gum are known, important sugar-trapping agents in the digestive tract. Xanthan gum, by itself, was found to help diabetics and weight watchers.[5,6]

Weight Loss The other area in which fiber has found popularity is in weight control. One of the most frequent problems encountered by people who try to lose weight is their inability to suppress or contain their craving for food. As a result, no matter what they do to deal with this problem, they end up frustrated, depressed and angry at themselves.

Several experiments have shown that fibers can be effectively used as natural suppressants of hunger and consequently aid in losing or controlling weight. Fibers do this in three ways.

One, when a soluble fiber like guar gum absorbs water in the stomach, it swells and turns into a viscous gel. This gives the individual who is trying to lose weight a sense of fullness. This sense of satiation will help the person to eat less. The same thing can be experienced with those fibers that are not water soluble. With these types, you might need to consume larger quantities to get the same effect.

Two, because fibers have a capacity for absorbing things in the stomach, fewer of the fattening food products, such as sweets, proteins and fats, have a chance to get absorbed in the bloodstream. This is consistent with what was stated earlier regarding the blood sugar stabilizing effect of fibers. When the sugar level in your body is stable, you feel less hungry.

Three, because fiber-rich foods take longer to chew and digest, people often eat less of them. When you combine this with the other two factors, you end up eating much less and ultimately lose weight.

In summary, considering that both cardiovascular diseases and colorectal cancers are some of the major killers in this country, eating plenty of fibers and less fat- and protein-rich foods will help you live longer. Losing weight is one of the major concerns people have in this country. When you give your body fiber-rich foods or supplements, you can effectively (along with other weight-reduction measures) deal with this problem as well. Constipation, high blood pressure, diabetes and environmental toxins are the other health problems that affect most of us at one time or another. By increasing our fiber intakes, we may be able to keep many of these health hazards at bay. It is reported that the average American consumes only 11-13 grams of fiber a day. According to the National Cancer Institute, our intake should be somewhere in the range of 20 to 30 grams a day.

CHAPTER 7
Fats and Oils, Including Cholesterol

Since both the number one and number two killers—heart disease and cancer, respectively—are caused largely by these organic substances, we will spend some time explaining the significance of fats and cholesterol in our food and bodies.

More than any of the foods discussed in the previous chapters, people have difficulty understanding fats because (1) they can be good or bad, (2) they come from many different sources and (3) there are many different kinds.

What are fats? In lay terms, fats are oils that are solid or have been made to become solid (like margarine) at room temperature. Chemically, fats are compounds that are made from carbon and hydrogen and little oxygen. Fats are assembled from long chain molecules called fatty acids and an oily alcohol called glycerol (see Figure E.1 on page 382). One glycerol molecule can take three fatty acids in tow. The resulting compounds, of which body fat largely consists, are called triglycerides.

Like proteins, fats can have functional and structural purposes. Functionally, fats can serve to transport fat-soluble vitamins (A, D, E and K) and essential fatty acids (discussed on pages 77-79). As an integral part of the cell membrane, fats also facilitate the movement of ions, nutrients, hormones and other organic molecules between the internal and external environment of a cell. Fats also contribute to the utilization of the B vitamins and their function in digestion, energy production, nerve health and mental well-being.

Structural fats, collectively referred to as lipids, include triglycerides, phospholipids and sterols, such as cholesterol. Triglycerides serve as the body's energy reserve, insulation and protection for vital organs. Phospholipids and cholesterol function as main components of cell membranes. The latter also serves as the precursor to many hormones (such as adrenal and sex hormones) and vitamins. Cholesterol is synthesized mainly from saturated fats but can also be made from glucose and aminoacid precursors.

What differentiates the various fats, or fats from oils, is the length and/or type of fatty acids attached to the glycerol base. (See Appendix E on page 381 for details on these differences.)

Saturated, Monounsaturated and Polyunsaturated Fats

Chemically, the difference between these fats is based on how many carbon sites in the fatty acid chain are occupied by hydrogen. If the acid chain contains the maximum number of hydrogen atoms, it is called *saturated.* If there are two adjacent carbons unfilled with hydrogen, enabling these atoms to form one double bond, that fat is called *monounsaturated.* When, on the other hand, there are many vacant sites in the chain so that multiple double bonds can form, that fat is referred to as *polyunsaturated.* (See Appendix E on page 382 for the chemical structure of these fats.) The structural variations among these fats lead to the differences in their physical characteristics and their significance to our health.

While saturated fats are solid at room temperature, monounsaturated and polyunsaturated fats are liquid (oil) at the same temperature. Saturated fats commonly come from animal sources in the form of meats and dairy products (red meat, cheese, butter, whole milk and lard). Some vegetable oils—such as coconut, palm and palm kernel oils—are also rich in saturated fats. Being dense, these fats are difficult for the body to emulsify (break down) and assimilate. Once inside the body, they often carry cholesterol with them.

Saturated fats have been implicated as one of the causes of major diseases, such as heart disease and cancer (prostatic, colon, breast, pancreatic and ovarian). When a sludge of fatty mass accumulates in the blood vessels, it impedes or blocks blood flow. This condition, besides depriving your cells and tissues of their vital nutrients, can lead to atherosclerosis, inner ear problems and stroke. Saturated fats are also one of the causes of high blood pressure, diabetes and immune-related diseases.

It is believed that saturated animal fats also contribute to osteoporosis—the hollowing of bones resulting from a loss or absence of calcium in the body. In the intestine, saturated fats combine with calcium to form insoluble soaps, which then pass through the feces. In this situation, to meet some of the critical demands (nerve impulse transmission, for proper functioning of the heart and skeletal muscles), the body begins to release its bone calcium reserves. If this continues for some time, it can lead to osteoporosis.

The other two fats—monounsaturated and polyunsaturated fats—are, theoretically, the best kind of fats for your health. The superiority of these fats over saturated fats lies in their ability to emulsify easily and assimilate into the body.

Their less compact or dense features (mainly the polys) enable the body to use them as building blocks for cell membranes and in the production of antibodies and certain hormonelike substances called prostaglandins. (See Appendix A on page 359 for more information on these substances.) Both of these fats are also known to aid in reducing cholesterol in the blood and in promoting good health.

Although all fats have a little bit of each type of fat, most have a predominance of one or two types. The monos, for example, are found largely in olives, rapeseed (source for canola oil), peanuts, almonds and avocados. Other foods, such as grains, vegetables, nuts and seeds, also have them but in lesser amounts. On the other hand, polys are found predominantly in corn, safflower, soybean, sunflower and cotton seeds and certain types of fish.

Because they are very stable molecules, monounsaturated oils are very good for cooking. They have a high resistance to temperature and oxidation. The polys don't have this property. These oils easily oxidize and degrade under high temperature and light and in the presence of oxygen. Their tendency to oxidize (break down) makes polyunsaturates bad for cooking. While in the body, these oils also tend to generate molecular fragments (or free radicals). (See the Chapter 4 discussion on free radicals.)

As mentioned in the discussion further ahead, polyunsaturates can have a *cis* or *trans* configuration. The difference has something to do with the way the hydrogen atoms orient themselves around the carbon atoms that have double bonds joining them in the fatty acid portion of a fat molecule. The cis-fatty acids are the ones normally found in nature. The trans are formed by partial hydrogenation of vegetable oils to create products like margarine and shortenings. As you will see later, these fatty acids are bad for the body.

Cholesterol

Perhaps there is no food substance other than cholesterol that has received wide press coverage, inspired fear in the hearts and minds of many and been held accountable for some of the major circulatory system diseases. These include stroke, angina, arteriosclerosis (hardening of the arteries) and atherosclerosis (accumulation of fat in the inner walls of the arteries). Yet cholesterol is a very important constituent of body cells. It serves as a precursor to vitamin D, as well as a number of important hormones and bile salts. It helps transport fats to various tissues.

In the body, cholesterol is primarily synthesized in the liver from a variety of foods, but mainly from saturated fats. All tissues of the body, including the brain and nerve cells, contain cholesterol. In foods, cholesterol is found mostly in egg yolk, dairy products and meats.

Despite people's fears, cholesterol is not such a deadly villain. It becomes a health hazard when too much of it oxidizes and accumulates in the blood. Cholesterol binds with saturated fats, which tend to make it bulky and sluggish. If you eat too many eggs, meats and dairy products, you increase the cholesterol and saturated fat levels in your blood. Often the end result is that these fats cling to the arterial walls and cause atherosclerosis, or they combine with calcium, leading to hardening of the arteries (arteriosclerosis). Both of these conditions can cause high blood pressure in the mildest cases, or stroke and heart attack in the worst.

To minimize these life-threatening situations, your body has a conveyor mechanism to transport cholesterol and triglycerides (saturated fats) away from the heart and blood vessels. These carriers, called lipoproteins (a combination of phospholipids and proteins), wrap around cholesterol or triglycerides and transport them to their destinations. These can be the cells where these fats and cholesterol can be used for fuel or structural purposes, or the liver, where they can be processed and excreted.

The combination of fats, cholesterol, phospholipids and proteins is often described by their weight or density. Since fats are lighter than protein, the higher the concentration of protein in a given lipoprotein, the denser it is. Hence, there are generally three classifications of lipoproteins.

Very low density lipoproteins (VLDLs) consist of predominantly triglycerides, 15%-20% cholesterol and a little protein. Low density lipoproteins (LDLs) may contain over 50% cholesterol, 20% protein and less than 30% phospholipids and triglycerides. High density lipoproteins (HDLs) carry over 50% protein, 20% cholesterol and 30% phospholipids and triglycerides.

From these three general characteristics, physicians often categorize VLDLs and LDLs as the bad guys and HDLs as the good guys. LDLs are "bad" because they tend to settle along the arterial walls and interfere with the free flow of blood and nutrients.

HDLs, on the other hand, do the opposite. They remove any fatty deposits from the blood vessels and deliver them to your tissues or to the liver so that it can excrete or convert them into bile salts. All the fat-soluble vitamins mentioned previously are also transported by HDLs. In times of shortage, HDLs can also be used for energy.

To reduce the cholesterol and fat level in your body, eat less, if any, dairy products and red meat. Also avoid coconut, palm and palm kernel oils. These oils are rich in saturated fats. Avoid fast-food outlets. Because of their heat stability and long shelf life, saturated fats are often used in food preparation in fast-food restaurants. Table 7.1 shows some of the age and risk factors for people with cholesterol problems (defined as milligrams per deciliter [mg/dl] of blood):

Table 7.1 Total Cholesterol

Age	Moderate Risk	High Risk
20-29	above 200	above 220
30-39	above 220	above 240
40+	above 240	above 260

The health risk associated with high blood cholesterol is not as simple and clear-cut as the figures in Table 7.1. There are many variables physicians have to take into consideration to properly diagnose a person's health problem involving cholesterol. Besides considering the total cholesterol levels as shown in Table 7.1, a physician may have to consider a patient's HDL, LDL and triglycerides levels. These types of fats, along with the ratio of total cholesterol to HDL cholesterol, are generally much better indicators of a person's health risk for coronary heart disease (CHD). In addition, a person's gender, family history, life-style, obesity status and other factors, such as high blood pressure, diabetes or a history of vascular diseases, are important and must be considered. Regarding CHD, men and postmenopausal women who do not take estrogen replacement are at a greater risk than any other groups in the population.

Table 7.2 illustrates a general guideline doctors use to describe a person's health condition concerning coronary heart disease. The total cholesterol and the LDL cholesterol figures are from the National Cholesterol Educational Program (NCEP) report.

Table 7.2 Cholesterol Types and Their Health Risk

Type	Acceptable	Borderline	High Risk
Total	below 200	200-239	above 240
HDL	above 45	35-45	below 35*
LDL	below 130	130-159	above 160
Triglycerides	below 200	200-400	above 400
Total/HDL ratio	below 3.5	3.5-4,5	above 4.5

*The acceptable value for women is greater than 55 ml/dl, and both sexes are considered at a high risk if their HDL figures drop below 35 ml/dl.
**These figures are based on fasting plasma triglyceride levels.

As mentioned above, although total cholesterol can be used as an overall guideline in assessing a person's heart disease risk, the ones often considered as better indicators are the HDL, LDL and triglycerides. The reasons for this are manifold.

Besides blood fat components, the other risk factors (gender, hypertension, diabetic condition and heredity) play important roles. To help us deal effectively with these risk factors and previously discussed problems, the National Cholesterol Education Program publishes a general guideline.[2] The following is a summary of that guideline.

1. If a person's blood cholesterol test is less than 200 mg/dl, the test should be repeated in 5 years.

2. If, on the other hand, the first test reading was found to be higher than 200 mg/dl, the test should be repeated and the average of the two numbers taken.

   If this number falls between 200 and 239 mg/dl, there are two situations to be considered:

   a. If the person has no coronary heart disease and has two, or fewer, other risks, the person can be given dietary counseling and the test can be done annually.

   b. On the other hand, if the person has coronary heart disease and has more than two additional risk factors, he/she should undergo lipoprotein analysis and this person's LDL level should be determined in order to take further action.

3. Any total cholesterol reading higher than 240 mg/dl is considered high risk, and the person should be treated as in 2b.

Similarly, readings of the LDL cholesterol should follow the above guideline. In a situation in which a person's cholesterol level is considerably higher than 240 mg/dl and if the aforementioned remedial steps fail, a combination of drug and dietary treatment is usually recommended. If you have a cholesterol problem or if you want to learn more about these treatments, contact your local clinic. Let's summarize.

From the discussion above, you can see that cholesterol is a mixed blessing to the body. Vitamin D and many hormones are synthesized from cholesterol. The cell membranes throughout your body are also made, in part, from cholesterol. On the other hand, because of its tendency to cling to the arterial walls and cause coronary heart disease and other circulatory disorders, cholesterol is one of the most feared food substances in our diet today. This problem is not beyond our control, however.

Cholesterol comes from two sources: from some cholesterol-rich foods we consume and from our liver, which synthesizes it mainly from saturated fats. By limiting your consumption of saturated fats and cholesterol-containing foods, you can minimize the incidence of heart attack and fat buildup in your circulatory system.

Thus, to avoid circulatory disorders arising from too much cholesterol and saturated fats, avoid cholesterol-rich foods or minimize your intake of them. As for cholesterol, the amount recommended by some health experts is less than 300 mg.ˑ If you are a typical American, you probably get over 40% of your calories from fat. This is far too much. (No wonder we have over 500,000 deaths every year from coronary diseases.) You should be able to get along fine with less than 20% fat calories.

Moreover, as you know, fat and fat-containing foods are everywhere. To lead a quality, long life, watch out for these foods. Increase your consumption of carbohydrates and fibers and exercise regularly. Exercises that stimulate the cardiovascular system, such as running, swimming, aerobics and cycling, are excellent mobilizers and burners of excess fat from your cells and circulatory system.

Essential Fatty Acids (EFAs) and Eicosanoids

Any discussion of fats would not be complete without talking about the star of all fats—the essential fatty acids and their associated derivatives called eicosanoids. The essential fatty acids which more specifically are known as omega-3 and omega-6* fatty acids, as you will see below, are very critical to the health and function of the body. A large part of their importance has something to do with eicosanoids, a group of hormone-like substances that are synthesized in the body from the essential fatty acids. Eicosanoids, as you'll also see below, are the genies that control many of the body's processes.

Essential Fatty Acids

Sometimes referred to as vitamin F because the body doesn't make them, essential fatty acids must be obtained from dietary sources. Although they have been found as structural components of cell membranes, their overall function in the body is more like vitamins—serving as co-factors of many biochemical reactions. Let's look closely at essential fatty acid's special characteristics and function in our bodies.

First, although they appear similar in chemical structure (see page 382), essential fatty acids are divided into two distinct classes, each containing molecules specific to that group. Hence, linolenic acid is a member of the omega-3 fatty acids and linoleic acid, which is sometimes called conjugated linoleic acid (CLA), belongs to the omega-6 fatty acids. From these two molecules the body makes a number of different compounds that have many health benefits. Thus, linolenic can give rise to *eicosapentanoic acid* (EPA) and *docosahexanoic acid* (DHA). Linoleic

---

* For those who are technically inclined, the numbers 3 and 6 in these fatty acids refer to the position of the first double bond in the fatty acid molecules. One end of these molecules contains a methyl group, the other, a carboxylic group. Hence, when we count the number of carbon atoms using the methyl group (the group that is non-reactive and therefore constant) as a reference point, we find the first double bond at the third carbon in the case of omega-3 and at the sixth carbon in the case of omega-6 fatty acid. See the molecular structure of these two acids in Appendix E.

acid can produce arachidonic acid and gamma linolenic acid (GLA). See table 7.3 for the food sources of omega-3 and omega-6 fatty acids.

Two, to manufacture the above compounds from their respective fatty acids, the body needs magnesium, zinc, biotin, vitamin B6, insulin and an enzyme called delta-6-desaturase. If your body has insufficient amounts of these substances and also contains high amounts of alcohol, cholesterol and saturated fats and chemical carcinogens, it cannot synthesize the aforementioned crucial compounds. (This information is illustrated graphically on page 358).

If, however, you are watchful of what you eat, you can also find the above fatty acid derivatives from certain foods. For example, arachidonic acids are found in meats such as turkey, chicken and red meat; and EPA and DHA are found in human milk, shellfish and other fish such as mackerel, salmon, menhaden, trout, sardines, anchovy and tuna; and GLA in evening primrose oil.

Three, essential fatty acids or rather their derivatives function as controllers of hundreds of physiological and biochemical process that take place in our bodies moment by moment. Here are some examples to illustrate this point. For instance, EPA

- lowers cholesterol and triglycerides in the blood.
- reduces blood pressure and, hence, minimizes the incidence of heart attack or stroke.
- thins blood out by making blood cells less sticky and by lowering blood's viscosity.
- helps reduce the incidence or the severity of migraine headaches.
- helps reduce the occurrence of inflammation for rheumatoid arthritis sufferers.
- helps the skin deal better with such problems as psoriasis, eczema, dermatitis and oiliness.

Furthermore, these fatty acids are important nutrients for the normal development of the brain cells and the nervous system as a whole. Mothers who breastfeed, for example, would be advised to include foods that are rich in the omega-3 fatty acid in their meals. Researchers, both here and in Japan, have shown that a

---

*Just to show you the amount of cholesterol found in some food, 3 oz. of calf's liver contains 331 mg; 1 egg yolk, 213 mg; 3 oz. of cooked beef or chicken, 76 mg; 1 cup whole milk, 33 mg; and 1 cup skim milk, 1 mg. (Source: USDA, *The Food Guide Pyramid.*)

deficiency of this essential fatty acid leads to poor mental development and, hence, to poor learning and memory in children.

Besides serving the body in some of the above areas, DHA is also important for the proper function of the retina and the brain cells.

Among the Omega-6 derivatives, GLA, found in evening primrose in high concentration, has been shown to serve equally impressive function in the body. It prevents hardening of the arteries, reduces the tension and discomfort experienced with premenstrual syndrome and fights cancer and diabetes.

GLA reportedly also increases sex hormone activities, lowers cholesterol levels and helps relieve pain and inflammation in the joints. It's also important in treating cirrhosis of the liver. It helps with immunity disorder and helps control the occurrence of candida albicans (yeast infection).

Furthermore, conjugated linoleic acid (CLA) helps mobilize fats from the storage sites while at the same time increase lean muscle mass. These fatty acids do this by increasing the availability of energy to the body and by activating certain enzymes that are responsible for the release of fat from its deposit sites.

Eicosanoids

Manufactured in the body from the essential fatty acids, eicosanoids are a group of short-lived, hormone-like substances that control a tremendous number of bodily functions—ranging from blood pressure, immune system competence, hormonal response to nerve impulse transmission and fat production to the growth and repair of tissues to thousands of other physiological and chemical processes in the body. Although grouped together under the same name, eicosanoids come in many different forms and have different functions in the body. For example, a subclass of eicosanoids called *prostaglandins* (see Appendix A for more information on these) increase the availability of oxygen to the cells and hence facilitate the burning of more calories. These eicosanoids, when available in sufficient quantities, also encourage the release of fat from its deposit sites while at the same time help increase its lean muscles. This piece of information is good news for those who want to lose or manage weight as well as for athletes who want to increase strength and build

---

*Barry Sears in his book, *The Zone,* says that the ideal proportion of the three major food groups should be; 40% carbohydrates, 30% protein and 30% fat. These proportions reportedly are important for the *maximum* production of a family of hormones called eicosanoids, of which prostaglandins (discussed in Appendix A) is one. Eicosanoids are localized hormones that have a tremendous influence on the proper function and health of the body.

mass. It has been found that this group of eicosanoids also improves the appearance of skin by increasing its water holding capacity and nails by making them less brittle.

In addition, prostaglandins regulate the function of involuntary muscles—gastrointestinal, ear, eye and heart muscles, controls the secretion of various bodily fluids and facilitates cellular division and repair. There are other classes of eicosanoids and these include thromboxanes (which causes platelets to aggregate thus allowing blood to clot, important during a cut or an injury), *protacylins* (which inhibits clotting and dilates vessels, important for cardiovascular health), *leukotrienes* (a bad eicosanoid which constricts vessels particularly around the bronchus causing difficulty in breathing) and *lipoxins* and *hydroxylated* fatty acids (which suppress the function of certain immune cells and create other disorders in the body).

By now you perhaps wonder where are eicosanoids made and how can we maximize the benefit of the good eicosanoids while at the same time minimize the bad ones. Presuming that you are properly nourished, eicosanoids are made by every cell in the body. With regard to the production of the bad and good eicosanoids, both are necessary but the key is to keep them in balance.* The best way to keep them in balance, according Barry Sears, author of The Zone, is by consuming sufficient amounts of the essential fatty acids and also by keeping carbohydrate to proteins and fat caloric consumption at 40%, 30% and 30%, respectively. This ratio reportedly is the best combination that keeps the good and bad eiconosides in balance, thus allowing the body to have the maximum benefit from these important substances. At the above ratio, the body will also be able to utilize the food one eats more efficiently hence minimizing fat storage and weight gain. According to Dr. Sears, the consumption of high carbohydrates food also leads to a high production of the bad eicosanoids and consequently to many of the unwanted health problems associated with these forms of the eicosanoids.

To receive the full benefit of prostaglandins, you need to supply your body with foods that are rich in the essential fatty acids. Table 7.3 shows a selection of food sources that are rich in omega-3 and omega-6 fatty acids.

---

* Because insulin and glucagon have opposing actions (a high level of carbohydrates leads to high production of insulin and also of the bad eicosanoids), which cause the body to store the excess as glycogen or fat. A low level of carbohydrates, on the other hand, causes the body to release glucagon which facilitates the conversion of glycogen into sugar and also cause the production of the bad eicosanoids.. This can lead to a vicious cycle which ultimately leads to gaining weigh and other complications.

Table 7.3 Sources of Omega-3 and Omega-6 Fatty Acids

Omega-3	Omega-6	Omega-3 & Omega-6
salmon	safflower	flaxseeds
trout	sunflower	pumpkin
mackerel	corn	wheat germ
sardines	sesame	canola
tuna	peanut	soybean
eel	avocado	walnut

Ideally, you want one food source that contains both the omega-3 and omega-6 fatty acids. In this case, flaxseed, pumpkin, wheat germ and canola are your best choices. Flaxseed is perhaps the richest source of all. (Please see Appendix B on page 361 for exciting information on this food of the ancient Egyptians and Babylonians. For a comprehensive fatty acid analysis see page 406)

The Problem with Fats

If fats are such an important part of our diet and our body, how and why do they turn against us? The answer to this question lies both in the quantity and in the quality of the fats we consume.

First, the standard American diet contains far too much fat. In terms of calorie consumption, the average American gets his/her daily calories as follows: 15% from protein, 20% from simple carbohydrates and refined sugars, 20% from complex carbohydrates and a whopping 45% from fats. This is a far cry from what is considered optimal: complex carbohydrates, 55%, fats, 20%, protein, 15%, and refined sugars, 10%*.

Food calories function to give you energy and to help you in the processing and transportation of nutrients throughout the body. Any extra calories that are not used for these and other functions are converted into and stored as fat. This conversion normally requires the expenditure of energy. While about 23% of the calories in other foods (i.e., carbohydrates and proteins) are used up in food conversion, an insignificant amount of energy is required to convert calories from fat into body fat.[3]

Second, on a gram-by-gram basis, fats have more than twice the calories found in carbohydrates and proteins. While fats contain 9 calories/gram, carbohydrates and protein hold 4 calories/gram each. So, if you see nutritional information on a food label that says 10 grams of fat and 10 grams of protein per serving, you'll know that the calorie content of the fat is 90, while that of the protein is only 40.

Third, a large percentage of the fat many of us consume has been physically and chemically altered. Such fat is hard for the body to process or assimilate, often interfer-

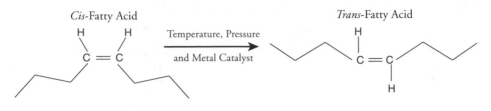

Figure 7.1 *Cis* and *Trans* Fatty Acids

ing or blocking the absorption or assimilation of normal fats that might exist in the diet. There are four common processes that contribute to such changes.

Hydrogenation This involves the addition of hydrogen under high temperature and pressure, in the presence of a metal catalyst, to polyunsaturated, often cheap vegetable oils, to convert them to solid or semisolid fats. The process is often partial hydrogenation—just enough to transform the oil to a thick consistency. The more hydrogen you add to these oils, the firmer the end product will be. Both margarine and vegetable shortenings are produced by this method.

Although hydrogenation improves the stability and shelf life of these products, it also changes the chemical structure of oil molecules from the biologically usable *cis* fatty acids to the useless and often toxic *trans* forms. In the body, the *trans* fats collect in the arterial walls and thus increase the cholesterol or triglyceride level in your blood. If they become incorporated into a cell membrane, they corrupt its physical and functional integrity. The hydrogenation process also creates many different molecular fragments, which, according to some scientists, have unhealthy consequences.

The *cis* configuration is a bent molecule, which makes it fluid and useful in the body. *Trans,* on the other hand, is straight, and it packs in a tighter, denser fashion—making it unusable in the body. (See Appendix E on page 381 for details.)

According to some experts, more than 60% of all the fats consumed in the U.S. are hydrogenated. No wonder there are so many cardiovascular-related diseases and deaths in this country.

Heat The commercial oils and margarine you buy in your supermarket have ordinarily gone through many different mechanical, chemical and heat processes after extraction from their vegetable or botanical sources. Each step of the process removes something valuable and adds something that is deleterious to human health. The manufacturers' objective is to improve shelf life, odor, flavor and color.

During the refining processes, many nutrients, such as calcium, magnesium, copper, iron, beta-carotene, vitamin E, chlorophyll and lecithin, are removed. The beta-carotene and vitamin E are the plant's own natural antioxidants. Moreover, the high temperature, sometimes in excess of 450 degrees, and a pressure of several tons per square inch change the chemical properties of the oil molecules.

Under these severe conditions, some of the fatty acids convert from the biologically beneficial *cis* to the harmful *trans* form. *Cis* fats melt at 55 degrees, while *trans* fats melt at 111 degrees. This difference becomes important when you compare them to the body temperature of 98.6 degrees. When you consume these two fats, the *cis,* being completely liquid, is readily available for the body's processes, while the *trans* form may sit in your arterial walls or in your tissues.

Trans fatty acids are very rare in nature, but they comprise about 15% in commercial oils, 30% in margarine and 47% in vegetable shortening.

Oxygen This life-supporting nutrient can cause just about the same damage to unsaturated fats as it does to most metals and plastics. In metals, it causes rust or tarnish. In plastics, it causes cracks and brittleness. With fats, oxygen attacks the double bond sites and creates peroxides or free radicals, causing them to go bad or rancid.

Besides the problem with obesity and complications with the cardiovascular system, there are two major problems with the consumption of too much fat, particularly polyunsaturated fat:

1.   The more fat you have in your body, the greater the chance for free radical or peroxide generation. This is not only from oxygen reacting with polyunsaturated fats but also from the interaction of the fats with other environmental agents (like smog, chemicals, exhaust, x-rays or cigarette smoke, or metals like iron, copper, nickel or lead.)

2.   Since oxygen readily interacts with these fats, you are depriving or limiting the availability of oxygen to your normal cells or tissue.

When these free radicals go unchecked, they speed up the aging of your body and increase the chance for succumbing to major hazards, like cancer or heart disease.

Homogenization Practically all the milk produced in the U.S. is pasteurized and homogenized. Pasteurization is the treatment of milk with heat to destroy bacteria, and homogenization is a process of reducing large fat globules into fine particles by passing pressurized milk through a small opening. This prevents the fat from settling at the top of a milk container.

There is growing evidence that homogenizing milk can contribute to heart disease.

This is because the fine fat particles, along with a noxious enzyme called xanthine oxidase, are absorbed into the bloodstream without being digested in the stomach. Once this enzyme is in the circulatory system, it attaches itself to the heart and arterial walls and begins digesting a membranous substance called *plasmalogen.*[4] Other fats and cholesterol rush to this site to cover up the tissue and save it from further damage. As this happens, more and more fats are attracted to this area, and what began as a protection to the tissue begins to interfere with the normal flow of blood. If the buildup continues and what is already there is not removed, the person could succumb to angina or stroke.

The other problem with milk is in its connection to osteoporosis. The incidence of osteoporosis is directly correlated with the level of milk consumption. In countries like the U.S., Finland, Sweden and Great Britain, where the consumption of milk is highest, there is a greater incidence of this bone-thinning disease.[5] Many other factors, however, may contribute to the higher incidence of osteoporosis in these countries.

Solutions

It's obvious from these last few pages of explanation that all fats have a certain level of health risk. Saturated fats and cholesterol can lead to cardiovascular diseases. The polyunsaturates are vulnerable to radiation, oxidation or free radical attack. This problem can often lead to cancer, heart disease and other degenerative conditions.

The best protection you have against these fats is to consume as little of them as you can. You should particularly watch for foods that are rich in cholesterol and saturated fats. These are dairy products, meats, eggs and tropical oils, such as coconut, palm and palm kernel oils.

The polyunsaturates like omega-3 and omega-6 fatty acids have many benefits to your health, so much so that these fatty acids are treated like essential vitamins and minerals. The best protection you have against free radical attacks or oxidation of these oils is the antioxidants such as vitamins A, C and E, phytochemicals, minerals and amino acids.

CHAPTER 8
Energy

People often say, "You are what you eat!" An interpretation of this may be, you are what you eat because your body is capable of converting the food you eat into energy and into the various tissues of your body. Inside your 60 trillion cells, chemical power plants, called mitochondria, produce 95% of the energy your body needs. This energy is extracted from the food you eat and temporarily stored in a chemical compound called *adenosine triphosphate (ATP)*.

As the continuous need arises, different enzymes in your body break down ATP to release the stored energy. It's this freed energy that enables your body to perform physical work (like muscle contraction), to transport ions and molecules in body fluids and to synthesize many organic compounds that build your cells and tissues. The following information is an overview of the process in which the body extracts energy from the food you eat.

During carbohydrate metabolism, starch and sugars are converted to monosaccharides (glucose, galactose, and fructose) by your digestive enzymes. These simple molecules are then absorbed by the intestinal wall to be distributed throughout the body. Of these three sugars, only glucose can be used by tissue cells. The others, galactose and fructose, have to be converted into glucose by the liver before they become useful to the body.

Your body can use only so much glucose at a time. With the help of insulin from the pancreas, any excess glucose (in a normal metabolism) is converted to glycogen and fat by the liver, muscles and fat cells. At any one time, a 150-pound man, for example, may have only about 40 kilocalories worth of glucose in circulating fluids. On the other hand, he may have as much as 600 kcal of energy stored in the form of glycogen and fat.

Whenever your body needs energy, glycogen is converted into glucose, which after a few biochemical reductions enters a series of biochemical reactions called the Krebs cycle. (See the discussion on page 91 and the illustration on page 378.) In the Krebs cycle, with the help of oxygen, minerals and vitamins, almost all the energy stored in glucose is harvested as ATP. ATP is the universal currency of free energy in our biological system. All the food you eat—carbohydrates, fats and some amino acids—end up in the Krebs cycle.

It's important to remember that glucose is also the main carrier of oxygen into the cells. This means that if the glucose level is dangerously low (as in hypoglycemia) your body will be deprived of not only immediate fuel but also oxygen, the life-supporting element. In effect, your cells will asphyxiate if your glucose level is severely low.

The road to providing your body with its daily fuel is not always a smooth one. Unless you are very careful in choosing your energy sources and watch your food intake, you could get yourself in trouble. This could range from feeling not quite up to par for the day to a chronic problem in which your health is compromised.

I am referring here to simple carbohydrates, such as sugar and honey, and processed foods, such as white bread and polished rice. These foods get digested and enter the circulatory system too quickly, and your sugar level shoots up sky high. Agents like coffee, tobacco, alcohol, other drugs and salt also disturb your blood sugar to make your day-to-day life uncomfortable.

Soon after they get into your bloodstream, these foods or substances can manifest themselves as irritability, nervousness, depression, fatigue and nausea. Often these are also followed by hunger and a craving for the same foods. These conditions can sometimes lead to severe problems such as obesity, hypoglycemia and diabetes.

The Problem with Sweets

Whenever you consume sweets like candy bars, table sugar, pastry or corn flakes, which are rich in sugar, they get absorbed quickly into the bloodstream. These foods don't often need much digestion. The moment they hit your stomach, some of them quite readily enter the circulatory system. As a result, the blood glucose level, which normally is kept within narrow limits, will suddenly rise and upset your well-being.

To alleviate this abrupt sugar surge into the bloodstream, the pancreas gland produces insulin. This hormone facilitates the absorption of glucose into muscle and liver cells to be used as fuel or converted to glycogen for storage. The secretion of too much insulin, however, can have the opposite effect. It will bring the blood sugar level so low that you start to feel hungry, fatigued and depressed and experience headaches.

In a healthy person, this problem will be reversed quickly by two hormones called epinephrine and glucagon. These hormones are secreted by the adrenal and pancreas glands, and they induce liver and muscle cells to convert the stored glyco-

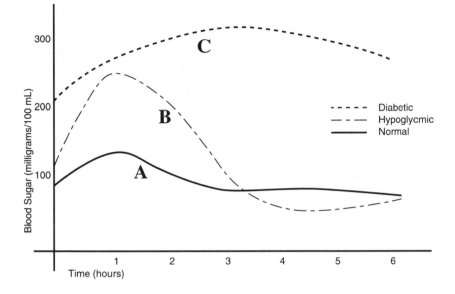

Figure 8.1 Blood glucose curves showing diabetic, hypoglycemic and normal conditions after a six-hour glucose tolerance test (GTT)

gen into glucose to bring up the blood sugar level to normal. Incidentally, the nervousness, restlessness or jitteriness one experiences after an intake of sugar-rich foods is due to the presence of large amounts of epinephrine in the blood. Epinephrine (also called adrenaline hormone) is a great stimulator of the nervous system, as in "fight or flight" situations, for example.

Testing for Your Glucose Tolerance

The standard method used to test how your body digests, absorbs and processes carbohydrates is called the glucose tolerance test (GTT). A GTT is normally administered after a person has fasted for several hours. In a case when the test is performed in the morning, the person taking the test would have been advised to eat nothing after supper. The next day, the individual is given a glucose solution to swallow, and every hour during the next six hours, the sugar level in the blood is monitored and the results recorded.

Although the results vary from person to person and from test to test, Figure 8.1 represents what the readings may look like after a six-hour run.

Curve A shows a normal GTT result, in which the glucose level starts within normal range (between 80 and 140 mg). It rises up a little and falls back to nearly where it started. Curve B, on the other hand, shows a classic case of hypoglycemia. The glucose level rises precipitously, only to fall rapidly to below the starting (fasting) level. Curve C sketches a severe diabetic condition in which the glucose level starts high and remains relatively high, even after the six-hour test.

It is important to bear in mind that although these were selected to show extreme variation from normal cases, both hypoglycemic and diabetic cases vary widely. They depend on the individual's tolerance level. "Normal" here is defined as the sugar level determined, after fasting, by the individual being tested.

GTTs provide a good test of how your body handles sugars (how steady or erratic your mental and physical energy will be). In a situation in which the sugar level rises and drops quickly, many bodily functions are disturbed: your heart, muscles, brain and nerves are sapped of their energy, and you will feel weak and tired.

The story with diabetics is somewhat different. As you will see below, these people suffer from the lack of insulin, which helps facilitate glucose entry into the cells, the body's most preferred fuel. With these people, the sugar accumulates in the blood until it gets eliminated in the urine. Consequently, a diabetic suffers from a lack of energy, excessive loss of water, which leads to constant thirst, and a depressed immune system, which leads to low disease resistance and poor wound healing.

The Other Culprits

Coffee

Coffee affects both diabetics and hypoglycemics significantly. First, the caffeine in coffee stimulates the secretion of epinephrine into the bloodstream. This in turn stimulates the conversion of glycogen into glucose. In diabetics, this new sugar exacerbates the already high glucose content in the blood. In persons who suffer from hypoglycemia, the new glucose production leads to the secretion of more insulin, which works to lower the glucose level. This leads to irritability, headaches, nervousness, anxiety and/or sleeplessness.

Caffeine-containing products, such as cola, chocolate, tea and drugs (like aspirin-containing drugs such as Excedrin and Bromo-Seltzer), have a similar effect on the body. Soft drinks like Coke and Pepsi also contain a considerable amount of sugar—containing as much as 8 teaspoons of sugar per 12 ounces of liquid. Similarly, one chocolate glazed doughnut can contain 6 teaspoons; a slice of chocolate cake with icing, 7 teaspoons; and a chocolate milk shake, 14 teaspoons of sugar.

Alcohol and Tobacco

Like caffeine, both alcohol and nicotine induce a rapid increase in blood sugar, but only to deplete it at an equally fast speed. All the classic symptoms of hypoglycemia (erratic behavioral patterns, anxiety, muscular twitches and unsteady hands and legs) are also present in people who are addicted to these substances.

Excessive consumption of alcohol and tobacco leads to many other health hazards besides hypoglycemia and mood swings. Too much alcohol, for example, suppresses appetite and interferes with the absorption of food from the stomach. This problem naturally deprives your body of many vital nutrients. It can also lead to liver diseases such as cirrhosis, hepatitis and liver cancer. Cigarettes can lead to many health problems, including lung cancer.

Other agents, like emotional stress, food allergies, nutritional deficiencies and salt are also well-known culprits of blood glucose imbalance in the body.

In summary, the consumption of simple and quickly absorbed carbohydrates (like white bread, sugar- and honey-based foods) has many short- and long-term consequences. The immediate impact on your health is the fact that every time you consume these foods you place your body under considerable stress. The rise and fall of your blood glucose level and insulin secretions can be devastating to your day-to-day mental and physical condition.

A temporary sugar glut in the body has compelled many people to bring harm to themselves and others. This problem has even been used as a defense in court cases. Do you remember the killing of George Moscone and Harvey Milk in San Francisco by Dan White in 1978? White purportedly had eaten sugar-rich Twinkies before he became berserk and went on a killing rampage. For the average person, it may not get this extreme, but emotional mood swings can still be quite dreadful.

In the long run, the sugar-insulin yo-yo syndrome can lead to complications in your pancreas gland. When you force this gland to manufacture large amounts of insulin to help curb excess sugar in the blood, it can finally rebel by either shutting down or producing too much insulin at the slightest increase of blood sugar. An overproducing pancreas can lead to hypoglycemia, while a corrupted, nonfunctioning one can cause diabetes.[1,2]

Diabetes can be a very disabling condition. A diabetic is like a sailor on the open sea who dies of thirst. The blood may contain all the glucose it needs, but there is no way of getting this important fuel into the cells in the absence of insulin. As a result, the body can literally starve. Particularly affected are the brain, kidneys, lungs, eyes and blood vessels. More than other organs or tissues, these body parts are highly dependent on glucose for their fuel and are literally destroyed over time if the entry of blood glucose into the tissues is not facilitated. Unless ways (like insulin injection) are found, blood glucose will continue to end up in the urine, unused by the body, and the body will continue to suffer.[3]

Bear in mind, though, that although diabetes is caused by a failing pancreas, the reasons for this are variable and include heredity, nutritional deficiencies, obesity and allergies. What is also important is that diabetes is a disease that afflicts over 12 million people and has been rising at the rate of 6% a year in this country.[4]

In short, if you prize a steady, stable and happy state of mind and body, you should avoid rapidly digested and easily absorbed carbohydrates such as white bread, sugar and honey-based foods. As you will see in Table 8.1, the foods that can provide you with a steady supply of glucose are carbohydrates, such as fructose, whole grains and legumes.

Glycemic Index

To determine the relative conversion of various carbohydrates into glucose and their absorption into the bloodstream, a form of measurement called the glycemic index was developed. With this method, the known glycemic values of various foods are your guideline. By knowing the glycemic indices of foods, you'll be able to choose those that can give you a steady flow of energy.

Table 8.1 shows a selected group of foods and their glycemic indices. The higher the glycemic index of a given food, the faster that food is broken down into glucose, and concomitantly, the faster it enters the bloodstream. For example, carbohydrates like maltose, glucose and corn flakes are bad because they are digested at a fast rate. All those foods that have low glycemic indices, such as fructose, legumes and some fruits, are good because they're processed slowly in the body. These foods can give you a sustained level of energy.

When you choose a food as an energy source, you may also have to consider its quality as a fuel. Sugars and grains are rich in carbohydrates, legumes in proteins and fruits and vegetables in fibers. Although you get the same calories from both carbohydrates and proteins, i.e., 4 calories/gram, carbohydrates are a cleaner fuel.

When a carbohydrate is completely burned in the body, its four by-products are ATP, carbon dioxide, water and heat. Proteins, on the other hand, produce, besides carbon dioxide and water, nitrogenous compounds that can be toxic to the body.

Table 8.1 Glycemic Index of Selected Foods and Sweets*

Sugars		Cereals		Legumes	
Glucose	100	Corn flakes	80	Beans—baked	40
Fructose	20	Oatmeal	49	—butter	36
Maltose	105	Shredded wheat	67	kidney	29
Sucrose	59			—soy	15
				Chickpeas	36
				Lentils	29
Grain Products		**Vegetables**		**Fruits**	
Bread—white	69	Beets	64	Apples**	39
—whole wheat	72	Carrots	92	Bananas	62
Rice—brown	66	Potatoes—instant	80	Orange	40
—white	76	—new	70	Grapefruit	26
Spaghetti—white	70	Yams	51		
—whole wheat	42				
Dairy Products					
Ice cream	36				
Milk—whole	34				
Yogurt	36				

*Source: Jenkins, D.J.A. Lente Carbohydrates: A newer approach to the management of diabetes. *Diabetes Care:* 1982; 44:364-368
**The sweet variety

From Table 8.1, even though soy (a protein-rich legume) has the lowest glycemic index, fructose, the next lowest, is a better fuel.

The difference in the glycemic index between bread and spaghetti is due to the added sugar in the bread. Although potatoes have a relatively high glycemic index, they also are a rich source of nutrients. This is the compromise you'll have to make with some of these foods.

The Krebs Cycle

When I was a child, my mother used to say, "Once food gets past a person's mouth, it's foreign." She was referring to the smell, taste, feel and even appearance most people relate to when it comes to food. It seems we could not care less for what happens to the food once it gets past our sense organs.

In actuality, food has no vitality for you until it ultimately reaches the Krebs cycle deep within the millions of cells in your body. Its significance for you to a large degree can only be captured once it enters this biological melting pot, also known as the citric acid or tricarboxylic cycle. Most people prefer to call it by the less pedantic term: Krebs cycle. It was named after Hans Krebs, who discovered it in the early 1950s.

All the foods you eat after absorption into the blood end up in the cells. Here, after a series of reactions, they enter the Krebs cycle. Krebs cycle is another series of reactions that takes place within the cell in tiny power plants called mitochondria. Here, oxygen combines with foods to produce the ultimate, important products: carbon dioxide, water, heat and the universal storage of energy, ATP. About 95% of the carbohydrate energy released takes place through this process. This energy is used to build proteins, to synthesize glycogen from glucose, to contract muscles when you exercise and to do hundreds of other similar energy-requiring processes.

Glucose is the preferred fuel, but in its absence, proteins, fats and even alcohol can be used as fuel to make ATP. Once in the cell, many more things can happen to the food you eat, depending on your body's need at any given moment. For instance, sugar can be used to make some amino acids, hormones or cholesterol, or it can be stored as glycogen or fat. Protein can be converted into fat or used to make sugar, which in turn can be used for any number of purposes. Fat (with rare exceptions) is the only food that cannot be made into sugar.

The point of all this is for you to remember that the Krebs cycle is the basis of your health's glory or demise. The accumulation of fat in the body, for example, is one of the most common health hazards in this country. The type of food you eat, your lack of physical activity and the Krebs cycle may have something to do with any extra weight you carry around. This may not sound revealing except for one fact: carbohydrates are your best ally in helping you to burn fat.*

According to one nutritionist, the "Krebs cycle can burn fat ... most efficiently and cleanly during physical activity *only when there is* enough carbohydrate present in the cycle at the same time."[5]

There is another advantage to having a sufficient amount of carbohydrates (particularly the complex or the slow-releasing types) in your system. These foods can help you prevent tissue protein breakdown. During strenuous exercise, once your

---

* The popular expression among biochemists regarding this is "fat burns in the flame of carbohydrate."

body has depleted its sugar level, it begins to reach for fuel elsewhere in the body—mainly your tissue protein. This is what you don't want to happen, since it will mean losing your muscle mass. For this reason, carbohydrates are often referred to as "protein sparing" foods.

PART V
Obesity and the Fat Content of Some Common Foods

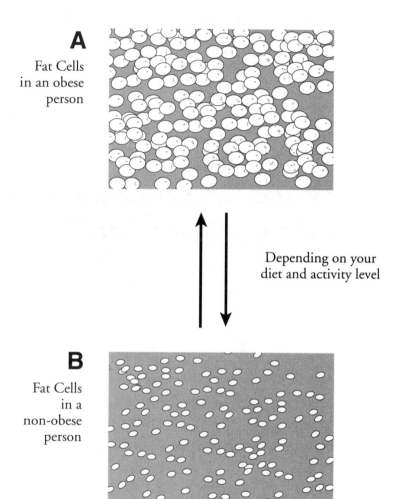

A
Fat Cells
in an obese
person

Depending on your
diet and activity level

B
Fat Cells
in a
non-obese
person

Figure 9.1 Although the number of fat cells in a person's body are constant, what determines whether or not one is obese is the amount of fat stored in these cells. Depending on a person's nutritional status and activity level, the size of these cells can change dramatically. Thus, as one consumes fatty and other high calorie foods and leads a sedentary lifestyle, these calories are converted and stored in the adipose or fat tissues of the body, causing these cells to literally balloon, as in the top illustration. On the other hand, when one watches what he or she eats and engages in a physical activity, the adipocytes lose their fat and become thin as shown in the bottom illustration. The following pages explain how these alternate processes can come about.

CHAPTER 9
Causes of Obesity and Possible Solutions

Crash or fad diets deprive the body of key nutrients, reduce lean muscle mass and put the body and mind under enormous stress. This type of dieting, ironically, is also the worst way to try to lose or manage your weight. This is because when important vitamins and minerals are scarce (as they are when you reduce your caloric intake), the body's metabolic processes will be depressed. As a result, not only will your body struggle to mobilize body fat to the mitochondrial furnace of the cell, but it will also have difficulty in efficiently processing the food you consume. As was stated earlier, this type of weight loss is psychologically and emotionally devastating to the individual. When the ordeal becomes unbearable, the person often abandons the program and goes on with life as usual.

The Roots of One's Weight Problem

Think about it. Save for a few exceptions, people don't just become too fat. Most often they bring it upon themselves. Here are some of the common reasons why people become overweight.

1. Consuming Too Much Fat

If you are a typical American, chances are you obtain over 40% of your calories from fat and fat-based foods. As much as this food substance is your body's secondary source of energy and offers more calories than similar amounts of carbohydrates and proteins combined, it is also one of the most easily stored substances in the body.

While nearly 25% of the calories from carbohydrates or proteins can be used to convert them into body fat, hardly any calories are expended to convert food fats into body fat.[1,2,3] In other words, your body has an "open-door" policy with regard to fats. Hence, as long as you consume too many grams of fat and you have a sedentary lifestyle, these fats simply roll in and get stored in your body tissues. To minimize this problem, experts recommend that you keep your fat calories to below 20% of your total calories.*

2. Consuming Too Many Refined Foods

Processed and refined foods such as sugar and white bread are some of the major culprits regarding the accumulation of excess body fat. Since these foods contain hardly any fiber, they get processed and enter the bloodstream quickly. Because the body's tolerance level for large quantities of sugar is low, this sugar is quickly brought to your body's cells. There, if not used for energy production, it will be converted into and stored as fat.

The consumption of sugar in this country is bad business. Just to show you how bad it has gotten, the per capita consumption of sugar has gone up from 19 pounds per year in 1970 to nearly 70 pounds in 1989.[5] This is an amazing 370% increase. Where do you think all that sugar ends up? Of course, most of it ends up in your fat cells. As you may know, there are many hidden and visible sugar- based foods. And the problem with an excessive intake of sugar is not limited just to the problem of obesity. You may also have to be concerned about dental cavities, hypertension, hypoglycemia and even adult-onset diabetes.

3. Sedentary Lifestyle

The average American not only consumes high-calorie foods but also exercises very little. The automobile is omnipresent, and walking even a few hundred yards to a neighborhood store may be viewed as walking a long way. A combination of high calories and no exercise means a higher conversion of those calories into body fat.

As you must know, exercise is one of the great mobilizers of body fat. When your body is at rest, it uses up minimal calories to run the basic bodily functions, such as respiration, digestion and circulation. This so-called basal metabolic rate has been shown to increase with exercise.[6,7] This means that those who exercise not only burn high calories during the activity but also increase their body's ability to burn fat when at rest. (See interpretation in Chapter 35.)

---

* The American Heart Association and the National Cancer Institute have recommended that we keep our fat calories to below 30% of our total calories.[4] But for those who have weight problems, experts recommend that fat calories be below 20%.

4. As You Age, Your Metabolism Slows Down

One of the great mysteries of nature is the process of aging. As our bodies age, not only do our skins wrinkle and lose their moisture and our hair thins out, but also the absorption of nutrients from the digestive tract and their metabolism in the cells are compromised. During this time, fat and other calories tend to collect in the tissues at a greater rate than when we were younger. This problem, of course, will cause us to be too fat along with becoming predisposed to degenerative diseases, such as heart diseases, cancer and diabetes.

Things We Can Do About Obesity

From the above discussion, you can see that obesity is largely associated with our consumption of high-calorie foods (fats and too many sweets) as well as from our body's improper utilization of the food we eat (because of a lack of exercise or slowed metabolism). You can also see that the long-term solution to this problem does not come from a crash or fad diet program. It is something we can accomplish by combining well-established weight management techniques with state-of-the-art nutritional ingredients and technology.

1. Reducing Your Caloric Intake

For a sedentary person, all calories (whether from carbohydrates, fats or proteins) can be fattening when consumed in high amounts. Particularly crucial, however, are those you get from fats. Fat calories, as mentioned above, are treated differently by the body than are other calories. Unlike the calories you get from carbohydrates and proteins, a quarter of which are used up before they turn into body fat, nearly all the fat calories that enter the body go directly into storage. In a country in which over 40% of our calories come from fat, the problem we have with obesity becomes readily apparent.

The best solution to this problem is, obviously, to reduce your daily fat calories to at most 20%, to eliminate or keep to an absolute minimum your daily consumption of sweets and to include regular exercise as part of your weight reduction effort. (You can be generous with your consumption of complex carbohydrates such as potatoes, pastas and brown rice. These foods can give your body a steady supply of energy.) If you are familiar with the traditional method of weight loss, you can see that the approach described above is revolutionary.

2. Managing Your Caloric Intake

Along with reducing your consumption of fats and sweets, you may also want to learn how to manage your daily calories. This is to say that although you now have lowered your caloric intake, unless you know how to properly distribute those calories through the day, you may have difficulty in achieving your new weight. Let's see what this means.

First, remember that any calories that are not used to run your basic bodily functions or your other energy needs are converted into and stored as fat. For example, let's say you have reduced your daily calories from 2,000 to 1,500. Unless you use these new calories wisely, you may not notice a great difference in your weight. How does this happen? Very simply.

Suppose you obtain a significant portion of the 1,500 calories from your evening meal. Since you are less likely to engage in physical activity at night, those calories not utilized by the basal metabolic process will end up in the fatty tissues. Once stored, fat calories are not readily available. (That is why, as discussed below, it takes at least four hours of walking at the rate of 3 miles an hour to lose a pound of body weight.)

Second, when you consume a large portion of your daily calories at night, you will have difficulty containing your hunger during the day and consequently maintaining or reducing your weight. How so? Once calories are stored, the body prefers to keep them for a "rainy day," so to speak. Thus, when the calories from the circulating fluids are depleted as a result of usage or storage, your brain sends hunger signals to the stomach, which you notice when you wake up in the morning or at other times during the day. Often what happens at such times is that you end up eating more at a meal or snacking more frequently on the wrong foods to satisfy the hunger. Neither of these options is going to help you in your weight reduction or maintenance efforts.

To circumvent this problem, you may want to consume a large portion of your 1,500 calories during the day. Since most of us are physically active during the day, we tend to expend a significant proportion of our caloric intake during this time. Thus, at dinner, you may want to have fewer calories but highly nutritious foods. Meals that are rich in protein, vitamins and minerals are preferable.

3. Using State-of-the-Art Nutritional Ingredients and Supplements

Very soon, much of our health and vitality, as well as the problem with obesity, may be in our own hands. In the past decade or so, advances in nutritional science and technology have opened the door to unique and exciting nutritional ingredients and technologies which, if properly used, may enable us to have greater control of our health and well-being.

Some of this may be in the area of weight management. For instance, substances like chromium picolinate and L-carnitine which you find in some supplements, are excellent mobilizers of your body's two major fuels: carbohydrates and fats. While chromium picolinate enhances your body's ability to efficiently process and burn sugar and fats,[8] L-carnitine specializes in rounding up fat molecules and dumping them into the mitochondrial furnace. With the availability of these nutrients in your food, less of the sugar and food fat will be converted and stored as body fat. Reportedly, these two substances not only aid you in burning fat but also may help to maintain lean muscle mass.[9] (See Appendix C on page 365 for more information on these compounds.)

Equally important in the metabolism of fats and sugars is the availability of key vitamins and minerals. In the previous paragraphs, very simplistic terms and analogies were used to describe the mobilization and burning of fats and sugar molecules. What actually goes on in your billions of cells to accomplish the conversion or mobilization of these substances is a very complex process involving millions of chemicals and chemical reactions. For these reactions to come to completion smoothly and efficiently, the availability of sufficient enzymes, minerals and vitamins is crucial.

It has been found that not only are minerals from our foods often poorly absorbed but also their absorption is reduced as we age. These problems limit the availability of key minerals in the cells to help them properly process the food you eat. To circumvent this dilemma, some companies chelate minerals with amino acids. Chelation is the process of wrapping metal ions with organic substances, such as amino acids, to increase their absorption. (See Appendix C for more.) With the availability of an "abundant" amount of key minerals, the body may now burn fats and sugars at higher rates.

4. Including Fiber-Rich Foods with Your Meals

(See the section "The Importance of Fibers for Your Health" on page 68 for details.)

5. Exercising Regularly

For losing or controlling weight, as well as for overall good health and a good mental outlook, exercise can make a world of difference in your life. As was briefly mentioned above and is thoroughly discussed in Chapter 35 on page 335, exercise helps the body burn fat during the activity as well as afterwards.

Through a process called lipolysis,[10,11] exercise encourages the release of fat molecules from their storage sites. This, according to experts, could go on for as long as 24 hours after exercise. Covert Bailey, author of *Fit or Fat*, says that exercise does this by inducing your cells to step up their production of the fat-burning enzymes. Thus, when you exercise regularly, you will increase the synthesis of these enzymes, which in turn will increase the burning of fat from your body. Aerobic exercises such as running, cross-country skiing, swimming, cycling and climbing stairs are excellent mobilizers of fat deposits. Furthermore, with exercise, you not only build strength and stamina but also increase your lean body mass.

Bear in mind, however, that unless you also include other weight reduction methods, such as taking the fat-mobilizing nutrients discussed above, the amount of poundage you shed through exercise alone over a short period of time can be frustratingly small. For example, to lose just one pound you may need to expend roughly 3,500 calories. This translates into five hours of walking* at the rate of 3 miles per hour or four and a half hours of running at 9 miles per hour.[12] Nonetheless, the best way to lose weight is to do it gradually. When you do it slowly, your body is unstressed and the loss can be permanent, as long as you don't overindulge in fattening foods and keep exercising.

What is the best exercise? For minimizing bodily injuries and for sustaining long-term weight loss, the low-impact types are often considered the best. These are swimming, cycling, walking, climbing stairs, low-impact aerobics, cross country skiing and weight lifting. High-impact exercises—such as downhill skiing, running or jogging, racquetball or basketball—can be stressful to an unconditioned body.

Regardless of the type of low-impact exercise you choose to pursue, bear this in mind: the frequency of the activity is more important than the length of the activity. This, in turn, is more important than the intensity of the activity.

Let me explain this further. Although almost all cells manufacture and store triglycerides (or fat), the ones that synthesize and store them the most are the adipocytes or fat cells (illustrated in Figure 9.1). When one is obese, as much as 95% of an adipocyte's volume can be occupied by fat. Hence, when you exercise,

---

* If you walked for 30 minutes every day at the rate of 3 miles per hour, over a period of a year, you could lose roughly 12 pounds.[13]

the triglycerides are broken down by the lipase enzyme and the free fatty acids diffuse out of the cells and enter the bloodstream which brings them to the working muscles where they are burned as fuel. As you increase your exercise, more and more blood will flow into the adipose or fat tissues, removing even greater fatty acids. The lipase enzyme is activated by a molecule called cyclic AMP (adenosine monophosphate) which in turn is regulated by the hormones, epinephrine, norepinephrine, glucagon and growth hormones. These hormones are secreted in greater amounts during exercise.

CHAPTER 10
The Fat Content of Some Common Foods

As discussed in Chapter 9, one of the major contributors to obesity is the consumption of fat and fat-based foods. There are many hidden as well as visible sources of fat calories. It is important that you know about them so that the next time you come in contact with these foods, you will know approximately the fat calories you are ingesting. Knowledge is indeed power, and by knowing what these fats can do to your body when taken in excess you will have the power to say no if you don't want them.

Tables 10.1 to 10.6 list some common foods and their fat content.

As you can see, the information that appears in the tables is fairly straightforward. There are a few subtle points we need to address, however, regarding the fat and other calories you find in these tables.

First, as you can see, next to each food item there appear three numbers. The first column shows the percentage of fat calories in each of these foods. The second column gives the amount of fat in grams. As you will see below, for your everyday use, this piece of information is what should concern you. The last column represents the number of teaspoons of fat in each of the foods listed. This measure is used to make it easy for you to visualize the amount of fat in a given food. You can't see percentages or grams in your mind, but you can "see" a teaspoon of something.

Second, besides considering the fat calories in a given food, you may need to consider the amount of other calories, particularly those that come from sweets. Calories from sweets, in addition to contributing to obesity can create havoc to your health. Because simple carbohydrates like table sugar and honey enter the bloodstream at a rapid rate after ingestion, they send your blood sugar level sky-high. This problem consequently leads to a series of unpleasant feelings. You may also need to be concerned about the possibility of hypoglycemia and dental cavities, especially if you consume sweets regularly. Simply put, a combination of high fat and sweet calories can have a double whammy effect on your body.

Third, regarding fat calories, as we said above, your main concern should be about the gram content of fat in a given food. Once you know the amount of fat in grams, you can quickly compute in your head the amount of calories your body has to deal with. We said elsewhere in the book that each gram of fat stores 9 calories.

Table 10.1

Food Source	% Fat Calories	Grams of Fat	Tsp of Fat
HIGH FAT FOODS'			
Dairy Products			
2% milk, 1 cup	38	5	1
Whole milk, 1 cup	48	8	1 1/2
Cheese, regular," 1 oz.	46-72	6-9	1-2
Cottage cheese, creamed 4% fat, 1 cup	38	10	2
Part-skim mozzarella, 1 oz.	56	5	1
Part-skim ricotta, 1/2 cup	50	10	2
Regular ice cream, 1/2 cup	48	7	1
Premium ice cream, 1/2 cup	60	16-20	3-4
Yogurt, whole milk, plain, 1 cup	45	7	1
Bread, Grain and Baked Goods			
Croissant, 1	46	12	2
Apple Danish, 1	50	13	2 1/2
Glazed doughnut, 1	50	13	2 1/2
Cracker, regular, 1/2 oz. (about 5 round crackers)	60	5	1
Cookie, small, (1/2 oz.)	59	3	1/2
Muffin, 1 medium	33-50	5-10	1-2
Fruit pie (e.g., apple, blueberry), 1 slice	40	18	3
Pecan pie, 1 slice	50	32	6 1/2
Meat, Poultry, Fish, Egg			
Chicken or turkey dark meat, no skin, broiled, 3 oz.	34-44	6-9	1-2
Fried chicken breast, 1/2	44	18	3
Fried drumstick, 1	51	11	2
Duck or goose, no skin, broiled, 3 oz.	50	10-11	2
Beef, 3 oz. broiled round tip, sirloin	32-36	5-8	1-1 1/2
Bottom round arm pot roast tenderloin	43	9	nearly 2
T-bone steak	45	9	nearly 2
Lean ground burger	66	18	3
Hard-boiled egg	68	6	1
Ham, canned, roasted, 3 oz.	61	14	nearly 3
Hot dog, 1	81	13	2 1/2

'Above 30% fat calories
"Includes cheddar, blue cheese, Monterey Jack, brie, etc.

But to simplify the conversion from grams to calories of fat, you may use 10 calories instead. Let's look at a few examples.

In Table 10. 1, for instance, one cup of whole milk contains 8 grams of fat. This figure translates into 80 calories. These fat calories represent 48% of the total calories found in one cup of whole milk. The remaining calories (52%) represent lactose (the

Table 10.2

Food Source	% Fat Calories	Grams of Fat	Tsp of Fat
Mixed Dishes			
Chicken pot pie, 8 oz.	51	31	6
Quiche, 6 oz.	72	48	nearly 10
Oils, Dressings, and Spreads			
Butter, 1 teaspoon	99	4	nearly 1
Oil, 1 teaspoon (corn, olive, canola, etc.)	100	5	1
Mayonnaise, 1 tablespoon	99	11	2
Reduced calorie mayonnaise, 1 teaspoon	77	3	1/2
Creamy salad dressings	90	6	1
Vinaigrette salad dressing (oil and vinegar), 1 tablespoon	100	8	1 1/2
Nuts and Nut Butters			
Nuts and seeds, 1 oz. (2-3 tablespoons)	73	15	3
Peanut butter, cashew butter, or other nut butter	75	8	1 1/2
VERY LOW FAT FOODS			
Dairy Products			
Skim (nonfat milk), 1 cup	0	0	0
Cottage cheese (uncreamed, dry curd, less than 1/2% fat)	7	1	1
Fat-free mozzarella, 1 oz. (Polly-O makes it.)	0	0	0
Free fat ricotta, 1/2 cup (Polly-O makes it.)	0	0	0
Nonfat yogurt, 1 cup (plain or flavored)	0	0	0
Nonfat frozen yogurt, 1/2 cup	0	0	1
Bread, Grains, and Baked Goods			
Bagel, 1	9	2	1
White bread, 1 slice	14	1	1
Whole wheat bread, 1 slice	13	1	1

milk sugar) and the proteins found in this milk. Let's look at some other foods.

Half a cup of premium ice cream could contain as much as 20 grams or 200 fat calories; a lean ground burger brings with it 180 fat calories, and a six-ounce slice of quiche contains a whopping 480 fat calories. Assuming that your daily caloric intake is 1,500 calories, these foods contribute roughly 12% and 30%, respectively, of those calories. In other words, unless you are very careful in your choices of food, you may end up frustrated with your weight management efforts.

Besides watching what you eat, there are a couple of things you can do to limit your

Table 10.3

Food Source	% Fat Calories	Grams of Fat	Tsp of Fat
Cereals*			
Cereal	10	1	1
Hot cereal, 1 cup cooked (oatmeal, Cream o' Wheat, etc.)	0-12	0-2	1
Grains			
Rice, brown or white, 1 cup cooked	4	1	1
Pasta, 1 cup cooked	6	1	1
Popcorn, air-popped, 2 cups	0	0	0
Baked Goods			
Angel food cake, 1 slice	0	0	0
Meringue cookie, 1	0	0	0
Graham Crackers, 1 rectangle	15	1	1
Legumes (Dried Beans)			
Beans,** cooked/canned, 1 cup	4	1	1
Meat, Poultry, Fish			
Chicken breast, no skin, 3 oz., broiled (no fat added)	19	3	1/2
Turkey white meat, no skin, 3 oz. cooked	17	3	1/2
Flounder, 3 oz. broiled (or other nonfatty fish)	11	1	1
Tuna, canned in water, 3 oz.	7	1	1
Shrimp, clams, crab, surimi, lobster, scallops, 3 oz., cooked without fat	9-15	1-2	1
Veal cutlet, broiled, 3 oz.	19	3	1
Fruits and Vegetables			
These groups of foods are generally low in fat, containing less than 1 gram of fat. One fruit that is rich in fat is avocado—it contains largely unsaturated fat.			
Salad Dressings			
Some of the known low-calorie brands are Hidden Valley Ranch's Take Heart Bleu Cheese, the Pritikin lines, Weight Watchers, or any of the Kraft Free dressings.			

* With no more than 1 gram per l-oz serving (e.g., Raisin Bran, All-Bran, Fruit Bran, Shredded Wheat, Fiber 1, Grape Nuts, etc.)

** All beans, such as pinto, kidney, garbanzo, lentil.

fat calorie consumption. One of these, as shown in Table 10.6, is to adopt certain food preparatory techniques. For example, by broiling instead of deep frying fish you can save almost 200 calories. Similarly, by using meatless in place of meat-based spaghetti sauce, you can eliminate 90 calories. And so on.

The other method is to include sufficient fiber in your daily meals. Fiber can aid in absorbing fat, thus reducing the calories that enter your circulatory system. It is reported

Table 10.4

Food Source	% Fat Calories	Grams of Fat	Tsp of Fat
LOW-FAT FOODS*			
Dairy			
1% milk, 1 cup	27	3	1/2
Low-fat yogurt, plain, 1 cup (made with 2% milk)	25	4	nearly 1
Cottage cheese, low fat, 1 cup (made with 2% milk)	17	4	nearly 1
Low-fat frozen yogurt or ice cream,** 1/2 cup	21	3	1/2
Bread, Grains, & Baked Goods			
Mixed grain bread, 1 slice	28	2	1
Corn tortillas, not fried	28	2	1
Meat, Poultry, Fish			
Meat, poultry, fish	30	4	nearly 1
Sea trout, broiled, 3 oz.	29	5	1
Swordfish, broiled, 3 oz.	24	3	1/2
Mussels, 3 oz. steamed	26-30	5	1
Beef: top round and eye round, 3 oz., broiled	10	2	1
Mixed Dishes			
Pasta with meatless tomato sauce: 1 cup pasta, 1/4 cup sauce***	10	2	1
Minestrone or lentil soup, 1 cup meat-free	0-28	0-4	1

* Those that contain 20%-30% fat calories.

** No more than 3 grams of fat per 130 calories.

*** Check labels: some tomato sauces contain higher fat calories than others.

that the average American consumes about 11-13 grams of fiber a day. This is a far cry from the 20 to 30 grams a day the National Cancer Institute recommends. Those who wish to increase their daily consumption of fiber may find the information in Table 10.5 helpful.

It is often said "living is an art." From what we have learned so far, living can be a science, too. In the long run, it is your understanding of the scientific bases of various foods and how they affect your health that will ultimately make a big difference in your life. Thus, to realize good health, good looks and longevity, you need to be a master of the foods you consume as well as of your health habits and practices. We hope the information covered in this book and these tables will contribute to your unfolding nutritional education.

Table 10.5

Food Source	Serving Size	Grams of Fiber
Cereals		
Wheat bran	1/2 cup	13.0
All-Bran extra fiber	1/2 cup (1 oz.)	13.0
Fiber-One	1/2 cup (1 oz.)	12.0
All-Bran	1/3 cup (1 oz.)	8.5
Oat Bran	1 cup	4.5
Raisin Bran	3/4 cup (1 oz.)	4.0
Cooked Legumes (Dried Beans)		
Kidney beans	1/2 cup	7.3
Lima beans	1/2 cup	4.5
Lentils	1/2 cup	3.7
Fruits*		
Apple	1	3.5
Pear	1	3.1
Dried prunes	3	3.0
Strawberries	1 cup	3.0
Bread, Grains, Pasta		
Whole-wheat spaghetti	1 cup cooked	3.9
Whole-wheat bread	2 slices	3.0
Air-popped popcorn	3 cups	3.0
Vegetables**		
Brussels sprouts	1 cup	4.6
Broccoli	I 1 cup	4.4
Green peas	1/2 cup	3.6

* The fruits listed in this category are considered the highest in fiber, but on the average, most fruits have at least 1.5 grams of fiber per serving.

** Similarly, most vegetables contain some fiber—at least 1 gram per 1/2 cup.

Menus

You probably expect a book of this kind to contain a few pages of menus. Besides the fact that I do not have any, I also happen to believe that most menus don't leave the pages they are written on. Menus may have their place in restaurants, in homes on special occasions or when someone has to follow a strict dietary regimen for a specific reason. Otherwise, for the average person and for everyday use, I think menus have very little practical value. Let's start with you. How many times have you used a menu to prepare your lunch or dinner? You just see what you

Table 10.6

Customary Cooking Method	Alternative (More Healthful) Cooking Method	Calories Saved	Fat Saved
Fried and Sauteed Foods			
French toast	Oven-baked French toast (2 slices), using egg whites only, baked on lightly oiled cookie sheets.	100	11 g
Sauteed vegetables	Steamed vegetables (1 cup); vegetables with spritz of lemon.	100	14 g
Deep fried chicken	Fried chicken, 1/2 breast w/out the skin and with egg white and butter. Cook chicken in shallow preheated lightly oiled baking pan.	124	10 g
Deep fried fish	Broiled 6 oz. fish, marinated in 1/2 teaspoon oil, lemon juice and herbs, and brushed with marinade during broiling.	190	20 g
Dressing and Sauces			
Spaghetti sauce	Meatless spaghetti sauce made without meat and with onions and/or garlic sauteed in 1/2 teaspoon olive oil (1/3 cup).	115	9 g
Hollandaise sauce	Hot oil dressing made by heating cheese sauce or fat-free salad dressing and pouring over vegetables with your favorite fresh herbs (1/4 cup).	125	10 g
Mixed Dishes			
Chili con carne	Meatless chili made by sauteing onions and other vegetables in 1/2 teaspoon oil, then adding beans and crushed tomatoes (1 cup).	171	14 g
Potatoes au gratin	Potatoes baked with cheese, parsley and lemon-juice sauce (heaping 1/2 cup).	215	23 g
Baked Goods			
Chocolate layer cake	Angel food cake made with egg whites, no oil or frosting	325	20 g

have in your refrigerator or food cabinet and prepare a meal, right? Well, that is what most people do.

If they decide to eat at home, most people in this country prepare their meals following their intuition, creativity or appetite. What is lacking, more than anything else, is proper education on the health aspect of the various foods we consume every day. For a long time, we have made the wrong choices in the purchase and consumption of foods so that we have become the victims of obesity and many degenerative diseases.

What we need now, more than fancy and elaborate menus, is a change in the emphasis of the type of foods we consume. We need to eat grains, fibers, fruits and vegetables instead of meats and dairy products and to drink pure water, fruit and vegetable juices or nonsugar soft drinks in place of alcohol or soda pop. Once we know which foods are considered healthful, we should have no difficulty making our daily meals from these foods. Let's go over what you know so far and see how you may be able to restructure your healthy meals.

From our discussion in Chapter 7, you know that most fats and oils are not good for you. And so, you should reduce or keep these foods to a minimum. According to experts, less than 20% of our daily calories should come from fats and oils. Particularly unhealthy are the saturated fats, such as those you find in meat and dairy products, and tropical oils, such as coconut, palm and palm kernel oils. Hydrogenated fats such as margarine and shortenings are equally unhealthy, at least at our current level of consumption.

You know that refined or processed foods, such as table sugars, white bread and white rice, are neither nutritious nor healthy for you. You should eliminate or minimize your consumption of these foods as well. Preserved, canned and frozen foods may often be nutritionally less valuable than fresh foods. On the other hand, organically grown whole-grain and fiber-rich foods are a much healthier alternative to many standard foods we obtain from local grocery stores.

Finally, to assist adequate nourishment, you should include quality vitamin, mineral and other food supplements along with your daily meals. These nutrients will act as your security blanket. Considering pollution levels and the stressful lifestyle most of us lead, vitamin and mineral supplements serve as a buffer to possible nutritional inequities.

Furthermore, during the day when you are physically active you may want to emphasize energy foods—e.g., complex carbohydrates such as pasta, rice and potatoes. For optimum nourishment you may also include light protein foods such as fish and the white meat of chicken or turkey. At night when you are at rest, your body needs protein, vitamins and minerals to build tissues and repair old ones. From this basic knowledge you should pretty much be able to configure your own meals.

Your morning meal should consist largely of carbohydrates, bearing in mind to include also fruits and vegetables and light protein foods, such as cereals,* oatmeal, wheat germ, whole-wheat bread, rolled oats or wheat bran. It is always good to

---

* With these foods make sure that you purchase those cereals that have no sugar added but have a sufficient amount of fiber in them.

stock a variety of these breakfast items so that you don't get tired of eating the same meal every morning. You might use skim or low-fat milk to prepare some of these foods. Instead of using sugar, you may want to use fruits like peaches, figs or banana slices in your hot or cold cereals. In addition, you may want to include an orange, a cantaloupe or half a grapefruit with any of these meals. For proper nutrition and balance, you may also want to add a protein food such as egg white and quality multivitamin supplements.

The key is moderation. You should prepare your meals according to the kind of physical activity you will facing you later in the day. If you have a sedentary job, you might want to eat just enough to tide you over until a midmorning snack or lunchtime. On the other hand, if your job requires physical labor, you might want to consume larger amounts of the complex carbohydrates. For balance you also want to include light protein foods such as beans, peas and or even white of the chicken. Rest for at least half an hour before you engage in your activity. This respite will give the body time to produce sufficient amounts of the necessary digestive enzymes and juices and enable it to proceed comfortably with the digestive process.

Your lunch menu should be decided according to the nature of your physical activity as well. If you are an office worker, you might want to eat a light lunch— consisting of soup, whole-wheat bread, fruits, vegetables and a glass of skim milk or water. On the other hand, if your job demands physical work, carbohydrate foods such as spaghetti, pasta with vegetables and a bowl of mixed fruit would be a good choice.

Consuming large amount of protein foods such as steak or even chicken can be cumbersome for lunch. Aside from the fact that these foods contain a considerable amount of fat, they are hard to digest. Thus, meatless proteins such as beans, lentils, peas or tofu can often be a better alternative to animal proteins.

For dinner you might want to eat lightly from carbohydrate foods and emphasize protein and protein-based foods. These can be fish, light chicken, turkey or tofu. In the long hours of the night, your body has plenty of time to process this type of food. Since the body uses fewer calories at night, you don't need to load up on too much carbohydrate. You may, of course, include quality fruit and vegetables with your meal. The vitamins, minerals and fibers often found in these foods are important digestive and metabolic partners.

Bear in mind that although the emphasis for your breakfast and lunch menu is on carbohydrate foods, for balance and optimum nourishment, you may want to include light protein foods such as egg white, fish and chicken. Likewise, for dinner even though the emphasis is on protein based foods make sure to include complex carbohydrates for optimum results.

That, in a nutshell, is what you need to know. As long as you know what to avoid, you can have a healthy menu at home or when you eat out. With these simple but important practices, the average person should have no problem in reducing a few pounds or maintaining his/her normal weight. Finally, remember that knowledge can give you not only power but also the freedom to choose a healthy and productive life.

PART VI
Vitamins

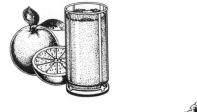

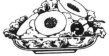
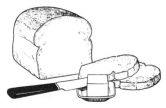
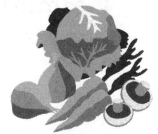

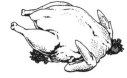
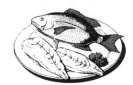
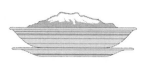
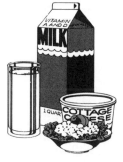
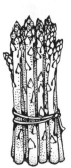

Vitamins: An Introduction

As briefly discussed in Chapter 6, vitamins are a group of organic compounds that have critical metabolic functions in the body. Vitamins are essential for the conversion of food into energy and the repair and growth of body tissues. In fact, all the carbohydrates, proteins and oils you eat would mean nothing to your body if you didn't have the necessary vitamins in your diet. Simply speaking, if you have a deficiency of one or more of the vitamins, your physical, intellectual and emotional activities will be all compromised.

Vitamins are divided into two major categories, those that are fat soluble—vitamins A, D, E and K—and those that are water soluble—vitamin C and the nine B complex vitamins. The fat-soluble vitamins require fat in the diet to be picked up by the lymphatic fluid and delivered into the bloodstream. You don't have to consume extra fat for this reason. What you obtain from your normal diet is usually sufficient.

Once in the body, any excess amounts of the fat-soluble vitamins are stored in the liver and the fat tissues of the body. Therefore, your need for this group of vitamins is not as frequent as for those that are water soluble, which get flushed out of your body with urine and perspiration. This latter group may stay, at the most, four days in the body. The only exception is vitamin B12, of which the liver stores in large enough supply to last you three to five years.

Vitamins are required in minute amounts. Although they don't become directly involved in metabolic processes (as fuel or structural components), they are responsible for the proper functioning of those processes as well as the general well-being of your body. Biochemically speaking, vitamins function as cofactors or coenzymes, enabling the various chemical processes in your body to take place efficiently and smoothly.

In this regard, vitamins resemble the oil or lubricating fluids in your car. Just as your car would begin to show problems and eventually come to a grinding halt if you didn't have a sufficient amount of lubricating oil in it, so would your body if you didn't give it the necessary vitamins. The absence or shortage of vitamins in your body can lead to deficiency symptoms. For instance, bleeding and easy bruising can be a sign of vitamin C deficiency, while listlessness, weight loss and heart failure can indicate a shortage of thiamine (vitamin B1).

With the exception of vitamin B12 and vitamin D, which can be synthesized by some animals, all the vitamins must be obtained from plant sources. Theoretically, if you choose your food from a wide variety of sources—whole grains, fresh vegetables and fruits and meats like liver and chicken—you should get all the vitamins and other necessary nutrients. This, according to several surveys, is far from being the norm. People in this country are nutritionally impoverished. There are several factors leading to this problem, including the food-processing industry, the lifestyles and habits of people and the long depleted soils. As discussed in Chapters 2 and 20, processing, canning and storing foods deplete or destroy nutrients. Added to this are the lifestyles and eating and working habits of people: skipping meals, eating on the run, working and living in stressful environments, smoking, drinking too much coffee and alcohol and consuming too much junk food.

If you are a teenager, a workaholic, an older person or an athlete or are pregnant, your need for complete and balanced meals is much greater than average. Just as a teenager or a fetus needs all the necessary nutrients to develop and grow properly, so does a workaholic or an athlete who depletes his/her body's nutrients from too much exertion. When one grows older or consumes excessive alcohol and coffee or when one is stressed, the absorption of nutrients from the intestine is compromised.

From national surveys, the most commonly deficient nutrients are vitamins A, C, D and E and the minerals calcium, potassium, magnesium, zinc, iron, copper, chromium, fluoride and selenium, as well as nearly all the vitamin B complex series. What is the solution to this dire problem?

The first thing you can do is watch what you eat and drink. Minimize or eliminate your intake of sweets, alcohol and coffee and select whole grains, fruits, vegetables and legumes as your primary foods and meats and dairy products as your secondary foods. If you feel you are not getting these foods on a regular basis, you may want to include quality supplements with some of your daily meals.

The following chapters can help you understand the significance of each vitamin in your health and factors that may aid or hinder their absorption through the intestinal wall.

CHAPTER 11
Fat-Soluble Vitamins

Vitamin A

There are two common forms of vitamin A. Beta carotene (a member of the carotenoid provitamins), which you find in yellow, red and green vegetables as well as eggs and dairy products, is the precursor of vitamin A. This form is the safest in terms of toxicity because once it gets into the body, the liver converts it into vitamin A as the need arises. You can consume a massive amount of beta carotene without having to worry about overdosing. The form of vitamin A found in fish oil and organ meats is known as retinol. Because it is fat soluble, if taken in excess for a prolonged period, it can build up in the body and become toxic.

Vitamin A is important for the health and appearance of your skin, hair and eyes and the lining of your digestive tract. It is also important for healthy formation of nails, bones and teeth and for growth and maintenance of tissues and organs. In addition, this important vitamin is involved in wound healing, as well as the healthy development and maintenance of intercellular tissues and mucous membranes. When you have sufficient amounts of vitamin A in your body, nerve cells transmit information faster, hence enhancing your ability to recall and think clearly.

Women who suffer from menstrual problems find vitamin A to be helpful in reducing flow and discomfort. For those who are pregnant, this vitamin contributes to full and healthy development of their fetuses. This vitamin is equally important for children and lactating women. A great antioxidant, vitamin A also helps fight infections and other diseases by strengthening the immune system.

A deficiency of vitamin A is often manifested as poor tooth formation and gum problems, susceptibilities to allergies and infections, night blindness and dry, scaly skin and hair. Furthermore, in children, vitamin A deficiency can lead to growth retardation and poor muscular and skeletal development. In adults, vitamin A deficiency can cause the mucous membranes of the mouth and the respiratory and gastrointestinal tracts to dry out. This can lead to a loss of taste and smell as well as vulnerability to colds and microbial infections.

Food Sources and RDA Requirements

As mentioned, all the colored vegetables, dairy products and organ meats, such as liver and kidney, beef and eggs are excellent sources of vitamin A. There are several reasons, however, why you can't depend on these foods as your main source of the vitamin.

Because of depleted farmland, most vegetables have low contents of vitamins and minerals. This means that if you rely entirely on food sources, you may not get even the RDA amounts to help you deal with low level needs. Several studies have shown that most Americans suffer from a deficiency of vitamin A.

To have the dosage necessary for some of the powerful effects of vitamin A, you may need to consume large amounts of the aforementioned vegetables. For example, to use vitamin A as a weapon against cancer and aging, you need to have a daily intake of four to five times the RDA. For most people, this is an impractical situation.

Finally, depending on your age, health and stress level, you may also need more of this vitamin to fortify you from infections and diseases or to assure your fast recovery from illness. As you age, the body also tends to generate more free radicals. This, combined with daily emotional or physical stress, can require larger amounts of this vitamin. Your best solution to this problem is to find a good supplement that can give you four to five times the RDA of vitamin A— preferably as beta-carotene.

Absorption Suppressors Alcohol, coffee, vitamin D deficiency and sometimes excessive iron.

Absorption Facilitators Vitamins C, D, E and F (the essential fatty acids), zinc, calcium and the vitamin B complex.

Vitamin D

Nicknamed the "sunshine vitamin" because it can be produced in the body with the help of the sun's ultraviolet light, vitamin D has several benefits to your health. These range from its function in the proper development of the skeletal system in growing children to the maintenance of adequate calcium levels in adult bodies to its use in the treatment of certain skin conditions and even to the suppression of some cancer cells.

There are ten different compounds that are grouped together as vitamin D, but the ones that are most important are vitamins D2 (ergocalciferol—found in plants such as yeasts and fungi) and D3 (cholecalciferol—found in animal products such as liver). Both of these vitamins can be formed in the skin and used by the body.

Historically, vitamin D deficiency has been linked to the malformation of bones in children and to the softening or hollowing of bones in adults. Vitamin D regulates the absorption and utilization of calcium and phosphorous—minerals responsible for the formation and development of strong bones and teeth.

The absence or lack of vitamin D in the body often leads to rickets in children and osteoporosis (hollowing of the bones) and osteomalacia (softening of the bones) in adults. Normally, these conditions can be avoided if one gets sufficient amounts of sunlight and minerals regularly.

Naturally, vitamin D is synthesized in the skin from the sun and cholesterol. After conversion into active form in the liver and kidneys, it enters the bloodstream where it functions as a hormone and a vitamin. As mentioned above, vitamin D promotes the absorption of calcium and phosphorous through the intestinal wall into the blood. When the availability of these minerals in the diet is limited or there are absorption problems, vitamin D induces the mobilization of calcium from the bones. This event can lead to osteoporosis or osteomalacia in adults if it occurs over prolonged periods.

In recent years, vitamin D has been found to help in the treatment of psoriasis when taken internally or used in skin lotions.[1] This white crystalline substance has also been shown to reduce the replication or duplication of certain cancer cells. Cancers that afflict the lungs, cervix, colon, breast and blood were shown to respond to vitamin D supplementation.[2] According to one study, people who spent a great deal of time indoors were more prone to get colon and rectal cancers than those who spent time outside.[3]

The absence of vitamin D in the body even seems to contribute to bilateral (both sides) deafness in humans. Since the cochlea in the inner ear is made up of bones, anything that affects the structural integrity of these bones (like increasing porosity) can affect the normal transmission of information from the outer to the inner ear. Although there has not been conclusive evidence to indicate whether vitamin D supplementation can help reverse the problem, preliminary findings show it to be promising.[4]

One thing to remember is the fact that as you get older, less and less of the available minerals will be absorbed by the intestine. By increasing your intake of calcium and phosphorous as well as vitamin D, you help minimize the problems associated with its deficiency.

Toxicity

Because vitamin D is fat soluble, it tends to collect in the fatty tissues of the body. When there are excess amounts of vitamin D in your system, calcium and phosphorous begin to accumulate in the wrong places—such as the blood vessels, the heart and even the lungs and kidneys.

The reported toxicity threshold is in the range of 500 to 600 mcgs/k of body weight per day[5] consumed over a period of several weeks. The resulting symptoms from vitamin D overdose vary from headaches, nausea, loss of appetite and thirst to excessive urination and lethargy.

Bear in mind that vitamin D toxicity can come only from food sources. It seems that the vitamin D produced in your body is monitored by keratin and melanin synthesis that block the ultraviolet rays.

Food Sources and RDA Requirements

The RDA requirement for vitamin D varies from 7.5 micrograms for infants to 10 micrograms for children, adults (up to 24 years of age) and pregnant and lactating women. For adults above 25 years of age, the dietary requirement for vitamin D drops to 5 micrograms.

Study after study bears out the fact that there is widespread vitamin D deficiency in the adult population in this country. This is another indication of the inadequacies of the RDA as a nutritional guideline. As you get older, your need for vitamin D, calcium and phosphorous is increased because of intestinal malabsorption and reduced exposure to the sun. With age, the body doesn't readily convert vitamin D into its active forms.

Fish such as salmon, herring, sardines and tuna as well as cod liver and fish oil extracts are good sources of vitamin D. Other food sources include egg yolk, liver, butter and fortified milk. Plants, in general, are very poor sources of vitamin D.

Absorption Suppressors Mineral oil.

Absorption Facilitators Phosphorus, vitamins A, C and F, choline and calcium.

Vitamin E

From its early discovery, vitamin E has been associated with something near and dear to everyone's heart: sex. Researchers who established the importance of this vitamin in our health also observed a correlation between the fertility of experimental animals and the presence of vitamin E in their diet. For example, rats that were fed food that lacked vitamin E failed to have offspring, but the reverse happened when they were given a diet with known sources of the vitamin. From this connection, early discoverers of this vitamin coined its scientific name: tocopherol. Tocopherol is a combination of two Greek words, *tocos* and *phero*, which means "childbirth" and 'to bring forth," respectively. For a long time, vitamin E has been dubbed as the 'sex vitamin" much to the wary minds of the researchers who came later.

Although you shouldn't expect to improve your sexual prowess by taking heavy doses of vitamin E, you can be assured that the reasonable level of the vitamin will enhance your fertility level. If you are a woman, you can also count on this vitamin to help reduce menopausal symptoms of "hot flashes" and headaches. If you are a man, you'll benefit by an adequate level of vitamin E in your diet; it plays a role in the proper functioning of the sexual glands.

Vitamin E is divided into several related compounds that, depending on their molecular structures are called alpha, beta, gamma, etc., tocopherols. There is also a synthetic version, which is prefixed as dl-tocopherol. The one that is natural and which people commonly refer to as vitamin E is the alpha-tocopherol. This is the most biologically active. The synthetic version is not as effective as the one that is natural.

The pure form of vitamin E is a yellowish oil that is very sensitive to light and oxidation. Vitamin E's primary function in the body is to protect the tissues and other vitamins such as A, C, D and F. Free radicals formed from unsaturated fatty acids and during metabolic processes have been linked to the genesis of various cancers and aging.

Vitamin E, by interfering with the damaging effects of these biological renegades, can help slow down the aging process and the onset of cancers in the body. For example, the testes and the brain cells are rich in unsaturated fatty acids. Vitamin E helps protect these organs from free radical damage and consequently can help prevent loss of fertility or brain tissue damage.

In other areas, vitamin E is found to help in the maintenance of healthy muscles and nerves as well as to protect the functional integrity of blood vessels. Your skin and hair and the lining of the mucous membranes also benefit from a proper level of vitamin E in the body. In addition, vitamin E was found to lower overall cholesterol levels while increasing the HDL (the good cholesterol) in the body. This versatile vitamin is also found to help in healing wounds and in improving circulation.

Vitamin E's Other Benefits

Vitamin E has many other important benefits, some of which are directly or indirectly related to its ability to fight free radicals. Our immune system, for example, declines with age, and it is believed that this is attributable to free radical damage to the immune cells. When you protect these cells by supplying an adequate amount of vitamin E and other antioxidants, you improve their effectiveness and protective power.

Vitamin E also helps protect the structural and functional integrity of red blood cells. Because this group of cells is critically involved in transporting life-giving oxygen in your body, the presence of a sufficient level of vitamin E in your blood will improve the efficiency and effectiveness of the red blood cells. This, in turn, will improve your energy level and well-being.

Those who engage in a strenuous physical activity (for example, athletes and construction workers) can greatly benefit from this vitamin. During physically stressful activities, the body produces many free radicals, and having a quality supplement along with regular meals can help protect the damaging effect of these harmful substances.

In addition, vitamin E is known to help with a host of other health-threatening situations. The aggregation of platelets that obstructs the normal flow of blood is one of the causes of heart attacks. Vitamin E has been shown to minimize this problem by keeping the platelets fully dispersed in the blood. One physician has used vitamin E to effectively control the fibrocystic breast disease, a precursor to breast cancer. A dosage of 600 I.U. of the vitamin was used in this particular experiment.[1]

This multipurpose vitamin has also been shown to help fend off the deleterious effects of some noxious chemicals in the air and damage from radiation and toxic industrial/agricultural chemicals, such as food additives, herbicides and insecticides. Vitamin E has also been shown to help with osteoarthritis, muscular dystrophy and something as common as tartar buildup on the teeth.

Women using birth control pills often hear of a common side effect: internal blood clots. This could lead to a serious heart problem if allowed to persist. The pill interferes with the adequate absorption of vitamin E into the intestinal tract. At higher doses of vitamin E, however, this problem was shown to be reversed.

What a Long-term Deficiency of Vitamin E Would Mean to Your Health

Unlike the other two vitamins discussed above, which have been associated with specific diseases when severe deficiency exists, no particular disease has been attributed to a lack of vitamin E. Nonetheless, a serious shortage of the vitamin does lead to a multitude of symptoms—from anemia (resulting from premature deaths of red blood cells) to the degeneration of the muscular, nervous and vascular systems, as well as to the atrophying of brain, spinal cord and endocrine glands.

It is now believed that a long-term, subclinical deficiency of vitamin E can also lead to cancer, heart disease, senility, premenstrual syndrome and even premature aging.

Food Sources and RDA Requirements

The current RDA requirements range from 3 milligrams for infants to 12 milligrams for breast-feeding women. As was stated earlier with the other vitamins, one needs to take considerably higher amounts than the RDAs to realize the full benefits of vitamin E. Some experiments used as high as 1,600 I.U. of this vitamin without any complications. Continuous usage of extremely high doses (in excess of 1,200 mg), however, has been reported to cause a number of ailments, including diarrhea, headaches, nausea and palpitations of the heart.[2]

There are a number of food sources for vitamin E. These include whole wheat, brown rice, oatmeal, rye, molasses, sesame and alfalfa seeds, potatoes, organ meats and nuts like almonds, walnuts and peanuts. Nearly all the green vegetables are other good sources, but the richest sources by far are foods such as wheat germ, cottonseed oil, soybean oil, sunflower seed oil, cottonseed oil and corn oils.

There are a number of reasons, however, why you would not get adequate levels of vitamin E from the above food sources. One, because a great percentage of the food in this country is processed, vitamin E is destroyed or eliminated during processing. What is available in processed foods is not sufficient to give the level of protection we discussed above, including fighting free radicals. As mentioned earlier, you need at least 600-1,200 mg of the vitamin to realize all its healing and protective benefits. Two, canning and long storage of foods, a common practice, can also destroy this rather fragile vitamin. Three, although vitamin E is found in greater quantities in oil-based foods, it is destroyed during the heat-extraction process. Cold-pressed oils tend to retain much of their vitamin E.

The Solution

In a word: SUPPLEMENT!

Absorption Suppressors Chlorine, heat, air-damaged oils and mineral oil.

Absorption Facilitators Selenium, manganese, phosphorous, vitamins A, C and F and the B-complex group.

Vitamin K

This vitamin is one of the unsung heroes because although its known function in the body is a critical one, it does not have the prominence or versatility of usage the other vitamins discussed so far have. Vitamin K, whose name was derived from the Scandinavian equivalent for "coagulation" (koagulation), has one primary but critical purpose in the human diet: it is responsible for stopping the flow of blood when you get cut.

Prothrombin is a precursor protein to thrombin, which enables the blood to coagulate and stops the flow of blood when you bleed. Vitamin K is the agent responsible for the synthesis of prothrombin in the liver and indirectly for blood clots.

There are three forms of vitamin K. K1 is derived from alfalfa. K2 is synthesized by bacteria within the intestinal tract of mammals, and vitamin K3 is man made and, functionally, has twice the potency of the natural forms.

Although vitamin K deficiency is relatively uncommon in adults, since the body can produce its own from the bacteria inside the intestine, newborns and infants experience vitamin K deficiency at a relatively high frequency. When the deficiency does occur, the associated symptoms are the appearance of blood in the stool, in urine and in vomit.

When the deficiency occurs in adults, it is usually a result of poor diet or the destruction of the vitamin K-producing bacteria in the intestine by antibiotics, barbiturates and sulfa drugs. Even aspirin, food, air pollutants and radiation can lead to the depletion of vitamin K in the intestinal tract.

In addition, since vitamin K is fat soluble, anything that interferes with the absorption of fats (such as poor production of bile and pancreatic juices, mineral oil, steatorrhea or celiac disease) can also interfere with the availability of the vitamin to the body.

Food Sources and RDA Requirements

Vegetables like cauliflower, cabbage, kelp and spinach are excellent sources of vitamin K. Soybeans, liver, egg yolk, fruits, cereals, yogurt, fish oil and dairy products are also known to have a sufficient level of the vitamin. Since your body naturally produces the vitamin, these food sources serve mainly as a security blanket.

For the first time, we now have an RDA for vitamin K. It ranges from 5 mcgs for newborns to 95 mcgs for lactating women. For other groups, see Table 1.1 on page 2.

Although there is no known full-blown toxicity from vitamin K overdose, a condition known as hemolytic anemia (resulting from excessive breakdown of red blood cells) has been observed in premature and low-birthweight infants.[1]

Absorption Suppressors. Mineral oil, aspirin, oxidized fats, x-rays and radiation.

Absorption Facilitators. None.

CHAPTER 12
Water-Soluble Vitamins

Vitamin C

From your health science classes, you probably remember a disease called scurvy that afflicted sailors in the British Navy until James Lind discovered the cure for it, the juice of citrus fruit. Scurvy is a vitamin C deficiency disease that manifests itself in a variety of ways, including hemorrhaging, gum inflammation, loosening of teeth, swollen joints, weakness, weight loss and difficulty in healing soft tissues after a bruise or trauma.

This disease is perhaps now no more than a medical curiosity, something akin to the bubonic plague, smallpox or cholera. When medicine was in its infancy and people didn't know much about health and nutrition, such afflictions were disastrous.

Today you hear more about the benefit of vitamin C and orange juice when you are sick with the common cold or the flu than you hear of its benefits in preventing scurvy. "Drink a lot of orange juice" is the classic response as soon as someone finds out about your malady.

Vitamin C's Role in Your Health

Vitamin C, also known as ascorbic acid, has many important and critical functions in your body. These range from lowering the incidence of cancer and heart disease to helping you cope with emotional and physical stresses. This nutrient is truly a wonder of nature. There is no other vitamin that contributes as much to the overall structural and functional integrity of your muscles, bones, teeth, skin and connective tissues as vitamin C. Simply put, if you had a severe deficiency of vitamin C, you could literally fall apart!

Collagen is the scaffolding protein that holds everything together from your connective tissues to your bones and teeth, to your skin and tendons. It will not function or form properly without an adequate level of vitamin C in your tissues. The adrenal, pituitary and thymus glands and the metabolically active tissues, like your muscles, also depend on the availability of vitamin C in the blood for their proper development and function.

Vitamin C also helps in the growth and repair of cells, blood vessels and gums. If you have a wound, a burn or a cold, vitamin C speeds your recovery from these maladies. By fortifying your immune system, vitamin C can also help your body protect itself against viral infections and many cancer-causing agents.

In addition, this wonder vitamin is known to help in alleviating stress by inducing the production of stress-reducing hormones in the body. For example, whenever you suffer emotional or physical stress, your body is drained of its vitamin C supply. Increased vitamin C intake during this time will help you cope better with your particular condition. Researchers have also observed the benefit of vitamin C in lowering blood cholesterol and triglycerides (fats) and the reduced incidence of clots in blood vessels. One British study showed that a high level of vitamin C significantly increases the HDL (the good) cholesterol while it lowers the LDL (the bad) cholesterol.[1] This role of the vitamin consequently reduces the occurrence of heart attack and stroke.

Vitamin C's Other Benefits

This great vitamin has many other roles in your health. For instance, sufficient amounts of vitamin C in your body will enhance your mental ability as well as improve your sleep patterns. The absorption of iron, calcium and certain essential amino acids from the intestinal tract, as well as the removal of toxic metals such as mercury, cadmium, lead and aluminum, is greatly aided by the presence of a sufficient amount of vitamin C in the body. Smokers and older persons have a higher need for vitamin C. Athletes and all those who engage in strenuous physical exertion will be benefited if they take a 500 mg - 1,000 mg of vitamin C before and after activity.

Do you have lower back problems? Are you recovering from surgery or trying to heal a wound? Take higher doses of vitamin C more frequently. Its ability to help in the formation of collagen plays an important role in speeding up the healing process as well as in strengthening your tissues.

Diabetics often suffer from easy bleeding and bruising because of weak and fragile capillaries. Vitamin C along with bioflavonoids, by strengthening the collagen matrix of these capillaries, helps decrease this problem.

People suffering from arthritis, fatigue, herpes or even schizophrenia find vitamin C to be very helpful in reducing the effects of their maladies. Vitamin C also improves fertility in both men and women and does a great job in mopping up the toxins and pollutants that may find their way into our bodies through the air, water and food we consume.[2]

Incidentally, smokers need more than the RDA amounts because each cigarette destroys 25-100 mg of vitamin C. Perhaps this is one of the reasons why smokers have such a high incidence of cancer. Carbon monoxide also has the same effect on vitamin C. For this reason, people who live in the city or in a polluted environment need to take extra supplements.

Some of the associated symptoms arising from vitamin C deficiency are swollen joints, muscular weakness, slow healing wounds, easy bruising and bleeding as well as low resistance to colds and infections.

How Much Vitamin C Is Necessary

For many of the above benefits, you need considerably higher than the RDA, which is 60 mg for adults. In many of the experiments that showed significant improvements, patients were given levels of more than 1,000 mg, and some as many as 3,000 mg daily.

Obviously, you are not going to get these amounts of the vitamin from your morning orange juice or even from vegetable sources such as broccoli, peppers, parsley, cabbage, tomatoes, brussels sprouts, collards and cauliflower. All these are known to be rich in vitamin C and may only help you to achieve the RDA. Because of vitamin C's water solubility, canning, cooking, soaking and storing these vegetables will further diminish their content of vitamin C.

If you are depending on frozen orange juice, chances are you may not even be getting enough vitamin C to meet the RDA. Vitamin C is highly oxidizable, and during processing and freezing much of the vitamin found in natural form is destroyed. Fresh fruits and vegetables are ideal, but to attain the beneficial levels (1,000 mg or more), you would have to consume a few dozen of such fruits or vegetables daily—obviously, not much of an option.

The Solution

The best solution to the above problem is to supplement. There are many supplements available. Both generic and brand name products abound at your local health food or drug store. You need to be watchful of the type of supplement you take, however. Some of the supplements you find in your local health food or drug store can be of poor quality and low potency. Regardless of what form (tablets or capsules) they come in, most of these supplements don't have even the RDA amounts.

As was discussed in Chapter 1, the RDAs are far from being sufficient to help us meet the many nutritional demands placed upon us daily. If you are physically active, a smoker or elderly or work at a stressful job, you'll need a considerably higher amount of vitamin C.

You also have to be concerned with the quality of the supplements. If tablets are pressed too hard or are constituted with fillers and binders that don't easily dissolve in the stomach, the vitamin C in them will simply pass through without getting absorbed by your body. Such tablets may also settle in the stomach lining while dissolving and cause local inflammation. Most manufacturers don't tell you what binders and fillers they use in their products. Look at the labels. Those suspended in natural cruciferous fibers are usually the better binders. Capsules are perhaps the best. You also may want to know with what the vitamin is formulated, i.e., whether it's an Ester-C®, which is one of the best forms of vitamin C or regular ascorbic acid, which is not as good. (See Appendix C on page 374 for some of the unique attributes of Ester-C.)

Food Sources and RDA Requirements

Your food sources range from citrus fruits, strawberries, tomatoes and cantaloupes to green and leafy vegetables, cauliflower and potatoes. The adult RDA for vitamin C is 60 mg.*

Absorption Suppressors: Stress, cigarettes, aspirin, cortisone and viral infections.

Absorption Facilitators All other vitamins, and minerals such as calcium and magnesium.

---

* Vitamin C is a harmless nutrient regardless of dosage. Its water solubility causes excess amounts to be flushed out of the system. One study reported that quantities of more than 10,000 mg (far more than anybody is likely to get) could result in kidney stones, but even this claim seems groundless. The possible side effects include gas, gastritis and diarrhea. Be aware that agents like cigarettes, aspirin, cortisone, antihistamines and barbiturates deplete your system's vitamin C.

The Vitamin B Complex: An Introduction

There are a total of eight B-complex vitamins. The B vitamins as a group have many important functions in the body. They are necessary for the conversion of the food you eat into energy, the building and repair of tissues, the transmission of nerve impulses, the metabolism and transportation of cholesterol in your blood and many other important biochemical reactions. In fact, your body's processes can be seriously compromised if you have a severe deficiency in even one of these vitamins.

Like the other vitamins covered in the previous chapters, the B vitamins function primarily as coenzymes in metabolic processes. Enzymes are highly specialized workers that cannot do their job effectively without help from vitamins and minerals. As an analogy, you might want to think of enzymes as engineers or architects and the B vitamins as laborers at a construction site. If anything of value is to be built or constructed, these two groups have to work in close cooperation. Just as laborers are needed to transport and deliver materials to the construction site, the B vitamins are needed for ferrying food molecules to reaction sites within the cells. Perhaps you can imagine how terribly slow and inefficient the project would be if the engineers or architects were not only to plan the design but also to actually pick up and deliver the necessary construction materials. What happens to your body if you don't have enough of the B vitamins is a lot more severe, but this gives you some idea of what could happen if you have a deficiency of the key B vitamins.

The carbohydrates, fats and proteins you eat will accumulate in the cells with very little happening to them. As a result, your nerves, brain and the immune system begin to malfunction and your overall health and appearance will be in jeopardy. Some of the symptoms could be subtle (if the deficiency is marginal), while others can be outright sickness.

The expressed symptoms of vitamin B deficiency can vary from mild depression, irritability, fatigue and forgetfulness to confusion, loss of muscular coordination, insomnia and nervousness. In an extreme case, coma and death can occur.

All the B vitamins are water soluble. This means they get flushed out of the body regularly. Unless you eat foods that are rich in these vitamins on a regular basis, your chance of being deficient in any of them is quite high. Any situation that encourages the loss of water will also remove these vitamins from the body.

More specifically, let's look at the individual vitamins in this group.

Thiamine (Vitamin B1)

Thiamine—also known as vitamin B1—serves as a facilitator in the conversion of sugar and starch into energy. Simply put, it is the spark plug that ignites these fuels to keep you going smoothly. Without a sufficient amount of this vitamin, partially "burned" carbohydrates (like pyruvic and lactic acid*) can accumulate in the body to cause muscle cramps and nervous and digestive system disorders. The health and appearance of your skin, hair and eyes also depend on having an adequate amount of this vitamin in your diet.

In general, any situation or process that requires the expenditure of very much energy will also require increased amounts of thiamine in the body. These can be such activities as athletic competition, mental concentration and surgery. Pregnant and lactating women also have a greater need for this vitamin. Alcoholics use up quite a bit of thiamine and, as a result, often suffer from a deficiency of this vitamin. The resulting symptoms involve loss of memory, confusion, lack of muscular control and delusion and, if severe, can even lead to paralysis and death.

The classic dietary disorder arising from thiamine deficiency is known as beriberi. It was first noticed in the Far Eastern countries where polished rice was the staple food among some of the natives. The most typical characteristics of this disease are a loss of appetite, fatigue, digestive disorders and feeling of numbness in the arms and legs. If deficiency persists, a gradual degeneration of the skeletal and heart muscles as well as of the nervous system will take place. Excessive fluid (edema) can also accumulate in the ankles and feet with thiamine deficiency.

In children, in its mildest form, thiamine deficiency can stunt growth and can impair their nervous system and learning ability. At its worst, beriberi can lead to a progressive hearing failure and death.

Food Sources and RDA Requirements

Some of the best sources of thiamine are organ meats (liver, heart and kidneys), beef, whole grains, eggs, beans and peas. Green vegetables such as spinach, broccoli, brussels sprouts and asparagus and dried foods such as raisins, prunes and nuts are also good sources of thiamine.

When you look at the list above, it seems that thiamine deficiency in this country should be nonexistent. You would think that there would be no problem get-

---

* See Figure D.1 on page 324 regarding these two molecules.

ting enough thiamine since it is found in such common everyday foods. Surprisingly, according to some of the national surveys, thiamine deficiency is among the most common deficiencies in this country.

Considering the fact that more than 60% of the food consumed is processed and that processing removes much of the nutrients, the high incidence of thiamine deficiency in the U.S. should perhaps come as no surprise.

Moreover, in such a fast-paced society where stress is an integral part of one's daily life, this vitamin can get depleted from the body quite easily. Coffee, alcohol and tea are some of the most frequently consumed drinks in the U.S. These beverages are the worst enemies of thiamine in the body. Since this vitamin is water soluble, daily loss can be quite high.

The RDA figures for thiamine are shown in Table 1.1, on page 2. Since there is no known toxicity of this vitamin, however, and there is a great need for it in our bodies, getting more than the RDA amounts may be of benefit.

Absorption Suppressors Alcohol, cigarettes, coffee, tea, stress, fever and surgery.

Absorption Facilitators. All the other B vitamins, manganese, vitamins C and E, sulfur and niacin.

Riboflavin (Vitamin B2)

Speaking in lay terms, riboflavin is the agent responsible for helping your cells to breathe efficiently by providing them with the correct mixture of fuel and air. Without this key vitamin, they would suffocate and operate sluggishly. Riboflavin is also the power behind the mobilization and conversion of proteins, fats and carbohydrates to energy and structural components.

Several of the intracellular enzymes, as well as the adrenal hormones and the other B vitamins, depend on riboflavin for their production and proper function in the body. In addition, this vitamin is important for the formation of red blood cells and antibodies that are part of your body's main line of defense. In some instances, B2 was found to help in removing toxic chemicals from the body.[1]

Since riboflavin is very important in the body's fundamental functions (the extraction of energy from foods and the utilization of foods for building tissues and other biochemical components), the lack of a sufficient amount of this vitamin can create major health problems. Biochemically, a deficiency of B2 can lead to a poor utilization of carbohydrates, proteins and fats. This means proteins (in the form of amino acids) will be excreted unprocessed, fats will accumulate in the wrong places (blood vessels, liver and kidneys) and carbohydrates will be burned sluggishly.

Often, the expressed symptoms of riboflavin deficiency are inflammation of the eyes, mouth, tongue and lips and skin conditions such as scaly, oily and dry spots around the nose, ears, hairline and eyes. In some instances, mental disturbances that manifest themselves as anxiety, depression and lack of concentration can be some of the other symptoms. The most typical examples of vitamin B2 deficiency however are amblyopia (poor visual acuity) and photophobia (abnormal sensitivity to light).

Food Sources and RDA Requirements

The best sources of riboflavin are dairy products, organ meats, fish, eggs, brewer's yeast, nuts, legumes, leafy green vegetables and whole grains. Riboflavin can be destroyed if exposed to light (but not heat), oxygen or acid.

The RDA requirements range from 1.2 to 1.7 mg daily, but lactating and pregnant women require slightly more than these amounts. Considering its importance in energy production, athletes, people who are physically active, sick people and stressed people can use substantially higher amounts of this vitamin.

Riboflavin deficiency is one of the most common vitamin deficiencies in this country. You may want to supplement your diet with a good source of this vitamin. As a water-soluble vitamin, riboflavin gets flushed out of your body in a short time.

Absorption Suppressors Sulfa drugs, estrogen, alcohol, coffee, excessive sugar and cigarettes.

Absorption Facilitators: All the B vitamins and vitamin C.

Niacin (Vitamin B3)

Niacin, or vitamin B3, has a multitude of functions. As a coenzyme, it functions in biochemical reactions that involve the metabolism of carbohydrates, amino acids and fatty acids. Niacin also plays an important role in the synthesis of sex hormones, cortisone, insulin and thyroxine. All these are essential in energy production and the metabolism of proteins, carbohydrates and fats and in dealing with stressful situations.

Niacin has also been found to be beneficial in lowering cholesterol and in improving blood circulation. Regarding its benefit in lowering cholesterol, niacin was shown to be more effective than clofibrate, a successful drug used in treating high cholesterol problems.[1] In other areas, niacin is necessary for the healthy functioning of the nervous and the digestive systems.

Several doctors, including one from Canada by the name of Abram Hoffer (who has been using niacin for over 20 years to treat patients with schizophrenia), feel strongly about the beneficial effects of this vitamin when given to certain mentally ill patients.[2] Another doctor, William Kaufman, has also used a form of niacin to treat patients who suffer from arthritis.[3] These treatments have not been without controversy, however. It's sufficient to say that this versatile vitamin is something you should enjoy having as part of your daily meals.

When you lack vitamin B3, the traditional deficiency symptoms are dermatitis, diarrhea and dementia (also known as the "3D's"). In dermatitis, exposed areas of the skin (such as the arms, legs, face and hands) become dry, scaly and itchy with dark pigmentation. The mucous membranes and the digestive tract will also be affected. The tongue may be swollen and bright red in appearance.

A malfunctioning gastrointestinal tract and a malabsorption of nutrients, which lead to diarrhea, are some of the other associated symptoms of niacin shortage in the diet. Symptoms associated with dementia are nervousness, irritability, depression, memory loss, sleeplessness and, in extreme cases, delusion, convulsion and death.

Pellagra was first noticed in the rural and poor areas of the South where corn was the staple food of the people. Since niacin can ordinarily be made from tryptophan (an amino acid), and corn is a poor source of tryptophan, those who lived mainly on corn suffered the worst. An exception to this are Mexicans, who consume lots of corn without any deficiency symptoms. This is because the lime water they use to soak the corn makes the tryptophan available for the body to convert to niacin.

Food Sources and RDA Requirements

The RDA requirements vary from 5 to 6 mg for infants to 18-20 mg for men and 13-15 mg for women. Add to these 2 and 3 mg of the vitamin for pregnant and lactating women, respectively. Niacin is not toxic except when taken as nicotinic acid and in doses over 100 mg per day. The resulting symptoms are itching and a burning sensation in the skin.

The best natural sources of niacin are milk, lean meat, liver, kidney, fish, poultry, eggs and legumes. Whole grains, roasted peanuts, dates and figs are also good sources of niacin. Eggs and milk have some of the highest concentrations of tryptophan and are the best, while processed foods like white bread and white rice are the worst. In this last group of foods, milling removes up to 90% of the niacin.

Absorption Suppressors Alcohol, coffee, sulfa drugs, sleeping pills, excessive consumption of water and sugar.

Absorption Facilitators All the B vitamins and phosphorus.

Pantothenic Acid (Vitamin B5)

Vitamin B5—also known as pantothenic acid or pantothenate—is an important nutrient that helps you cope with all kinds of stressful situations. These could be emotional, like the loss of a loved one, or physical, like athletic competition. It could also be environmental stress, such as cold weather, pollution or confinement in unusually crowded places.

Pantothenic acid enables you to withstand any of these situations because it stimulates the adrenal cortex to produce the hormones necessary for you to deal with stress. These are your "fight or flight" hormones, and they depend greatly on pantothenic acid to function effectively.

To show the importance of B5 in dealing with stress, three groups of rats were given "excess," "standard" and "less than the standard" amounts of the vitamin and made to swim in cold water until they became exhausted. Interestingly, those that were given "less than the standard" amount swam for only 16 minutes, those that were fed the "standard" amount swam for 29 minutes and those that were given the "excess" amounts swam for an amazing 62 minutes.[1]

In a different experiment, which tested deficiency response in humans, subjects who were fed a synthetic diet with B5 antagonist agents in it showed mental, physical and psychological disturbances within a few weeks. These varied from fatigue, irritability and loss of muscular coordination to vomiting and total exhaustion.[2]

Metabolically, pantothenic acid's function in the body is in the conversion of sugars, proteins and fats into energy. In fact, pantothenic acid is a precursor (the raw material) of coenzyme A—a very important molecule needed by every cell in the body during energy production. Pantothenic acid is also essential in the synthesis of antibodies, hemoglobin, cholesterol and bile acids. Neurotransmitters like acetylcholine and sphingosine also depend on vitamin B5 for their production and function.

In other areas, pantothenic acid is also known to help heal wounds and reduce the incidence and/or the adverse effects of allergies and radiation. According to some researchers, this vitamin may even help alleviate the pain and stiffness in joints that is associated with rheumatoid arthritis.

Although this should not lead you to rush out and buy a jar full of B5 supplements, in some animal experiments, pantothenic acid was shown to prolong life by as much as nearly 20%.

Food Sources and RDA Requirements

Some of the known sources are whole grains, all organ meats, brewer's yeast, chicken, eggs, saltwater fish, nuts, potatoes, milk, legumes and green vegetables. You might consider obtaining these foods as fresh as possible. Canning, cooking and storing, as we have said often, remove many of the valuable nutrients, including pantothenic acid.

The National Research Council (RCA) recommends from 5 to 10 mg of the vitamin for adults. To get the most of its beneficial effects (like reducing the pain associated with rheumatoid arthritis) you may be advised to take doses of more than 500 mg a day. There are no known pantothenic acid toxicities.

Absorption Suppressors Alcohol, coffee, sleeping pills, sulfa drugs.

Absorption Facilitators Folic acid, vitamin C and all the B vitamins.

Pyridoxine (Vitamin B6)

Pyridoxine, or vitamin B6, is perhaps the most versatile and highly beneficial vitamin of the B-complex group. In women, it helps minimize birth defects and alleviate PMS*-related problems such as moodiness, depression and irritability. This important vitamin is also known to benefit those who suffer from arthritis, heart diseases, cancer and diabetes as well as those who have asthma, anemia and seborrheic dermatitis. The list goes on.

Biochemically speaking, pyridoxine enables the body to convert foods such as fats, proteins and carbohydrates into energy. These foods, in turn, are responsible for the health, growth, repair and proper functioning of your tissues and organs. For example, many of the amino acids that are used in the repair and building of tissues are also important precursors to many of the brain chemicals (neurotransmitters) that control your memory and thoughts, as well as your moods, appetite,

---

* PMS stands for premenstrual syndrome. Somehow, the premenstrual syndrome seems to deplete the vitamins women get from their normal meals.

sexual desires, sleep and breathing patterns. Pyridoxine is the key vitamin that controls the conversion of these amino acids into neurotransmitters.

An insufficient amount of this vitamin in a person's diet could lead to nervousness, irritability, confusion and depression at the least, or convulsion, mental retardation and even death at worst. A salient example of this is what happened to babies who were fed an infant formula brand called SMA in the early 1950s. For no apparent reason, babies who were on this formula went into sudden convulsions. Curiously, when these babies were fed a different formula or milk, their maladies disappeared. It was later discovered that what was missing in the SMA formula was pyridoxine.

Adults, particularly the middle aged, pregnant women, PMS sufferers and those who are on the pill, sometimes experience a neurological disorder that affects their hands.* It is called carpal tunnel syndrome. The associated symptoms are pain, numbness and a tingling sensation in the hands. People who have rheumatoid arthritis also have this problem. In some studies, when such people were given pyridoxine, their condition was reduced or eliminated.

People with diabetes and cancer also seem to have a greater need for B6. Tests have shown that these people have a low level of the vitamin. For some unknown reason, their conditions seem to use up most of the B6 they get from their normal meals.

Pyridoxine's importance in diabetes and heart disease is largely due to its function in collagen formation. Collagen is the structural protein found in the heart and skeletal muscles, blood vessels and others tissues. When you have a strong heart and durable blood vessels, you can minimize some of the problems associated with heart failure. The red blood cells and immune cells also depend on vitamin B6 for their production and proper function.

In other areas, pyridoxine is the key nutrient involved in the conversion of tryptophan to niacin. Niacin is the parent molecule to vitamin B5. As was discussed earlier, niacin is one of most powerful vitamins and is involved in a multitude of reactions in the body.

In addition, pyridoxine helps remove or reduce the side effects of toxins like those in cigarettes and certain chemicals and drugs such as those used for sedation and psychiat-

---

* It is reasoned that somehow, in the presence of the pill or with rheumatoid arthritis or hormonal changes, pyridoxine's effectiveness has been blurred or that the body needs this vitamin in higher amounts.

ric treatments. This versatile vitamin even has a place in dentistry. In one study, children taking supplements of the vitamin had a 40% reduction in tooth decay when compared to those who were given placebo or "dummy" pills.[1]

Food Sources and RDA Requirements

The RDA figures range from 0.3 mg for infants to 1.6 and 2.0 mg for women and men, respectively. The requirement for pregnant and lactating women is about 2.2 mg. These may be far too low, however, to get all the beneficial effects of this great vitamin.

To cite an example, in one experiment when animals were fed a diet that consisted of a pyridoxine level found in the normal American diet, they had more tooth decay than those that were supplemented.[2] As mentioned above, individuals with certain health conditions have a higher need of pyridoxine. Furthermore, the many physical and emotional stresses people experience daily raise the requirement of this nutrient. As a solution to all these problems, you need to include top quality vitamin B6 supplements with your daily meals.

One word of caution: although pyridoxine has not been shown to have toxic side effects, daily doses of over 2,000 mg could lead to some neurological disturbances.

Good food sources are organ meats, whole grains, soybeans, poultry, fish and yeast. Cabbage, bananas, potatoes, prunes, avocados, peas and green peppers are also well-regarded sources. Poor sources range from refined and processed food to egg white, lettuce and milk.

Pyridoxine is soluble in water, so much so that the longest it can stay in your body after you consume this vitamin is eight hours. Thus, canning and cooking pyridoxine-containing foods in water can deplete a major portion of the vitamin. Fiber-rich foods also tend to trap the vitamin and make it unavailable for absorption by your system.

Absorption Suppressors Alcohol, contraceptives, cigarettes, light, fiber, radiation exposure and coffee.

Absorption Facilitators All the B-complex team, sodium, vitamin C and magnesium.

Folacin

Folacin, also known as folate, folic acid or vitamin M, is part of the B vitamin group. Although it doesn't have the versatility or the prominence of vitamin B6, folacin has a few known crucial functions without which life would not be possible.

The first one of these is its role in the synthesis of proteins and the genetic materials DNA and RNA. Of course, without these two, life would not be possible. In this regard, you might say that folacin is life itself. From the moment of conception to your death, folacin is necessary for cell division and replication. It is also necessary for the repair and maintenance of your body, enabling you to look and feel your best.

Human life begins from the union of two cells: an egg and a sperm. After several divisions of the genetic materials and differentiation, the whole organism comes to being. The process of cell division is continuous from conception to birth and adulthood.

Think of the basal cells of your skin, hair and nails and those cells that line the nasal passage and digestive tract. All these cells are continually born and replaced after they reach maturity. The cells of the male reproductive organ and the immune system also continuously divide to replace those that are dead or dying. Cell division goes on in other parts of the body as well but at a slower pace.

This means that if you want to have beautiful skin, hair and nails and overall good health, you need a sufficient amount of folic acid in your diet. The production of red blood cells in the bone marrow and the synthesis of the oxygen-carrying hemoglobin greatly depend on folic acid.

A deficiency of this vitamin leads to a rather tongue-twisting condition called megaloblastic anemia. When the red blood cells are born in the bone marrow, they go through several stages of development. Megaloblasts are abnormally large cells that never went past one of those stages due to folic acid deficiency. This could also happen when there is a vitamin B12 deficiency.

The nervous and immune systems are also affected by a folate deficiency. Ordinarily, brain and spinal fluids contain the highest concentration of folic acid. This is because, among other things, folic acid serves as a coenzyme for the synthesis of norepinephrine[*] (a hormone/neurotransmitter) and methionine (an amino acid that serves

---

[*] Norepinephrine is also produced by the medulla of the adrenaline gland. Its primary function there is to constrict small blood vessels and to increase blood pressure and flow through the arteries while slowing the heart rate. It's secreted largely in fright, fight, flight situations. In the brain, norepinephrine increases alertness.

as an antioxidant in the brain). Regarding the immune system, a low level of folic acid tends to affect the production and activity of the immune cells.

The expressed symptoms of foliate deficiency are irritability, forgetfulness, weakness in legs and feet and poor reflexes. Some of the other symptoms include depression, numbness in the extremities, insomnia, paranoia and dementia. Because of these correlations, doctors have used large doses of folic acid to ameliorate certain congenital conditions such as some forms of retardation, schizophrenia and other psychological disorders. A sore and inflamed tongue, weight loss, digestive disturbances and diarrhea are also common with people who lack a sufficient amount of folic acid in their diet.

In other areas, folic acid has uses in dealing with hypoglycemia (low blood sugar), psoriasis, gingivitis and even heart disease.

Food Sources and RDA Requirements

Not surprisingly, folic acid deficiencies are very common, particularly among pregnant and lactating women, alcoholics and the elderly and in those who use all kinds of drugs, including the prescribed, and contraceptives.

The RDA for folic acid varies from 25 mcg for infants to 400 mcg for pregnant women. The interesting thing is that although the RDA for adult males and females is 200 mcg and 180 mcg respectively, what people often end up getting, due to poor absorption, is only 20% to 50% of these figures.

You must also realize that up to 90% of the vitamins contained in foods are destroyed during cooking, storing, canning and processing. Thus, considering that the RDAs on the whole are marginal and high losses can be encountered during food preparation, your consumption of folic acid should be much greater than the RDA figures to assure yourself of good health.

Folic acid is found in many different sources. These include dark green vegetables (broccoli, cabbage, asparagus, collard greens, etc.), beets, cauliflower, whole grains, yeast, orange juice, beans and peas, organ meats, wheat germ and others. Folic acid has no known toxicity.

Absorption Suppressors Alcohol, drugs, stress, coffee, intestinal bacterial infections and cigarettes.

Absorption Facilitators All the B vitamins, biotin and vitamin C.

Cobalamin (Vitamin B12)

Vitamin B12, or cobalamin as it's sometimes called, is unique of all the vitamins in that it contains a mineral (cobalt). Vitamin B12 is also unique in another way: it is the largest and the most complex of all the vitamins, and it comes strictly from animal sources. (See page 396 for its molecular structure.)

In the human body, cobalamin has so many crucial functions that if you didn't have this vitamin for a prolonged time, you could encounter a serious health problem. For example, the syntheses of proteins, DNA and RNA cannot be adequately accomplished without this vitamin. Cobalamin is also important for the development and proper function of nerve cells and red blood cells. Like folacin, B12 is intimately involved in the health and development of the fetus.

In children, B12 promotes growth and enables them to have better appetites, memory and concentration. In adults, B12 functions as a provider of energy by enabling them to properly metabolize proteins, fats and carbohydrates. Cobalamin also has fortifying functions in the nervous and immune systems, for a deficiency of this vitamin can lead to mental disorders and susceptibility to diseases.

Cobalamin is required only in extremely minuscule amounts—something like one millionth of a gram. Even so, there is a fatal disease called pernicious anemia associated with the deficiency of this vitamin. The related symptoms are irritability, disorientation, nervousness, impatience, forgetfulness, poor muscular coordination, a sore and inflamed tongue, lethargy, weakness, depression and diarrhea.

One group who can be prone to pernicious anemia is strict vegetarians. As we said above, cobalamin is the only vitamin that comes from an animal source. However, even these people are not entirely without help if they watch what they eat.

Certain seaweeds, like spirulina, kombu and wakame contain organisms that synthesize the vitamin. Artificially, this vitamin can also be made by growing yeast (like brewer's yeast) in a cobalt-rich medium. Unpasteurized milk, fermented soybean (miso) and soybean paste (tempeh), tamari soy sauce, fish and pickles can also be a good source of the vitamin. Then, of course, there are supplements you can take.

Another group that can be affected by B12 deficiency is people past middle age. As you get older, not only do you have problems with malabsorption, but you also have more frequent gastrointestinal disturbances that can lead to deficiency symptoms of certain vitamins, including B12.

Sometimes, deficiencies can result even if you are taking a sufficient amount of a vitamin. For example, the absence of cofactors—calcium for vitamin D and iron for vitamin C—can cause vitamin deficiency symptoms. Vitamin B12 requires one such cofactor known as an "intrinsic factor," an organic substance produced by the stomach that assists in the absorption of B12 in the intestine. Depending on your health, with age, the secretion of the intrinsic factor can be diminished.

Interestingly, some of the crankiness, depression, nervousness and even psychosis that sometimes comes about with old age is thought to be nothing but a result of B12 or other vitamin deficiency. There exist many documented cases in which patients with unexplainable mental disturbances were treated with cobalamin injections. (Please bear in mind though that every time you have the above symptoms, it is not necessarily because you have a vitamin B12 or other vitamin deficiency.)

If you eat a well-balanced diet and are healthy, you may not need to worry about deficiency problems. This water-soluble vitamin manages to stay in the body for a long time: up to five years. The liver serves as a storehouse for B12. Be that as it may, this vitamin has no known toxicity.

Food Sources and RDA Requirements

Other than the vegetarian sources mentioned above, for carnivores, liver, kidney, beef, pork and lamb are very good sources. In addition, fish such as mackerel and herring, oysters, clams, eggs and tofu contain sufficient amounts of cobalamin.

Although vitamin B12 survives moderate cooking, agents such as acids, alkali and light can easily destroy it. This means that it would be of great benefit to you to minimize exposure of the aforementioned foods to those destructive elements.

The RDA for this vitamin range from 0.2 mcg for infants to 2.0 mcg for adults, with extra requirements for lactating and pregnant women. Supplements up to 2,000 mcg are available.

Absorption Suppressors: Cigarettes, alcohol, coffee, estrogen, sleeping pills and laxatives.

Absorption Facilitators: All the B vitamins, inositol, vitamin C, calcium, sodium and potassium.

Biotin (Vitamin H)

Biotin is one of those quasi-vitamins that is not well understood. It is required by the body, yet the body can make some of its own with the help of bacteria in the intestinal tract. There are also definite, though not common, deficiency symptoms associated with biotin, which therefore make it an essential vitamin.

Like most of the B vitamins, biotin plays an important role in the metabolism of proteins, fats and carbohydrates. The synthesis of proteins, fatty acids and nucleic acids is also aided by the availability of this vitamin in the blood. As a coenzyme, it assists many enzymes to perform their duties effectively.

Those glands directly involved in the metabolism of carbohydrates, such as the thyroid and adrenal glands, as well as the skin and the nervous system, are also the beneficiaries when there is sufficient biotin in the body. Sufficient amounts of biotin contribute to healthy skin, hair, nails and muscles.

Unless you have an intestinal disorder or eat a very restricted diet, which includes the consumption of raw eggs, your suffering from a biotin deficiency is unlikely. There are many sources of biotin, and as mentioned above, your body also produces its own. In the event you wonder what is wrong with raw eggs, a protein-carbohydrate compound called avidin (found in egg white) combines with biotin in the intestine and renders the vitamin unavailable to the body. When you cook eggs the heat deactivates avidin.

The resulting symptoms when deficiency occurs are many, but some of the obvious ones are severe skin abnormalities such as eczema and seborrheic dermatitis, loss of appetite, anorexia, depression, fatigue, numbness of the hands and feet, insomnia and anemia. Other symptoms such as improper function of the heart, high blood cholesterol, muscular pain and increased susceptibility to infections and diseases can occur.

Food Sources and RDA Requirements

Many plant and animal foods contain biotin, so much so that it is believed that the average American gets between 150 and 300 mcg of biotin per day. Some of the common food sources are organ meats, pork, beef, whole wheat, brown rice, nuts, fruit, molasses, cheese, milk, chicken, soybeans, fish and eggs.

The RDA requirements range from 10 mcg for infants to 100 mcg for adults. Bear in mind, however, that although these requirements are less than what people are thought to get every day from their meals, you should not be lulled into believing that everything is fine with you regarding this vitamin. Even though we don't know a great deal about this vitamin (since it is relatively new), there is also evidence to show that people such as alcoholics, the elderly, pregnant women and athletes often have inadequate levels of biotin in their systems.[1]

There is no known toxicity of biotin.

Absorption Suppressors: Alcohol, raw egg white, coffee, sulfa drugs and antibio-tics.

Absorption Facilitators: Folic acid, B2, B6, niacin, B12, pantothenic acid and vitamin C.

Inositol

This is another of those B vitamins not completely studied. According to prelimi-nary findings, inositol is believed to have a number of benefits. These range from its role in enhancing the appearance of the skin, hair and nails to its function in the metabolism of fats and cholesterol. The nervous system and vital organs like the liver, heart and kidney, as well the skeletal muscles seem to benefit from inositol as well.

This new member of the B family has also been shown to enhance nerve impulse transmission (thus giving you good muscular coordination) and aids in suppressing cancer of the bladder. Since the brain is one of the areas where there is a high concen-tration of inositol, this vitamin purportedly has a calming or sedative effect during anxiety. In the circulatory system, inositol helps minimize the accumulation of fat in the liver and blood vessels.

Food Sources and RDA Requirements

Some of the best sources are organ meats (heart, liver, beef brain, lungs), canta-loupe, grapefruit, oranges and cabbage. Raisins, peanuts, cooked beans, limes, green beans, whole wheat bread, nuts and brewer's yeast are some of the other sources.

Since it is new, the RDA for it has not been figured out yet. In practice, doses ranging from 100 to 500 mg are being used by some doctors. There is no known toxicity with inositol.

Absorption Suppressors: Coffee, alcohol, excessive sugar, antibiotics, food process-ing, sulfa drugs and estrogen.

Absorption Facilitators: All the other B-complex vitamins, phosphorus and linoleic acid.

Choline

Here is another inadequately studied, borderline vitamin. Choline is classified as part of the B-complex. Because the body can make some of its own choline and there are no known deficiency symptoms associated with it, it has so far been relegated to a quasi-vitamin status. Be that as it may, what choline does in the body and the kinds of diseases it has been linked to would make you think twice before you disregard this nutrient and assume it is a nonessential vitamin.

Choline's primary function is as a precursor to acetylcholine, a very important chemical messenger in the brain involved in memory and thought processes. Choline is also used as a structural component by nerves and brain cells. Myelin, the sheath that covers and protects nerve fibers and the membranes in brain cells, is composed of phosphatidyl choline. Elsewhere in the body, choline is involved in the metabolism and transportation of fats and in the proper functioning of the gallbladder and the thymus gland. It is also good for hair.

Regarding its role in memory and thought processes, choline is the raw material from which acetylcholine is made. Acetylcholine serves as a transmitter of electro-chemical signals from one nerve cell to another. This relaying of information across a synapse enables you to think clearly and retrieve stored information quickly. There are many neurotransmitters like choline in the brain. Any abnormalities that lead to an imbalance of these chemicals can lead to depression, confusion, and aggressive and compulsive behaviors, including excessive drinking, substance abuse and eating disorders.

Such degenerative diseases as Parkinson's disease, tardive dyskinesia and Huntington's disease (all of which are characterized by loss of muscular control that leads to tremors and shaking) are often observed in some elderly people and are believed to have nutritional bases. Alzheimer's disease is also one of those degenerative diseases affecting memory in this group of people.

Several experiments performed to test the effect of choline on patients suffering from Alzheimer's disease have shown some promising results. A similar test done on college students, though not conclusive, was found to be encouraging.[1] Although all these are preliminary studies and we should not draw any conclusion from them, the fact that there could be a nutritional basis for many of our ailments is a tantalizing fact that should make all of us be selective in what we eat.

Food Sources and RDA Requirements

Most foods contain only a tiny amount of choline. The best source is lecithin—found mostly in seed oils, soybean oil, brewer's yeast, flax, whole grains, cereals, legumes, egg yolk, liver, green leafy vegetables and fish.

There are no established RDA amounts for choline. Some nutritionists believe

20 to 300 mcg would be optimal for both men and women. The average diet is thought to contain many times more than these figures. Choline has no known toxicity.

Absorption Suppressors: Alcohol, coffee, cigarettes and excessive sugar.

Absorption Facilitators: Linoleic acid, inositol, vitamin A, folic acid and all the B-complex vitamins.

Para-Aminobenzoic Acid (PABA)

You probably have seen PABA more often on sunscreen products than on food labels. For many years, PABA has had a reputation as one of the best chemical compounds for protecting you from the sun's cancer-causing ultraviolet rays. Now, its use as a vitamin is getting more attention than its former role.

PABA, or paraaminobenzoic acid, is categorized as one of the B-complex vitamins, albeit a quasi one. There has not been extensive, controlled research done on PABA to show its essentialness. What is known so far, however, is sufficient to include it in food ingredients.

PABA, like all the other B vitamins, works as a coenzyme for the breakdown and utilization of proteins. For example, with pantothenic acid, PABA is purported to restore or delay graying of hair. PABA also helps bacteria in the gastrointestinal tract in their production of folic acid and in the bone marrow with the formation of red blood cells. In other areas, PABA has been found useful as an antioxidant protecting tissues from ozone—a damaging, poisonous gas found mostly in the upper atmosphere.

Aesthetically, PABA is known for its function in maintaining healthy skin and hair and in retarding wrinkle formation.

Food Sources and RDA Requirements

The best food sources of PABA are liver, kidney, brewer's yeast, wheat germ, molasses and whole grains. There are no RDAs for PABA, but some nutritionists recommend 25 mg and up for most common uses. There is no known toxicity for PABA.

Absorption Suppressors: Sulfa drugs, coffee and alcohol.

Absorption Facilitators: Vitamin C, folic acid and all the B vitamins.

PART VII

Minerals

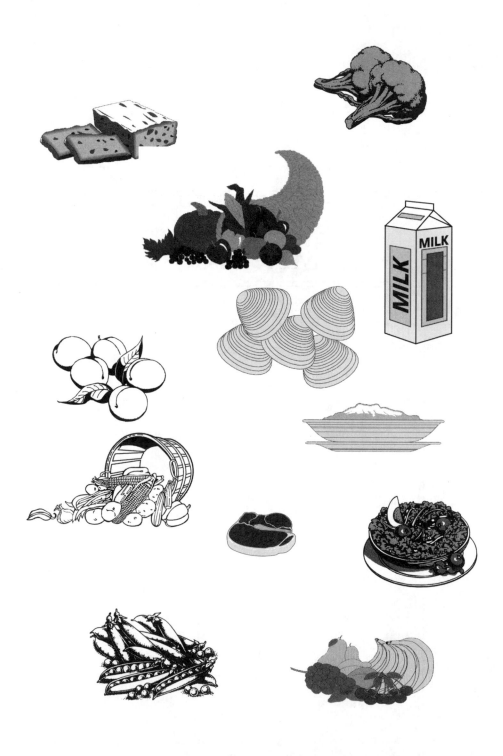

Minerals: An Introduction

Like vitamins, minerals have many crucial functions in our bodies. Whether serving as structural components and cofactors of many biochemical processes or functioning as electrolytes, minerals are some of those essential nutrients you can't live without. If you don't get all the necessary minerals for a long time, your bones and teeth begin to disintegrate, your heart and skeletal muscles become weak and your brain malfunctions.

There are many different minerals found in the body, but over 70% of these consist of calcium, phosphorus, sodium, potassium, magnesium, chlorine and sulfur. These are called macro (or bulk) nutrients because your body uses them in large amounts. In our discussion of individual minerals, in this group all but chlorine and sulfur will be covered. There are no known deficiency symptoms associated with chlorine and sulfur.

The others that are needed in small amounts (the so-called trace elements) are chromium, manganese, zinc, iron, molybdenum, iodine and selenium. Bear in mind, though, the quantities have nothing to do with their essentiality. The trace elements are just as important to the body as the macro minerals. Be aware also that there are still other trace elements found in the body, and they include cobalt, fluorine, nickel, silicon, vanadium, tin, and bromine. In fact, you can pretty much expect to find nearly every element found in the earth's crust in the body, albeit in tiny amounts. By weight, minerals account for about 4% of your body mass.

When you think of minerals as structural components, perhaps what you think of is calcium, because for years milk commercials have touted it as the mineral that strengthens your teeth and bones. Phosphorus and magnesium do the same, but you probably have never seen commercials about these minerals or iron, which is very important for the synthesis of hemoglobin, a critical life-supporting protein.

There are many other minerals (although in smaller amounts) that are part of the skeletal system, body tissues and fluids. What you also don't hear about are these minerals' roles as cofactors of many enzyme systems and their function as electrolytes that regulate your heart rhythm or thought processes. Furthermore, minerals are essential for the maintenance of acid-base neutrality and the regulation of body fluids across cell membranes (also known as osmotic pressure).

Before we discuss the individual minerals, let's briefly define a few terms.

What Are Cofactors?

Cofactors are similar to enzymes, and they help other components (like enzymes) speed up certain chemical reactions and bring them to completion. For example, calcium is a cofactor in the synthesis of blood-clotting protein, and chromium helps the hormone insulin to bring sugar to the cells. Without each of these minerals, bleeding cannot be stopped and sugar cannot be metabolized. Copper is another mineral that serves as a cofactor for several enzymes in the body. The generation of energy from fuel and the formation of elastin, collagen and melanin (the skin and hair pigment) all need the availability of copper to the enzymes that accomplish these processes. Copper is also involved in the synthesis of superoxide dismutase (SOD - the powerful antioxidant enzyme that protects the body from the aging and tissue-damaging effects of oxygen free radicals). Manganese and zinc are also involved in this.

In short, the hundreds of metabolic processes that convert proteins, carbohydrates and fats into energy, water and carbon dioxide in your body, or those that catalyze the synthesis of muscle tissues, hormones and countless other biological molecules, are dependent on minerals. Even the absorption of food from the intestine and into the individual cells is facilitated by minerals. For instance, sodium and magnesium assist in the uptake of carbohydrates. Calcium assists the absorption of vitamin B12. The enzymes that catalyze the breakdown of food in your stomach and intestine also use minerals as their cofactors.

What Are Electrolytes?

An electrolyte is a substance, or a group of substances, that dissociates into two (positively and negatively) charged ions when melted or dissolved in water. For example, when you dissolve table salt in water you get free sodium and chloride ions. Such ions are often capable of conducting electrical charges or impulses. There are many other minerals and organic molecules that have this property (see Table 12.1 on page 156). In the body, these substances serve as regulators of fluids (osmotic pressure) between the internal and external environment of the cells. Minerals are also important in the maintenance of an acid-base balance of body fluids and in the conduction of electrical impulses along nerve fibers.

In your body, there are three defined spaces or compartments: intercellular (exist inside the blood vessels), intracellular (found inside the cells) and interstitial (spaces outside the blood vessels and between cells). The distribution of water and nutrients among these spaces is regulated by a process called osmotic pressure. In this process, particles or fluids move across a semipermeable membrane from where they are highly concentrated to where there are fewer of them or none at all. On the basis of this simple principle, food is able to get past the intestinal wall into the bloodstream and be delivered to various tissues and organs. In turn, waste material is removed from the blood by the kidneys and lungs.

Minerals also facilitate in the conduction or transmission of nerve impulses along a nerve fiber. If you recall from your biology classes, a nerve cell consists of a body, a long tubelike structure (axon) and tiny fingerlike projections called dendrites. The transmission of a nerve impulse along the axons and dendrites (nerve fibers) is accomplished by a change in the electrical properties of the fluid that bathes the nerve cells when stimulated by the impulse.

This change, which creates a temporary electrical charge on the cell membrane, is caused by the exchange of sodium and potassium ions across the cell membrane when stimulated by a nerve impulse. This process facilitates the transmission and propagation of the nerve (electrical) signals down the axon. At the juncture of the dendrites and the next neuron are tiny gaps called synapses.

Acetylcholine is the chemical that serves to bridge these gaps so that the electrical impulses can continue their journey to the next series of nerve cells. In less technical terms, this means that when you have healthy and properly functioning nerves, an abundance of acetylcholine and the necessary minerals, you can think clearly and remember things more quickly.

Similarly, the contraction and relaxation of muscles are influenced by the presence of an adequate amount of certain minerals in the fluids that bathe these tissues. Calcium, for example, is responsible for the muscle contraction, while sodium, potassium and magnesium are necessary for its relaxation. The proper functioning of all the body muscles, including the heart, depends on these minerals.

It is apparent from the above information that anything that upsets the balance of minerals in your body severely compromises your health and well-being. Tetany, for instance, is a muscular condition characterized by spasm and twitching of the face, feet and hand muscles. This problem is often caused by a drop in the calcium level in the body fluid (due to an improper functioning of the parathyroid gland), calcium deficiency or rickets. Calcium rigor is a condition induced by an excessive presence of the mineral in the blood. Similarly, magnesium deficiency can lead to muscle weakness, depression and disturbance of muscular contraction.

Table 12.1 Major Electrolytes Found in Body Fluids

	Extracellular Fluid (from blood plasma) mEq/l	Intracellular Fluid (in muscles) mEq/l
Positive ions		
Sodium (Na+)	145	10
Potassium (K+)	5	150
Calcium (Ca++)	3	2
Magnesium (Mg++)	2	15
Total	155	177
Negative ions		
Chloride (Cl-)	105	5
Bicarbonate (HCO3-)	25	10
Phosphate (PO4 ---)	2	
Organic Acids	6	120
Proteins	17	42
Total	155	177

mEq/l = milliequivalents per liter
Source: J. R Robinson, "Water and Life," *World Review of Nutrition and Dietetics.*

Minerals also influence the alkalinity of the bile and the acidity of the stomach juices as well as the acid-base balance of the blood. The proper strength of the bile and stomach juices is important for efficient digestion and processing of food. Blood acid-base neutrality, which must be kept within a pH range of 7.35 to 7.45, is also important. Any deviations from these values can lead to acidosis or alkalosis, conditions that arise from an increase in the acidity (lower than pH 7.35) or the basicity (higher than pH 7.45) of the blood.

The mineral salts, or rather, the electrolytes generated from them, play a major role in monitoring the movement of fluids in the different body spaces. For example, an increase in electrolyte concentration on one side of a semipermeable membrane raises the osmotic pressure on that side of the membrane. This differential in osmotic pressure encourages fluid to move from low to high electrolyte concentration. This movement of fluid between the two sides of the membrane will go on until the osmotic pressure is even on both sides.

From the above synopsis you can see that minerals are a very important part of your health. You should provide your body with sufficient amounts of these nutrients daily to experience good health and well-being. Since minerals are water soluble, they don't get stored in the body unless they are part of tissue structures like calcium and phosphorus in the bones and teeth. Moreover, the body tissues are constantly broken down at varying rates, and you need to have all the necessary nutrients to help rebuild or repair them.

In the body, electrolytes control much of the fluid movement across the capillaries into the cells, and vice versa. The biological significance of this is that water and other nutrients are able to get into the cells. Any major increases or decreases in the electrolyte concentration will cause a shift in the homeostasis of the body.

Now let's discuss the individual minerals.

CHAPTER 13
Bulk Minerals

Calcium

Calcium is the king of all minerals. It is the most abundant and the most fundamental mineral nutrient in the body because our teeth and skeletal system are built largely from this mineral. Calcium, in addition to being important for the proper functioning of the muscles, including those of the heart, can help facilitate the reactions of many metabolic processes in the body.

The enzymes that catalyze the conversion of food into energy and body tissues and those involved in blood clotting all require the presence of a sufficient amount of calcium in the blood. The absorption of vitamin B12 from the intestine and the synthesis and breakdown of the neurotransmitter acetylcholine are also aided by this mineral.

We receive many other benefits from calcium. Calcium can help lower blood pressure. It can help prevent colon cancer and heart disease. For women, the most important of all its functions is in deterring the onset of osteoporosis and osteomalacia. In other areas, calcium is known to block the absorption of poisonous metals like strontium, cadmium and lead. As was discussed in the previous pages, calcium's role in nerve impulse transmission and muscle contraction is equally important to the health and well-being of an individual.

About 30% of bone is a rather flexible and porous material composed of collagen, mucopolysaccharide, carbohydrates and glycoprotein. These substances are formed during fetal development, and shortly after birth they begin to gain hardness as calcium compounds are deposited in the porous collagen matrix. For the next 20 years or so, the whole human skeleton forms and grows by this gradual deposition of calcium in the bones and teeth. In the end, the body can accumulate roughly 2 1/2 pounds of the mineral. About 99% of the calcium in the body is located in bones and teeth. The other 1% circulates in the bloodstream.

Bear in mind, though, that calcium deposition is never a one-way process. During the growth process and throughout life, bone (and therefore calcium) is continuously resorbed and rebuilt to replace older, stressed bone. Bone is also broken down when there is a drop of the mineral found in the blood. For survival, the presence of an adequate amount of calcium in the blood is more important than having strong bones and teeth.

There are quite a few factors that limit the availability of calcium in the blood. One of these is simply not having enough calcium in your diet. The other may be not getting enough sunshine or vitamin D (which helps in the absorption of calcium). It may also be that you have a problem with your parathyroid gland, which produces hormones that regulate the calcium level in the blood. Your emotional state, the amount of exercise you get, the level of phosphorus in your blood and the acid-alkaline balance in your digestive system also determine calcium absorption.

Other interfering factors are the consumption of too much protein, cereals, vegetables and fruits like rhubarb, cranberries, spinach and beets and tea. These foods contain chemical compounds called physic acid and oxalic acid that combine with calcium in the gastrointestinal tract, thus making it unavailable for absorption. Vomiting, diarrhea and even excessive fat and fibers can be some of the other culprits. When too many of these agents are limiting the availability of the mineral, microscopic segments of the bone begin to break down to release more calcium to meet such life-sustaining needs as keeping your heart beating.

The most common of the above situations is not having enough calcium in the diet. Milk is often the best and easiest source of calcium, but most people don't drink milk once they are past their formative years. The estimated optimal daily requirement for calcium ranges from 1,000 to 1,500 mg. To meet these requirements, you may need to drink four to six glasses of milk a day. There are two problems with this option.

One, the average adult does not commonly drink even one glass a day, let alone four to six. Two, drinking this much milk a day can bring along with it the problem of excess calories, saturated fat, cholesterol and too much protein. All of these are thought to encourage the loss of calcium from the bones as well as the incidence of other health-threatening diseases.

As a result the average adult American doesn't get even half of the adult RDA (800 mg) a day. Add to this the fact that on the average, only 35% of that amount gets absorbed into the blood. In some cases, some nutritionists think that it might even be as low as 2%. The requirement for lactating and pregnant women and those under 24 is 1,200 mg. A quick computation will tell you that 35% of the RDA for lactating and pregnant women is 420 mg; and 35% of the general adult RDA is 280 mg. Considering that the average person can lose up to nearly 400 mg of calcium a day, this figure is not even sufficient enough to replace what is being removed from the bones daily.

No wonder, then, that some nutritionists call osteoporosis a 20th-century epidemic. It is a very subtle disease causing the bone to become thin and brittle like a pane of glass, and neither x-rays nor regular blood tests can show its existence. It takes a loss of 35% to 40% bone mass before it becomes apparent. It is estimated that roughly 20 million adults in this country suffer from osteoporosis, and these figures are double what they used to be over 30 years ago.[1] Certainly calcium deficiency is not the only cause of osteoporosis, particularly in menopausal and post-menopausal women (see Chapter 30 on page 304), but it is important to remember that chronically low levels of calcium in the diet will undermine the structural integrity of your skeleton.

Two more factors that can contribute to osteoporosis are the overconsumption of phosphorus and the undersupply of magnesium in the body. These two minerals are integral parts of the bones and teeth. For the body to use calcium properly, phosphorus and magnesium must combine with calcium in the right proportions. While the required calcium to phosphorus ratio is 1:1, that of calcium to magnesium is 2:1. Any deviations from these figures often lead to an improper utilization of calcium.

As you may well be aware, phosphorus-containing foods and drinks are available everywhere in Pepsi, Coca Cola, some meats, canned foods, cheeses, salad dressings, bread and many other processed foods that use phosphate compounds as preservatives. As a result, the average American consumes far too much phosphorus, exacerbating the already bleak problem concerning calcium consumption and absorption. Incidentally, whole milk is said to have a 1:5 calcium-to-phosphorus ratio, and for this reason some experts advise us not to rely solely on whole milk as the calcium source. Low-fat milk, on the other hand, is supposedly a much preferred alternative.[2]

The case with magnesium is more a problem of undersupply. Far too many people in this country get less than 50% of the recommended levels of magnesium. As a result calcium absorption and utilization are affected.

The incidence of osteoporosis is 400% greater in women than men. By the age of 70, the average woman can lose up to 25% of her bone mass. The shrinkage in height and the hunched back so characteristic of some older women (and, to some extent, older men) are a result of more bone breakdown than bone formation, for whatever reason (mineral deficiency, lack of hormones, etc.). For most women, it usually begins by about age 35, although some say even at a younger age, and continues into old age. There are several reasons advanced for the difference between men and women regarding calcium loss.

One of these reasons is the drop in the production of the hormone estrogen as women get past menopause. It is believed that this hormone helps prevent the net loss of calcium from the bones while it encourages its formation. Another reason is low calcium intake and poor absorption. During pregnancy women have a tendency to use up the calcium from their bones to meet the needs of the fetus as well as their own needs. Moreover, women lose a lot of blood during their reproductive years, and this tends to rob the calcium store in the bones and set the stage for osteoporosis in later years.

Another very common disease associated with calcium deficiency is one that affects the teeth and the alveolar (jaw) bone that supports them. It's called periodontal disease, and it affects over three-quarters of the people in this country. This disease is a slow one that becomes more apparent as a person ages. It is said that 50% of the population loses some teeth by the age of 60.

Please bear in mind there are also other causes of periodontal disease. These include the growth and action of bacteria on food debris that collect under the gum, which turns into a hard plaque. If left untreated, this condition eventually grows to become gingivitis. Later, as it spreads under the periodontal membrane and the alveolar bone, it causes the teeth to become loose and ultimately fall out. This often is a prelude to chronic periodontal disease.

Besides preventing or reducing the incidence of osteoporosis and periodontal disease, calcium has been shown to help in lowering cholesterol levels (particularly the LDL). Calcium is also believed to prevent colon cancer. In one study, the administration of 1,200 mg of calcium daily for three months to people who had colon cancer showed a reduction in the growth of the cancer. In addition, calcium was found to help normalize high blood pressure. In one study where patients were given 1,500 mg of calcium carbonate supplement daily for an extended period, they were shown to have a significant improvement in their blood pressure.

Food Sources and RDA Requirements

The best food sources for calcium are dairy products. Others include soybeans, salmon, sardines and green vegetables, such as cabbage, collard greens, kale and broccoli. Peanuts, dried beans, walnuts, sunflower seeds, oysters, clams and shrimp are also good sources of the mineral.

The RDA for calcium starts at 400 mg for infants and goes to 1,200 mg for young adults and pregnant and lactating women. Considering the low level of absorption and high rate of daily loss, some experts think that these figures are misleadingly low. Raising them by 50% may help reduce the onset of osteoporosis and other diseases. You may wonder if it's necessary to drink six glasses of milk each day to meet even the RDA for calcium.

Your alternative is, of course, to find a good supplement. In the marketplace, calcium supplements come in many different forms. There are tablets made from bonemeal (crushed bones) and dolomite (naturally found in the earth as calcium-magnesium carbonate). Then there are calcium gluconate and calcium lactate, which come from vegetarian and milk sources, respectively. These two are known to be safer and better absorbed than dolomite or bonemeal supplements, which can contain lead contaminants. Don't forget that the RDA of 1,200 mg means 1,200 mg of *elemental* calcium: 1,200 mg of calcium gluconate contains only 9%, or 108 mg, of elemental calcium. So be careful to calculate your calcium supplement needs, bearing in mind that it must be the amount of elemental calcium you need.*

Absorption Suppressors Excessive amounts of fat, vegetable derived acids like physic, oxalic and tannic acids, stress and lack of exercise, vitamin D and magnesium.

Absorption Facilitators Vitamins A, C and D, iron, manganese, magnesium and phosphorus.

Toxicity It is reported that the consumption of over 2,000 mg of elemental calcium for a prolonged time could lead to hypercalcemia, which in infants can lead to mental disorder. In adults, it can contribute to atherosclerosis (hardening of the arteries due to calcium and fat deposits).

Phosphorus

Since phosphorus is the second most abundant mineral in the body, it is only logical that we discuss phosphorus as our next essential mineral. In the bones and teeth, phosphorus is found at a 1:2 ratio with calcium. The amount found in these tissues is roughly 80% (or 560 grams). The other 20% is distributed throughout the body, fulfilling many other metabolic as well as biochemical requirements.

Some of its roles are the production and storage of energy, the synthesis of

---

* Here are some common calcium compounds and their elemental calcium percentages: Calcium glubionate contains 6.5%, calcium gluconate 9%, calcium lactate 13%, calcium citrate 21%, calcium acetate 25%, calcium carbonate 40% of elemental calcium. Hence, in the above example, 9% of 1,200 mg of calcium gluconate contains only 108 mg of calcium. You can use the above percentages to compute elemental calcium in a supplement that contains these calcium compounds.

nucleic acids (DNA and RNA) and the metabolism and transportation of fats, proteins and carbohydrates. It is also an integral part of the cell membrane and a number of enzyme systems. The function of the heart and kidneys and the growth and repair of cells, as well as the assimilation of niacin, are aided by phosphorus. Additionally, this versatile nutrient serves as a buffer in body fluids. This relates to the maintenance of neutrality in these fluids in order for the body to carry out its numerous metabolic processes efficiently.

Because phosphorus has so many critical functions, you would ordinarily be concerned about its adequacy in your diet. As it turns out, this is one of the few minerals you need not worry too much about. Phosphorus is just about everywhere. If anything, most of the concern is that we may be getting too much of it. This is because whenever there is excess phosphorus, calcium absorption is depressed while the latter's resorption (its removal from the bone) is increased. Therefore, if osteoporosis is a major concern to you, watch what you eat and drink.

Food Sources and RDA Requirements

The RDA for phosphorus ranges from 300 mg for infants six months and under to 1,200 mg for young adults and pregnant and lactating women. Phosphorus deficiency is not common in men. It's important to remember, however, that to maximize its benefit as a structural component, you need to take an equal amount of calcium with it. Like calcium, phosphorus is constantly resorbed from the bones and teeth.

Legumes, milk and milk products, poultry, meat, fish, whole grains, bonemeal, nuts and seeds are all good sources of phosphorus. There is no known toxicity associated with phosphorus, and the only known deficiency is in animals that graze on phosphorus-poor land.

Absorption Suppressors An excessive intake of iron, magnesium, aluminum and white sugar.

Absorption Facilitators Calcium, thiamine and vitamin E.

Magnesium

Magnesium is the third most abundant mineral in the bones and teeth, and its content in these tissues accounts for roughly 60% of the mineral found in the body. Its function in these tissues is clearly to produce strong, hard bones and teeth.

The remaining 40% of the mineral is found in cells and extracellular body fluids, where it is involved in so many critical functions. In the cells, it facilitates the production of energy as well as its release from ATP—the universal carrier of energy in the body. This energy is used to synthesize proteins and nucleic acids (DNA and RNA), to transport nutrients around the body and to perform many other functions. A number of enzyme systems depend on magnesium for their function and activation.

Magnesium's role in the muscles is purely "mechanical" but a very important one nevertheless. It enables these tissues to relax, while calcium (magnesium's antagonistic partner) empowers them to contract. It is evident that life could be quite miserable without a sufficient amount of this mineral in your body. As you can see below, magnesium deficiency can be quite harrowing, too.

Magnesium also assists nerve cells to conduct electrical impulses efficiently. This feature of the mineral enables you to think quickly and clearly and maintain a well-balanced and integrated body and mind.

In addition, magnesium has other healthful functions you might appreciate knowing about. These range from its role in the maintenance of your heart and normal blood pressure to fighting kidney stones, diabetes and osteoporosis. Magnesium's importance for keeping a healthy heart has so far not been fully understood. It has been found that people who live in areas of the world where the water's content of the mineral is high have less incidence of heart attack than those who live where the magnesium content in the drinking water is low. The scientific basis of this information has yet to be fully explored.

Its function in controlling blood pressure seems to stem from the fact that it helps keep the blood vessels in proper working condition. Just as you need a flexible and elastic water hose to accommodate any changes in water pressure, you need blood vessels that have similar properties. Magnesium is able to relax not only the blood vessels but also the tissues that surround them. This dilating and relaxing effect helps you maintain normal blood pressure.

In other areas, magnesium helps diabetics by increasing their tolerance for sugar. In women with PMS, it helps reduce the tension and depression that is often associated with this malady. Its significance in minimizing osteoporosis is related to the fact that it's an integral part of bones and teeth. When used with the vitamin pyridoxine (vitamin B6), magnesium can be an effective treatment for kidney stones. This excruciatingly painful complication often results from a lodging of crystallized calcium oxalate in the urinary tract. It's believed that magnesium helps keep the offending compound fully dissolved in the urine. Food sources of oxalic acid (the precursor to calcium oxalate) are rhubarb, leafy vegetables and coffee. If you are susceptible to kidney stones, it helps to avoid these substances.

Magnesium has also been used in treating certain mental disturbances such as schizophrenia, nervousness, insomnia, depression and similar conditions. During diuretic therapy (administered to help patients remove excess fluids), magnesium is one of the minerals that gets depleted. During this time it's important that you take extra amounts of the mineral to keep its normal presence in the body fluids.

Although there reportedly exists no magnesium deficiency in this country, the average daily magnesium intake of Americans is not something one can write home about. In a nationwide survey, it was found that 50% of Americans get less than two-thirds of the RDA of magnesium.[1] Certain groups such as alcoholics, bulimics, diabetics and those that use certain therapeutic drugs are known to have low levels of magnesium in their bodies.

When magnesium deficiency does occur, the experience can be quite dreadful. The associated expressed symptoms vary from muscle weakness, irritability, confusion and dizziness to outright convulsions, tremors, delirium and even seizures and coma. These are, of course, extreme situations. What may be common, however, are the marginal or subclinical conditions. You feel there is something wrong with you, but you and your doctor can't figure out what it is. Such subtle symptoms may serve as a clue to your dietary magnesium imbalance, for otherwise there are plenty of food sources that can provide you at least the minimum amount of magnesium. What you want, of course, is maximum health and well-being, and this is where supplements come in handy.

Food Sources and RDA Requirements

The best sources of magnesium are meat, dairy products, fish, tuna, molasses, soybeans, nuts and seeds. Other good sources are brown rice, honey, bran, oatmeal and green vegetables. Remember, anytime a food is processed, it loses its mineral content—in some cases as much 90% of it.

The RDA starts at 40 mg for up to six-month-old infants and goes to 355 mg for lactating women. (See Table 1.1 on page 2.)

While we are talking about requirements, it's important to discuss briefly the importance of magnesium to athletes. Because this mineral is involved in energy generation and utilization, as well as in muscular activities, athletes around the world have come to realize the beneficial effects of magnesium and magnesium supplements. So, whether you are a football jock, marathon runner or weekend jogger, make sure you have plenty of the mineral in your diet. Studies have shown that people who engage in intensive physical activities utilize oxygen more efficiently when they have extra magnesium in their foods.

Absorption Suppressors Alcohol and diuretics.

Absorption Facilitators Calcium, phosphorus, vitamins B6, C and D and protein foods.

Potassium

The majority of the body's potassium—nearly 98%—is found in the cells. It serves to maintain the osmotic pressure (fluid balance) as well as the acid-base neutrality of the cell. Potassium also functions as a cofactor to many enzyme systems that are involved in the breakdown of energy-providing foods (carbohydrates, proteins and fats). The synthesis of proteins and the conversion of glucose into glycogen (the tissue's stored fuel) are also accomplished with the help of potassium.

Together with sodium, potassium enables the heart to work in a steady, regular rhythm. Potassium helps you to think clearly by facilitating the transportation of oxygen to the brain.

In other areas, potassium is involved in nerve-impulse transmission and muscular contraction. It works antagonistically with sodium, which is found predominantly outside the cells. As was explained previously under "Electrolytes," in the presence of a nerve impulse, the potassium from within the nerve cell migrates outward, thus altering the electrical potential of the cell and allowing the impulse to be transmitted down the axon. This is critical for the proper functioning of the brain and the rest of the nervous system.

Potassium's role as a muscle relaxer, along with magnesium, is equally important because some of the life-sustaining muscles—such as the heart, intestinal and respiratory muscles—won't function effectively without a sufficient amount of potassium. Magnesium and potassium enable your heart to beat steadily and rhythmically.

Potassium has also been found to alleviate hypertension or high blood pressure in some cases. To the 50 million people who suffer from hypertension this may be a little bit of good news. The mineral sodium is very common in the American diet, and this mineral also has a high water retentive capacity that can lead to high blood pressure. Since sodium and potassium are antagonistic partners, the presence of a large amount of the latter tends to normalize the former. In this regard, the presence of high amounts of calcium and magnesium also have a blood pressure-lowering effect.[1]

The explanations advanced for potassium's effectiveness in lowering sodium are manifold. One, because the two minerals compete for reabsorption in the kidneys, the higher the potassium in the renal fluids the less sodium will be reabsorbed (i.e., it will leave more sodium to be eliminated). Two, potassium's muscle-relaxing effect enables blood vessels to dilate and thus helps lower blood pressure. Catecholamines are a group of stress-induced chemicals that are capable of increasing blood pressure. Potassium can reduce the secretion of these hormones.[2]

One little caveat relating to this effect of potassium on blood pressure is the fact that it's somewhat controversial. Some scientists have questioned the efficacy of the mineral on hypertension, although there are those who believe that it has an influential role. The research that is being done in various labs will, one would hope, prove it one way or the other, but until then there is nothing wrong with being optimistic about what potassium does for this particular purpose.

There are roughly 250 grams of potassium in an average-sized body, and any substantial drop from this level usually leads to serious health problems. The first associated symptoms of potassium deficiency are general muscle weakness, irritability, confusion, pulse irregularity, lethargy, loss of appetite, muscle cramps and constipation. In severe cases, paralysis, a drop in heart rate and even death can occur.

Food Sources and RDA Requirements

The estimated RDA for potassium is 500 mg for six-month-old infants, 700 mg for one-year-olds, 1,400 mg for age two to five, 1,600 mg for age six to nine and 2,000 mg for teenagers and adults. Certain drugs, as well as excessive sweating can cause a substantial loss of potassium. For this reason, and the fact that potassium has a beneficial effect on hypertension, the NCR suggests that a daily intake of up to 3,500 mg can satisfy the need for the mineral.

Amounts of more than 25 grams consumed on a daily basis, however, can lead to acute toxicity. Sometimes kidney failure or other complications such as infection or severe acid-base imbalances can be the cause. Some of the associated symptoms are confusion, lethargy, weakness and paralysis of muscular tissues. One could also experience an erratic heartbeat, which, if prolonged, can lead to cardiac arrest. Some of these symptoms are similar to what happens when there's a deficiency of the mineral.

Potassium is found in many foods, such as legumes, vegetables, fruits, meat and milk. Bananas, potatoes, broccoli, cantaloupe, dried apricots, peanuts, avocados and lima beans are some of the great sources of the mineral. Remember, however, that potassium is one of those minerals that is lost in cooking water. For this reason, steaming or microwaving the foods is strongly recommended.

Absorption Suppressors Coffee, alcohol, sugar, diuretics, stress and cortisone laxatives.

Absorption Facilitators Vitamin B6, sodium and magnesium.

Be aware, also, that any substantial drop in your potassium level because of the aforementioned suppressors can be the cause of many of your mood changes. Coffee drinkers, alcoholics and sweet eaters often become hyper or jittery. This may be due to the loss of potassium from the blood as much as from the effect of these products on your system.

Sodium

Sodium is potassium's antagonistic partner. Most of the body's potassium is found inside the cells. Most of sodium bathes the outside of the cells. (See Table 12.1 on page 156.) This relationship is the key to their function in tandem to coordinate muscle contraction and nerve impulse transmission, which are important for the mechanical movements of the body parts, as well as for processing thoughts.

By itself, sodium's primary purpose is to regulate the in-and-out flow of fluids and nutrients from the cell in a process known as the "sodium pump." Sodium is also involved in the transport of carbon dioxide and amino acids across the cell membrane and intestinal wall. Because sodium causes high water retention, it saves the body from total dehydration—particularly in arid environments.

However, because of sodium's ability to pick up water, a large intake of it can lead to high blood pressure—at least partially so because there are some researchers who think that there should at the same time exist low levels of other minerals for this to happen. Minerals such as magnesium, potassium and calcium, when they exist in higher amounts, tend to neutralize the hypertensive effect of sodium.

Because American food is rich in sodium and the salt shaker is omnipresent, one should have very little concern with sodium deficiency. The concern most people have is of overindulgence. Besides the salt shaker that you find close at hand in every restaurant and at every dining table, there are many hidden sources of sodium. These can be cured meats, cheese, canned soups and vegetables, luncheon meats, etc.

In very rare instances, such as starvation, sodium malabsorption and diarrhea, deficiency may occur. The symptoms associated with sodium deficiency are loss of concentration, impaired carbohydrate metabolism, muscle weakness, dehydration and collapse of blood vessels.

The toxicity correlated with high sodium intake is the increase in blood pressure and excessive accumulation (edema) of fluid that can lead to swelling in ankles and feet, as well as buildup of fluid within the chest cavity and other tissues around the body.

Food Sources and RDA Requirements

The estimated RDA ranges from 120 mg for infants under six months to 500 mg for teenagers and adults—and on the average, roughly 280 mg for children over one year but younger than ten.

Food sources vary from various canned and frozen foods (soups, ice cream, olives, sauerkraut, ketchup, etc.) to eggs, meats, shellfish, carrots, beets, dried beef and bacon. There are other hidden sources like baking powder, soy sauces, mono-sodium glutamate (MSG) and several others that are used as preservatives, such as sodium sulfate, sodium nitrate and nitrite.

Absorption Suppressors None known.

Absorption Facilitators None known.

CHAPTER 14
Trace Elements

Chromium

One of the many amazing things about life and biochemical processes is how imperceptibly small things can contribute to health and well-being when available or become detrimental to health and life itself when absent. The mineral chromium is perhaps one example of this. This mineral is one of the micronutrients. That means the amount of chromium used by the body daily is so small (less than a pinch) that you think it should make no difference whether or not you have this mineral at all.

I have news for you. Without chromium, life could literally come to a clanking and sluggishly grinding halt. This shiny mineral's number one job is to help insulin bring glucose to your cells. As has been discovered, without chromium, blood sugar can never enter the cells. Glucose is very important as a fuel and for many biological processes. Your brain cells are entirely dependent (save for a few exceptions) on glucose for fuel, and they need chromium just as much as insulin to absorb and metabolize their fuel.

So what does the absence of chromium mean to you? Well, the first sign is that you start to feel lethargic and fatigued. If uncorrected, this can lead to depression, hypoglycemia and even diabetes. *Glucose tolerance* is the term used to describe your body's ability to process and metabolize sugar. Many adults in this country have very low glucose tolerance—some even being diabetic or borderline diabetic.

This is even more common in the older generation, because as one gets older, one's ability to absorb and metabolize nutrients decreases. Although we cannot say that chromium deficiency leads to diabetes, there are many instances where diabetics* were helped by being treated with chromium supplements.

In other areas, chromium also facilitates the metabolism of fats and proteins as well as the synthesis of genes (RNA and DNA). Studies with both human and animal subjects have shown that chromium deficiency can contribute to the accumulation of fat in the blood vessels, which can lead to atherosclerosis and other circulatory disorders.

Other conditions associated with low levels of chromium in the blood are high cholesterol and high blood pressure. In animal studies, these conditions were treated

---

* Particularly those diabetics who are insulin-dependent.

with chromium supplements.

In one study, when rats were given a low-chromium diet, their growth was stunted and they died sooner than average rats. Those that were given extra supplements of chromium, however, lived considerably longer, grew better and were healthier. All these studies indicate that chromium is indeed vital to health and longevity.

There are a variety of inorganic chromium supplements. But the one that is known to be highly absorbable is chromium picolinate. Picolinate is an organic molecule that acts as a carrier or transporter of chromium ions across the intestinal wall. In addition to increasing sugar metabolism (particularly important with hypoglycemics and diabetics, as well as the elderly), chromium picolinate is found to reduce fat and cholesterol levels in the blood. Because of its ability to mobilize and metabolize fats, chromium picolinate may be an excellent supplement to those who wish to lose weight.

Food Sources and RDA Requirements

Brewer's yeast, meat, poultry, shellfish, corn oil and whole grain cereals are good sources of chromium.

The RDA for this nutrient has not been formulated. The National Research Council (NRC) has yet to devise a method that quantifies the "active" chromium in food. Nonetheless, based on research findings, anywhere from 50 to 200 mcg/day has been suggested by the NRC. Some nutritionists have recommended as high as 300 mcg/day. Because there is no known chromium toxicity, even higher amounts would be tolerable.

Absorption Suppressors. None.

Absorption Facilitators. None.

Copper

As you read and learn more about the various minerals mentioned in this book, you come to realize how much a part of the earth we are and how much the content of the earth's crust is a part of us. Copper is one more earthware that contributes to our health and well-being. It's not one of the most studied minerals, but what is known about it so far is pretty impressive.

Unlike calcium, iron or phosphorus, when you think of copper's benefit to health, you probably draw a blank. Perhaps the most you have heard about it is its role in traditional folklore, where arthritic people wore copper bracelets to alleviate their pain. As you can see below, copper actually does help in relieving arthritis.

Besides relieving arthritis, copper has many benefits, one of which is the production of energy from the food you eat. Copper is part of many enzyme systems that are involved in this process. Indirectly, copper is involved in the absorption and distribution of oxygen around your body. Considering life can cease within minutes without oxygen, this mineral is important to your health and well-being. Let's see how copper works in this area.

The hemoglobin in the red blood cells is what carries oxygen to all the tissues of the body. Iron, which gives blood its characteristic color, is very important for the formation of hemoglobin, and copper is largely responsible for the absorption of iron from the intestine. Without iron, the oxygen conveyor system can be quite weak and fragile. Incidentally, copper also combines with plasma protein to form ceruloplasmins. It's believed that ceruloplasmins protect hemoglobin and the red blood cells from free radical damage.

One of the most potent antioxidant enzymes is superoxide dismutase (SOD). Copper is also an integral part of this enzyme, which protects us from the savagely dangerous singlet oxygen free radicals. Free radicals are known to be one of the major causes of cancer and aging. In this connection, you may say that copper has an indirect (as part of SOD) anticancer role.

From both human and animal studies, copper has been found to lower the blood serum cholesterol while raising the HDL cholesterol. Regarding osteoarthritis, copper helps to relieve pain by reducing tissue swelling. The pain-relieving effect of copper bracelets on certain types of arthritis was experimentally verified by a double-blind* study.[1] The researchers in this experiment discovered that body perspiration can dissolve tiny amounts of elemental copper and cause it to seep into the skin, where it can have healing effects on the affected tissues.

Copper is also good for your skin and hair. It is involved in the formation and development of the fibrous proteins, such as collagen and elastin, found throughout your body but largely concentrated in the skin. The production of your natural sunscreen (melanin), as well as water, during energy-producing reactions in the cells also depends on the availability of copper in your body.

The amino acid tyrosine is a key nutrient for the formation of melanin, and copper facilitates its use in the synthesis of the pigment. The absence of the mineral in the body leads to skin and hair discolorations. How sharply discerning are your taste buds? Well,

---

* A situation where neither the experimenter nor the patient knows what treatment is being administered in the study.

copper can help them work better, too.

Some of the other deficiency symptoms (although rare in humans) seen in animal studies include increases in blood cholesterol, anemia, malfunctioning of the nervous and reproductive systems, weakening of blood vessels and poor development of the skeletal tissues. Some deficiencies observed in humans involved infants. For example, those infants who were fed only cow's milk had a copper deficiency. The expressed symptoms were malformation of the bones and hair follicles (causing hair to grow rough, twisted and kinked), and disorders that afflicted the circulatory and nervous systems.

Food Sources and RDA Requirements

Perhaps one of the reasons there are no widespread deficiencies of copper, although subclinical or marginal ones may occur, is because there are many common food sources of the mineral. These are all meats, almost all seafoods, whole grains, nuts, legumes, chocolate and mushrooms. If you live in an area where there is hard water or use copperware in your cooking, chances are you get a certain amount of copper from these sources as well. Copper pots, however, are deadly in interaction with vitamins C and E and folic acid.

Be aware that there is a certain amount of toxicity associated with excessive intake of copper. Some of the symptoms of this effect are mental and sleep disorders and increased blood pressure. Those who cannot metabolize copper (Wilson's disease) can suffer from jaundice and cirrhosis of the liver (a result of free copper deposition in the liver).

The adult RDA for copper ranges from 2 to 3 mg/day. Some nutritionists think this is less than half of what it should be. For infants up to 12 months old the RDA amounts range from 0.4 to 0.7 mg/day.

Absorption Suppressors Excessive amounts of zinc, vitamins C and E and Folic acid.

Absorption Facilitators Iron, cobalt.

Toxicity Excessive intake of copper

Iodine

So far as we know, this is perhaps one of the few minerals that has limited but very important functions in the body. Iodine's primary function is in keeping the thyroid gland healthy. Thyroxine and triiodotyrosine, the two hormones produced by the thyroid gland, depend on iodine for their formation. These hormones regulate the body's energy-producing processes. For instance, thyroxine's major role in the body is maintaining a satisfactory rate at which the body converts food into energy. The significance of this is great.

First, when you have an efficient metabolism it means your cells are using more fuel and oxygen and you'll have less fat storage in the body. This will also influence the synthesis of proteins and hormones as well as many other biochemical compounds that have a direct influence on the replication of cells, development, growth and health of the individual.

Second, cretinism is an iodine deficiency disease that afflicts children in areas of the world where there is insufficient iodine in their diet. The characteristic symptoms of the disease are mental retardation and poor, dwarfed muscular and skeletal development. The skin also becomes dry, rough and coarse with iodine deficiency. Cretinism is normally a congenital condition caused by a lack of iodine in the mother's diet. Unless an infant is treated with iodine supplementation right after birth, the damage will be permanent and irreversible.

Third, in adults, goiter is the most common condition that results from iodine deficiency. Although now rare in this country, it affects over 200 million people worldwide. The classic symptom of goiter is an enlargement and protrusion of the thyroid gland, which is in the throat area. Goiter is a result of an overstimulation of the thyroid gland (because it is trying to compensate for the absence of iodine). Goiter is an often painless, but nonetheless unattractive appendage. If caught early, goiter can be treated with iodine supplementation.

Be aware, however, that the lack of iodine may not be the sole reason for goiter or cretinism. Other factors such as a lack or malfunction of the enzyme responsible for the synthesis of thyroid hormones, food and chemical goitrogens (agents that induce goiter), such as are found in turnips, peanuts, cabbage, spinach, strawberries, radishes and rutabagas, can sometimes be the cause.

Food Sources and RDA Requirements

Seafoods such as fish and seaweeds (kelp) and plants and vegetables that grow in an iodine-rich soil are your best sources for this mineral. When buying table salt at the store, you can choose either iodized salt or plain salt. If you buy noniodized salt or only use small amounts of iodized salt, you might consider using iodine supplements.

The RDA for iodine is from 40 to 50 mcg for infants under one year old, 70 to 120 mcg for those between one and ten, and 150 mcg for teenagers and adults. Pregnant and lactating women require 175 and 200 mcg, respectively.

There is no known iodine toxicity from normal foods. As supplements you can take up to 1000 mcg/day without any fear of toxicity. The thyroid gland has a built-in mechanism by which it maintains normal production of the hormones even in the presence of excess iodine. Extremely high doses, 10 to 20 times the above figures, can lead to simple skin rashes, abnormal breathing, headache and iodide goiterism.

Absorption Suppressors. None.

Absorption Facilitators. None.

Iron

As we have seen so far, many vitamins and minerals are needed to maintain the human body's health and keep it properly functioning. It seems the more you learn about the benefits of one vitamin or mineral, the more important or beneficial that vitamin or mineral appears to be compared to any you have studied or read about so far.

When you read about the benefits of iron to your health, it will seem to you that this must be the most important of all the micronutrients you have studied thus far. In reality, one essential nutrient can't be more important than any other, because in the long run the body can be severely affected by the lack of any one of these nutrients.

Iron is one of those minerals (or nutrients) you would think is so important that you couldn't live without it. That seems a valid perception because the availability of oxygen (the breath of life) to the various tissues in the body is dependent on iron.

The hemoglobin in the red blood cells is a four-part protein molecule that contains four atoms of iron. The iron atoms combine with oxygen molecules when you breathe air. Without iron, there is no oxygen for the tissue cells to burn the fuel and provide you with energy. In effect, there's no life. We said elsewhere in this book that you can live without food for up to five weeks but only a few minutes without oxygen. In this regard, iron is perhaps the most essential of all nutrients.

Perhaps you will never be in a situation in which your body will be totally devoid of iron, but what can often happen is that if your body doesn't have enough iron it won't operate at its optimal level. Iron-deficiency anemia is one of the most common conditions that affects people in this country and elsewhere in the world. In one study, 88% of college women in this country were found to be deficient in iron.

The characteristic symptoms of iron-deficiency anemia range from weakness, fatigue and pale complexion to headache, irritability, forced breathing during exertion and cracks at the corners of the mouth. Some of the other conditions arising from iron deficiency are apathy, listlessness and loss of appetite for normal food. Strangely, those who suffer from a severe lack of iron may have a craving for nonnutritious foods (pica) such as grass, clay, stones, ice or clothing. Children who are deficient in iron will have difficulty in concentrating, reading and solving problems. They also tend to be cranky and have little interest in activities.

Iron is important for the conversion of tyrosine to dopamine, one of the brain chemicals necessary for thought processes. Thus, iron not only brings oxygen to the brain but also helps the brain to work better.

How Does Iron Deficiency Come About?

After the epithelial cells of the intestinal tract, red blood cells have the highest turnover rate in the body. While the epithelial cells are replaced every three or four days, red blood cells can live up to three or four months. Every second, there are about 4 million births and roughly the same number of deaths of the red blood cells. Because these cells are in a fluid medium, they also tend to be lost quite easily through bleeding or menstruation. During its lifetime, a red blood cell makes roughly 75,000 trips between tissues and the lungs.

Red blood cells are made up largely of hemoglobin—each cell containing approximately 300 million of these globular substances, each of which contains four iron atoms. Given that the body has all the other nutrients necessary for the synthesis of the hemoglobin protein, iron will therefore be the only limiting factor for the adequate formation and maturation of red cells in the bone marrow.

Although nearly 90% of all the iron from dead cells is reused, the other 10%, and that which gets lost through bleeding or menstruation, will have to be replaced through the diet or supplements. Incidentally, a small percentage of iron is also lost through sweat, urine, dead skin, hair and nails.

To make matters worse, the iron you get from ordinary food sources such as vegetables, beans, cereals and fruits is the least absorbed. Reportedly, only 2% to 10% of the iron in these foods gets metabolized by the body. Because of this, and the aforementioned problems, iron is one of the most commonly deficient nutrients in the human body. Yet iron is vital to life.

Iron deficiency is indeed prevalent in this country. Those who are most frequently affected are women of child-bearing age, teenagers, children, some infants, the elderly and certain economically disadvantaged people. Let's look at each group individually.

Teenage girls and premenopausal women suffer the most from iron deficiency because they lose much iron during the menstrual cycle. Some of these people, particularly the teenagers, are finicky eaters and don't get well-balanced meals. Because pregnant women produce a large volume of blood and share their iron with the fetus, women who bear children often have a problem with iron deficiency anemia. Lactating women can lose as much as three grams of iron a day.

It has been found that both men and women runners, as well as other athletes, have problems with a low level of iron in their blood. In some cases, as many as 50% of them were found to be borderline anemic.

After they are born, infants have just enough iron to last them a few months, and unless they are fed iron-rich nutrients they, too, are vulnerable to iron- deficiency anemia. Getting a sufficient amount of iron is particularly important to infants and children because the proper development of their bodies and brains depends on the availability of sufficient oxygen to their tissues. Children who have iron deficiency have difficulty concentrating, memorizing, reading and solving problems.

While economically disadvantaged people have iron deficiencies from not getting well-balanced meals, the majority of the elderly suffer from this malady largely because of insufficient absorption. As mentioned above, iron is one of the most poorly absorbed nutrients. To make matters worse, the elderly will have even less of it because of a lowered absorption rate. The elderly also tend to suffer more frequently from internal bleeding, such as caused by ulcers, and external bleeding, such as caused by hemorrhoids, increasing the loss of iron.

The absorption of iron in the digestive tract is also limited by such interfering factors as calcium, phosphates, zinc and plant-based organic substances, such as phytates, and oxalates found in cereal husk. Tannic acid (found in tea), egg yolk and aspirin are also found to be common antagonists to iron absorption. On the other hand, vitamin C and chelating agents, such as amino acids and other organic compounds, increase the absorption and utilization of iron.

Finally, bear in mind that in addition to the formation of red blood cells, iron is used for other functions in the body. Roughly 25% of the total iron found in the body is used in enzyme synthesis and as part of organic molecules that are closely involved in the production of energy. Another 5% is found in *myoglobin,* a protein-iron complex used as a reservoir of oxygen in the liver and muscle cells. This is nature's backup arrangement that helps you weather any temporary shortage of oxygen supply.

In addition, iron helps strengthen the immune cells. The deleterious effects of toxic metals (such as cadmium, lead and mercury) are minimized when you have a high intake of iron. The syntheses of large proteins like collagen and other tissue fibers are facilitated by iron-rich enzymes. Iron is also important for absorption and utilization of all the B vitamins.

Looking at it from the aesthetic point of view, iron enhances your skin, teeth and nails. It is important for the formation of healthy bones and tissues. Iron helps you to cope better during times of mental or physical stress.

Food Sources and RDA Requirements

Pregnant women with a need for 30 mg of iron have the highest RDA requirements. Then come lactating women and females from 11 to 50 years old, with 15 mg. The requirement for children up to ten years old and for adult males above 19 years of age is 10 mg. Teenage boys need 12 mg.

Although adult males reportedly lose about 1 mg of iron a day from their total body reserve of 1,000 mg, females, who often have much less (200 to 400 mg), lose up to roughly 2.5 mg of iron a day. This is why the requirement for women is much higher. Even then, as it has already been mentioned, women have the worst time with iron deficiency.

At one point or another, between 25% and 50% of menstruating women and up to 60% of pregnant women are deficient in iron.[1,2] According to one government survey, as many as 35% of infants were found to be deficient in iron. In another survey, 30% of the infants born to economically disadvantaged families were found to be anemic, while another 25% were shown to be deficient in iron.[3]

It seems, therefore, that considering the low absorption and the wide prevalence of iron deficiency in this country, we need to consume considerably higher than the RDA amounts to meet just the RDA figures for iron. It is reported that a person consuming a well-balanced meal can get about 6 mg per 1,000 calories consumed.

For men who consume up to 2,500 calories a day, meeting the RDA seems to be no problem. What is not accounted for, however, is how much of that 6 to 15 grams is actually being absorbed. Women who consume less (1,700 to 2,000 calories) get even less iron. This means both men and women can use iron supplements to live a healthy and energetic life.

Some of the excellent food sources are liver, kidney, heart, red meat, eggs, fish and clams. In addition, wheat germ, oysters, nuts, molasses, leafy green vegetables, beans, poultry, oatmeal and dried fruits are good sources of iron.

As we said earlier, the problem is with absorption. In general, the iron you get from meat sources is better absorbed than the iron you get from non-meat sources.

You should have very little concern about iron toxicity. In very rare situations, excessive iron could build up in the soft tissues, such as the liver and spleen, to cause some complications. This condition, known as hemochromatosis, results mainly from excessive deposition of iron in the aforementioned tissues. Alcoholics and people with chronic liver problems are sometimes predisposed to the condition.

Absorption Suppressors Excessive zinc, coffee, phosphates, phytates, oxalates and tannic acid.

Absorption Facilitators Folic acid, copper, cobalt, manganese, vitamin C and vitamin B12.

Molybdenum

This tongue twister is relatively new to the human dietary scene, although it has long been known to be essential for plant growth and development. It is often added to steel and iron to give them hardness and strength, and as a food supplement, it may do just about the same for you.

In legumes, molybdenum is one of the two key minerals (the other is cobalt) used to catalyze the fixation of nitrogen. Its benefit for human health has gradually been establishing solid roots. Some of these involve the metabolism of iron (important in the production and growth of red blood cells), the prevention of certain cancers and even the health and appearance of your teeth. Regarding molybdenum and cancer, here's an interesting story.

In one Chinese province, the incidence of esophagus and stomach cancers was found to be the highest in the world. It was later discovered that such disproportionate rates of death from these cancers had something to do with a lack of molybdenum in the soil. By adding molybdenum to the soil, scientists were able to reduce deaths associated with the cancers.

In connection to its importance to teeth, studies have shown that molybdenum helps minimize the occurrence of dental cavities, possibly by promoting the retention of fluoride in the teeth.

Molybdenum has been found useful in removing certain food preservatives that often accumulate in our bodies and become toxic. The sulfites are common additives used by the wine, restaurant and food-processing industries. Perhaps the most common food products containing sulfites are the salad accoutrements (dressings, etc.) and processed foods (bread, cakes, etc.). Often the symptoms resulting from sulfite buildup are diarrhea, nausea, asthmatic disorders and, in extreme instances, loss of consciousness and death. Molybdenum activates sulfite oxidase—the enzyme that destroys sulfite food additives.

The formation of urine, as well as the removal of toxic metabolic by products like aldehydes, is also aided by molybdenum.

Food Sources and RDA Requirements

Molybdenum is most commonly found in leafy vegetables, whole grains (barley, wheat, oats), legumes (beans, soybeans, lentils) and sunflower seeds. Please remember that the amount of molybdenum in these foods depends on the soil content of the mineral where they were grown and how much they have been spared by food-processing companies.

The estimated RDA ranges from 15 mcg for infants to 75 mcg for young children (up to age six). For older children and adults, it ranges from 75 mcg to 250 mcg, respectively. There has not been molybdenum toxicity reported in humans. In animals, however, growth retardation, weight loss, diarrhea and muscle wasting have been observed.

Absorption Suppressors: None known.

Absorption Facilitators: None known.

Selenium

Perhaps there is no better nutrient than selenium that can illustrate the relationship between the absence of a well-balanced diet and the incidence of major diseases such as cancer and heart disease. This element, which for a long time had been considered toxic for human consumption, has in recent years been elevated to an "essential nutrient" status. Now, for the first time, we have the RDA values for selenium.

Selenium's importance, for both human and animal health, is so great that in the areas of the world where there is little selenium in the soil, diseases like cancer, muscular dystrophy, heart disease and several other degenerative conditions prevail. From the depths of mainland China to the far reaches of Turkey and Finland to the heartlands of

America, scientists have found uncanny correlations between the occurrence of heart disease, cancer and other afflictions and low levels of selenium in the soil.

One disease stemming from a selenium-poor region in Turkey, where the peasants suffered and died from weak and scarred hearts, is called Keshan's disease. It was later discovered that it afflicted children in China as well. The Finns, as shown in Figure 14.1 on page 183, have the worst incidence of heart disease. This is correlated quite well with their low level of selenium intake compared with other nations. To bring this home, similar heart problems are seen in the "stroke belt" of Georgia and the Carolinas, as well as in Ohio, Vermont, Texas, New York and Indiana.

For a long time, this geographically specific occurrence of cardiovascular disease and cancer was a mystery to scientists. It was only in the past decade or so they discovered a connection between the low level of selenium in the soil and the frequency of heart disease in these specific areas. With this discovery came the resolution; in China, for example, Keshan's disease has now been virtually eliminated through the use of selenium supplementation.

Figure 14.2 on page 184 shows the distribution of selenium in American soils. Depending on where you live, it will be important for you to have access to foods that are grown in selenium-rich soils or to take supplements as a protective measure. (See also Figures 4.3 and 4.4 on pages 49 and 51, respectively. These graphs show the relationship between the selenium level in the diet and the incidence of cancer and heart-related diseases.)

Together with the above, selenium's value to human health lies in its ability to fight free radicals and retard the process of aging. Selenium can do this by itself, as part of the enzyme glutathione peroxidase, or in conjunction with vitamin E. Of course, as a team these two nutrients are very powerful in protecting the body from free-radical damage. The parts of the body that are susceptible to free radicals, particularly those produced from the oxidation of fats, are the cell membranes and the contents inside the cells, like the DNA and RNA, mitochondria and other organelles.

Selenium is found throughout the body, but the organs that seem to have the greatest concentration are the liver, kidney, heart, testicles, spleen and pancreas. Besides its ability to help prevent cancer and heart disease and in moving toxic metals* (i.e., cadmium, mercury, lead, aluminum) out of the system, selenium is found to reduce problems associated with dandruff and acne and keeps the skin elastic and youthful.

---

* Some of the physical symptoms of these metals are irritability, depression, mental retardation, fatigue and headaches.

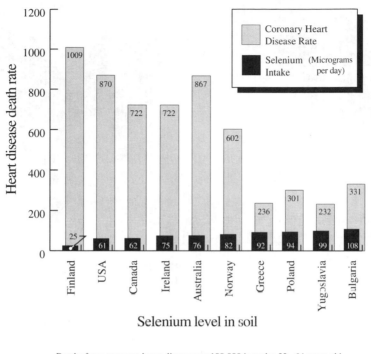

Deaths from coronary heart disease per 100,000 in males 55 - 64 years old
in the countries shown above

Source: Ambau drawing based on data given in Passwater, Richard, Ph. D.
Selenium as Food and Medicine, Keats Publishing, New Canaan,
Ct., 1980, p. 54.

Figure 14.1 World heart disease rates vs. selenium intake.

Menopausal women find selenium to be helpful in alleviating hot flashes, palpitations, stress and emotional disturbances that come as a result of hormonal changes in the body.

Food Sources and RDA Requirements

Food sources of selenium range from whole grain foods (wheat, barley, rye) to fish (tuna, herring, shellfish) and organ foods (kidney and liver). To a limited extent, green vegetables, brewer's yeast, asparagus, tomatoes and peanuts may also contain selenium. Bear in mind, though, that all these depend on the selenium richness of the soil in which the products are grown.

The current RDA requirements for selenium range from 10 micrograms for infants to 75 mcg for lactating women. Many researchers feel that these values are far below

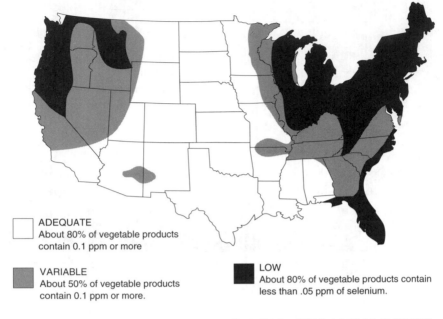

ADEQUATE
About 80% of vegetable products
contain 0.1 ppm or more

VARIABLE
About 50% of vegetable products
contain 0.1 ppm or more.

LOW
About 80% of vegetable products contain
less than .05 ppm of selenium.

Source: Data from USDA Technical Bulletin No. 758 (1967)

Figure 14.2 Geographical distribution of selenium in the U.S.

what they should be for the body to have optimal protection from the myriad of substances that attack the tissues every second. From their research, many scientists believe that we need to have as many as 250 to 350 mcg of the mineral daily.

In those areas of the country where the incidence of cancer and heart diseases is less frequent, the average daily dietary intake of selenium was reported to be over 100 mcg. Selenium is absorbed at over 90%.

Absorption Suppressors None.

Absorption Facilitators Vitamin E.

Manganese

Manganese is one of the most prevalent micronutrients in nature, yet the body tissues use very little of it. Although it is found to be essential and has many important functions in the body, the Food and Nutrition Board of the National Research Council (NRC) has not yet made manganese a nutritional requirement. This is primarily because there has not been, according to the NRC, "a practical way for assessing manganese status" and because of the abundance of manganese in food sources.

You don't have to wait until the NRC comes up with an RDA for manganese to appreciate its importance to your health. Manganese is involved in many different biochemical processes. These include its role in the synthesis of mucopolysaccharides—a group of complex carbohydrates used as structural components of tendons, bones, cartilage and ligaments. As a cofactor of many enzyme systems, manganese is also involved in the synthesis of proteins, collagen fibers, fatty acids and cholesterol. The proper functioning of mitochondria is aided by the presence of manganese.

The digestion of protein and the formation of urea (a by-product of protein breakdown excreted in the urine) are facilitated by manganese. The synthesis of thyroxine, the key hormone made by the thyroid gland used to stimulate the production of energy in the body, is influenced by manganese. This versatile mineral is involved in reducing the symptoms associated with diabetes, convulsions and epileptic seizures, as well as those in schizophrenia. Manganese facilitates blood clotting and insulin utilization. The efficacy of this mineral with all these conditions was observed in both human and animal studies.

Manganese plays a role in keeping the immune system healthy and in reducing the effect of certain free radicals. Superoxide dismutase (SOD) is a key antioxidant responsible for neutralizing the singlet oxygen free radicals. Manganese is one of the minerals that make up SOD. Without manganese, the enzyme would not be formed and the free radicals could have a field day in your body and immune system.

Although there are no outright deficiency symptoms associated with manganese in humans, in animals a variety of conditions have been observed. These range from skeletal deformities, growth retardation and poor glucose tolerance to neuromuscular disturbances that resulted in epileptic seizures and convulsions. Animals that were fed a manganese deficient diet had offspring that were poorly developed.

Like iron, manganese is responsible for the production of dopamine from tyrosine. This chemical is important for the proper functioning of your brain. It's involved in thought processes, emotions and muscular control. This is why manganese supplementation seems to help children who have poor muscular coordination and learning and speech problems.

Food Sources and RDA Requirements

As mentioned, there is no RDA requirement for manganese primarily because it has not been fully studied. However, there are amounts that have been suggested as enough for the proper functioning of the body. The RDAs range from 0.3 to 1.0 mg for infants to 1.0 to 2.0 mg for children from one to ten years old. Teenagers and adults can use from 2.0 to 5.0 mg of the mineral per day.

There is very little toxicity associated with manganese except to those who work in industrial and mining environments. In these cases, excessive amounts of the mineral can collect in the lungs and other tissues in the body where it can cause anorexia, cramps in the legs, headaches, apathy and even impotence. In an advanced situation, more severe neuromuscular conditions such as muscle tremor, rigidity and a loss of spontaneous movement can occur. In some cases, the afflicted cannot modulate their voices or show facial expressions.

The best natural sources of manganese are organ meats, meats, nuts, whole grains, peas and beans, beets and egg yolks. Leafy vegetables, seaweed, oatmeal, avocados and dry fruit also have a significant amount of manganese.

Absorption Suppressors: Excessive intake of phosphorus and calcium and phytates.

Absorption Facilitators Vitamins B1 and E.

Zinc

Zinc's name may start with the last letter of the alphabet, but what it can do for your health is absolutely *numero uno*. There are roughly 2 to 3 grams of zinc in a human body, but those areas that have the highest concentrations include the eyes, liver, kidney, bones, muscles, hair and the male reproductive organs (prostate and seminal fluid). Zinc is a remarkable mineral that has many important functions in the body.

For starters, zinc works as a cofactor in at least 40 enzyme systems in humans (as many as 59 have been reported, including those in animals). All these enzymes have very specific functions, and without zinc many of the biological processes would be in serious trouble. For example, the synthesis of DNA and RNA—two substances critical for the growth and replication of cells—is dependent on enzymes that use zinc.

Several other enzymes that help digest food in the stomach and small intestine and those that break down sugar and fat molecules in the cells are also dependent on zinc. Alcohol dehydrogenase breaks down and detoxifies alcohol (including methanol and retinol). This enzyme is necessary because alcohol will become toxic when allowed to accumulate in the liver and other tissues. The breakdown, or removal, of carbon dioxide from the cells and body fluids is also accomplished by a zinc-dependent enzyme. Imagine what these two substances would do to the body if allowed to collect—a very dangerous and explosive situation would ensue.

From a less technical point of view, here are some of the other things zinc can do for you. Let's start with the skin, hair and nails. The basal layer of the epidermis, the papilla of the hair and the matrix of the nail are among the fastest reproducing tissues of the body. Since zinc is very important for replication, growth and repair of the cells, the health and appearance of your skin, hair and nails will depend as much on the level of zinc in these tissues as on the level of other essential nutrients.

To cite another example, how fast and how well a wound can heal are greatly influenced by the amount of zinc present in your body. In one study, surgical patients who were given zinc supplements healed on the average twice as fast as those who were not supplemented. In another study, zinc sulfate was used to dramatically reduce scars left from a chemical treatment of acne.

Acrodermatitis enteropathica is a congenital and often fatal disorder affecting the hands, feet, mouth, scalp and anal areas in infants. The skin in these areas is characterized by red and ulcerated rashes and hair loss. Acrodermatitis is caused by the body's inability to absorb zinc. Sometimes similar symptoms can result when an infant is switched from breast-feeding to a formula that may be lacking zinc. For years, this disease was a mystery. Now doctors can successfully treat individuals who suffer from acrodermatitis with zinc supplements.

Another area where the absence of zinc has a profound impact is on the reproductive system of both sexes and on the subsequent offspring. It was mentioned earlier that the reproductive organs are some of the areas where zinc is found in high concentration. Since zinc is very important for reproduction of strong and healthy cells, and since sperm cells are some of the fastest duplicating cells, the availability of a sufficient amount of the mineral will determine the proliferation, maturity, health and fertility of the sperm cells. In this case, zinc deficiency can lead to a retardation of sexual development in teenagers and young adolescents and perhaps even in impotence or sexual dysfunction in adult men.

Zinc deficiency in a pregnant woman could have many complications, including miscarriage. For the baby, it could lead to mental retardation or physical deformity. In one animal study, zinc-deficient female rats showed nearly a 100% incidence of birth defects. These varied from severe complications with the nervous system of their offspring to physical deformities such as clubbed feet and cleft palates.

Some of the other manifestations of zinc deficiencies are loss of appetite, taste and smell. There may be complications in the eyes that lead to color blindness, inflammation of optic nerves and the formation of cataracts. Zinc seems to be critical to the activation and proper function of vitamin A—the nutrient that is often associated with the eyes. Zinc deficiencies elsewhere in the body also seem to lower the body's stress response and affect its ability to fight infections or cope with toxic foreign elements such as alcohol, heavy metals and air pollution.

Zinc is truly a remarkable mineral that has beneficial effects on blood circulation, rheumatoid arthritis and sickle cell anemia. The health and proper functioning of the prostate gland and of the skeletal, nervous and immune systems are aided by the sufficient availability of zinc in the body.

Millions of germs, bacteria, parasites and viruses seek entry into the body every day. Within the body, certain cells may tend to become cancerous, and toxins may build in tissues to threaten the health and well-being of an individual. These elements, to a large degree, are put in check or neutralized by the body's own defense forces.

Although most of the body's defenses are born in the bone marrow, they reach maturation elsewhere in the body. For instance, the B-cells, which produce antibodies, develop in the thymus gland, the spleen, lymph nodes and the intestinal wall. T-cells develop in the thymus gland, and after maturity they migrate into other locations such as the spleen, lymph nodes, blood and liver, where they are needed to deal with any potential foreign agents. It seems zinc is intimately involved in the proliferation and maturation of all these cells, as well as in the health of the organs and tissues that produce them.

Both animal and human studies have shown that the immune system is one of the first areas to be affected by zinc deficiency. People who took zinc supplements had fewer infections. Those who had an infection such as the common cold or were recovering from surgery and took supplements regained their health faster than those who were not taking supplements. AIDS is probably the worst communicable disease of the twentieth century. Researchers have found that those who succumbed to the disease were sometimes found to have a low serum level of zinc.

Food Sources and RDA Requirements

Zinc is one of those minerals that does not store well in the body. If you are sick, recovering from surgery or undergoing mental or physical stress, some of the zinc stored in your body can be used up. Moreover, this mineral is easily lost from the body through sweat and in the feces. In a hot climate or during strenuous exercise where there may be excess sweating, the loss of up to 3 mg/day is reportedly common. This means that considering its multipurpose function and your body's inability to store it, you need a regular intake of the mineral to keep your body healthy and strong.

The RDA for zinc ranges from 2 to 5 mg for infants and up to 30 mg for pregnant women. Children from 1 to 10 years old need 10 mg, while females and males above 10 years old require 12 and 15 mg, respectively. The recommended intake for lactating women is 15 mg.

The best food sources are meats, poultry, wheat germ, brewer's yeast, eggs, pumpkin seeds, liver, legumes, nonfat dry milk, whole grains, herring and oysters. Speaking of oysters, perhaps now you know why they are erroneously considered aphrodisiacs. Other foods such as vegetables, fruits, potatoes, onions, carrots and nuts may also have zinc, albeit in low levels.

The levels of zinc in various plants vary depending on the mineral content of the soil they were grown in. Most of the farmlands in this country have been depleted a long time, and as a result not many people get the RDA amounts of zinc. Moreover, processed foods, particularly grains, can lose up to 80% of their zinc.

There are also absorption problems you have to be concerned with. It's reported that zinc uptake by the intestinal walls could vary from 20% to 80%. It all depends on the food sources and factors that might interfere with its absorption. For example, the zinc in meats is better absorbed than that in cereals. Phytates in cereal fibers can interfere with absorption. Drugs such as diuretics and oral contraceptives can inhibit zinc absorption. High intakes of alcohol and calcium are some of the other culprits. On the other hand, vitamin A, copper and phosphorus are good absorption facilitators.

Zinc is a relatively nontoxic mineral. When up to 150 mg/day of zinc was given to individuals for a certain period, no toxicity was observed. It seems that the body has a way of monitoring zinc intake—stepping up its absorption of the mineral when it's low and eliminating it when there is more than enough. A very large dose, say 300 mg at one shot, can cause vomiting.

Absorption Suppressors Phytates, diuretics, oral contraceptives, high intakes of alcohol and calcium.

Absorption Facilitators Vitamin A, copper and phosphorus.

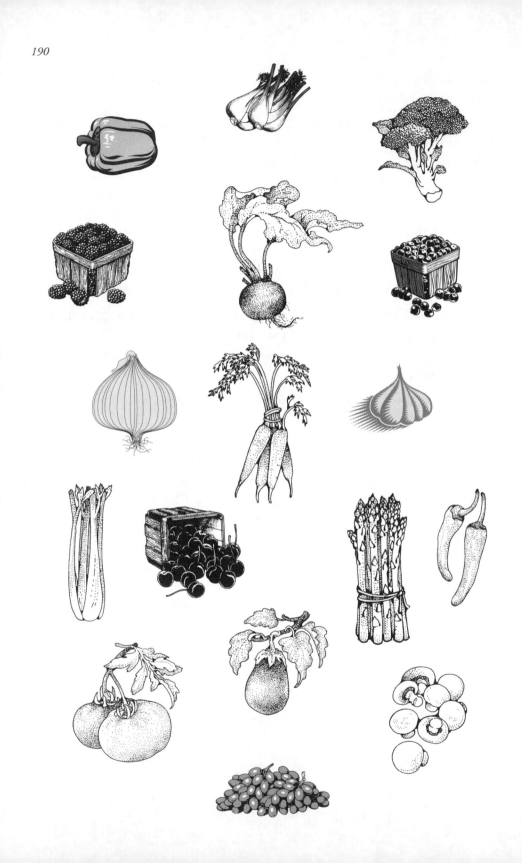

CHAPTER 15
Phytochemicals

We've heard it from our mothers, nutritionists and some doctors about the importance of consuming vegetables and fruits daily. We are also cognizant of Hippocrates' famous dictum: make food thy medicine and thy medicine thy food. We even find a reference in the bible about the significance of vegetables in our health and appearance. During the reign of Nebuchadnezzar (about 6th century B.C.), Daniel along with other young men was recruited to be trained and eventually enter the king's service. When he began his training, one thing was not quite right to Daniel: the food and drink being consumed at the royal court. Daniel said to the chief official that he would not defile himself by indulging on the royal food and wine.

When the official, for fear of punishment, demanded that Daniel comply with the existing dietary practice, Daniel challenged him by asking the guard whom the chief official had appointed over him and his colleagues to instead feed them vegetables and water for ten days and compare their appearance with those who consumed the royal food and wine. The guard agreed to do so, and after the ten days, Daniel and his colleagues indeed "looked healthier and better nourished than any of the young men who ate the royal food." From then on, the guard took away the royal food and gave the men vegetables and water for their meals.

From early on we have been indoctrinated about the benefits of fruits and vegetables, but until recently, neither we nor our educators knew about the real benefits of these groups of foods. Even nutritionists, when they recommended that we eat a balanced diet, often did so that we would obtain enough vitamins, minerals, carbohydrates and proteins for sufficient energy and to adequately build and repair tissues. Beyond these basic but important functions, to most of us, the idea of eating a balanced diet as a way to prevent disease, enhance one's memory, improve one's appearance or increase one's life span has never been a consideration.

Now thanks to the advancement of science, we are discovering that grains, fruits and vegetables are a storehouse of substances that hold the key for our day-to-day well-being as well as for long-term health. These substances are called phytochemicals and are found locked in the green, red, yellow, orange or blue of the fruits and vegetables we consume daily. In fact, it's these substances that give flowers, autumn leaves, and various fruits and vegetables their distinct colors.

Also called "phytonutrients," "designer foods," "medicinal foods," "neutraceutical foods," "physiologically functional foods" and "pharma foods," phytochemicals are not nutrients, at least so far as we know, but are organic compounds that have a tremendous influence in the biochemical and physiological processes that take place in our bodies. We will talk about the specific compounds and their functions in our bodies later, but for now let me give your some general comments.

One, as mentioned, phytochemicals are not nutrients and are not converted into tissues or used up as fuel by the body. There are no known deficiency symptoms associated with them if we stop taking them, although, as you'll see later, opportunistic disease may take over in their absence. From research that has been conducted around the world, phytochemicals play crucial roles in our bodies. These range from minimizing the incidence of cancer and heart diseases to improving with conditions that come with aging, such as arthritis, inflammation of the joints and loss of memory and concentration, to the slowing of the aging of the body itself.

Two, although potentially there can be found millions of phytochemicals in plants, the ones that are known so far number only several thousands. James Duke in his book, *Handbook of Phytochemical Constituents of GRAS Herbs and Other Economic Plants,* has cataloged 3,000 phytochemicals extracted from 1,000 plants. Depending on the effect they have on the body, these compounds can be either GRAF (generally regarded as food), GRAS (generally regarded as safe) or GRAP (generally regarded as poisons or medicinal.)

Three, phytochemicals are found scattered throughout the plant kingdom. But some plants, fruits or vegetables may have a higher concentration of one kind of phytochemical than another. This variation in the phytochemical constituents of plants is the reason for the recommendation to consume a wide variety of fruits and vegetables.

Four, the phytochemicals discovered so far function by serving as antioxidants, helpers of other antioxidants (such as vitamins A, C and E) and by blocking or interfering with processes that lead to disease conditions in our bodies. All these happen at a biochemical and physiological level, and hence the impact they have on our health can be profound.

Finally, phytochemicals are not always single compounds. There can be many variations of the same compound* or substance, and for this reason, it's often suggested that we eat whole foods as opposed to relying on supplements that contain only the active principle of these compounds. Of course, supplements when available and are of good formulation can some times serve as nice stand-ins for some of these phytochemicals found in these foods.

Specific Phytochemicals, Their Food Sources and Functions in Our Bodies

To understand and appreciate the importance of phytochemicals, we need to begin with the amazing world of cellular operations. It's what happens in the cells that determine who we are as humans: young, middle-aged, old, sick or healthy. As you know, the cell is the fundamental unit that when duplicated (sort of) 60 trillion times forms the human body.

Hence, if we understand what goes on in a cell, we can pretty much understand what goes on in the rest of the human body. To illustrate this point and how phytochemicals play a role in our health, wellness and longevity, we'll need to understand what an ordinary day is like in the life of a cell.

An ordinary day in the life of a cell, assuming you have properly nourished it, involves the conversion of food molecules into energy, body tissues or thousands of other substances that take part in the operation of the cell and the rest of the body. During these processes, there can also be many agents that interfere with or hinder the normal operations of the cell, including threatening its very existence. Hence, part of a cell's daily task is housekeeping or maintaining order so that it can function continuously and comfortably. But how does the cell manage its house maintenance job, and what specifically are the agents that can damage the cell or disrupt its operation? How does the food we eat, particularly fruits and vegetables give us protection against those substances or agents that threaten the life of the cell and the rest of the human body? Let's answer each of these questions.

Some of the agents or substances that can be deleterious to the cell can come along with the water, air and food we consume. Considering the level of pollution in our environment, the different chemicals that are added to foods as preservatives, coloring or bulking agents and fruits and vegetables that are often treated

---

* For example, beta carotene comes in six different versions. Similarly, Vitamin E has six forms. So, eating foods that contain all these different forms of the vitamins is now believed to have greater benefits than just one or two of the active components..

with pesticides, herbicides and other chemicals, it comes as no surprise that our bodies are at constant threat from these various elements. Internally, just the normal metabolism (the process of food utilization by the body) and everyday stress can also produce substances that can be toxic or damaging to the body. Many of these, as discussed in Chapter 4, are free radicals.

Scientists have discovered that free radicals and many of the extraneous substances that we get from outside sources can lead to degenerative diseases such as cancer, cardiovascular diseases, diabetes, Alzheimer's, and other illnesses that afflict us in this country.[1]

Fruits, vegetables, grains and seeds can give us protection because they contain phytochemicals that interfere with or block certain processes that may lead to diseases. They do this either by serving as antioxidants to free radicals, by inhibiting certain enzymes that facilitate the formation of diseases such as cancer or by whisking out of the cell those chemicals or substances that are going to be deleterious to our body. Almost all of these substances, as you'll see below, are found in the dark green, yellow, red, orange or blue variety of the vegetables and fruits. Let's see what these foods are, what substances they contain and how they function in our bodies.

Berries, citrus fruits, cherries, grapes and grape seeds. This group of vegetables is a great source of a class of water-soluble phytochemicals called bioflavonoids. Important contributors to the vivid colors* we see in fruits, vegetables and flowers, in your body, these compounds may likewise bring you vibrant health, good looks and longevity. Let's see how and why.

One, sometimes referred to as vitamin P, bioflavonoids function as helpers of vitamin C and as important contributors to the health, function and integrity of the capillaries (the smallest of blood vessels). Because it's these tiny tubes that ultimately deliver nutrients and oxygen to all the cells of the body, you can see the significance of these phytonutrients to the health and appearance of your body. This can range from the smoothness and elasticity of your skin to improved circulation, greater resistance to bruising to enhanced memory and visual acuity. In fact, the "P" in the vitamin name stands for *permeability factor*, because, bioflavonoids enhance the transference of nutrients across the blood vessels to the various cells in the body.

---

*Incidentally, while bioflavonoids represent the blue, red and some yellow pigments, the carotenoids account for the orange and yellow of the fruit, vegetable and flower colors.

Two, as co-workers of vitamin C, bioflavonoids contribute to the health and function of the body wherever vitamin C is involved. This benefit varies from the neutralization of free radicals to building and strengthening of the collagen matrix of your skin, gums and bones to helping alleviate cold and flu symptoms. Those who suffer from asthma, allergies, arthritis and bursitis may also benefit from bioflavonoids.

Three, because they can function as antioxidants and also help recycle vitamin C that may have been destroyed by free radicals, bioflavonoids may help protect the body against cancer, heart diseases, reduced memory and other degenerative conditions.

There are reportedly over 20,000 bioflavonoids registered in *Chemical Abstracts*, but a few well-studied ones that you may want to be familiar with include hesperidin, rutin, quercetin, pycnagenol and catechin. Hence, for example, catechin helps reduce histamine release and hence helps with those people who have allergic reactions; quercetin can help with inflammatory responses such as those experienced by people who have arthritis or suffer from injury, bursitis and asthma, and rutin is important in maintaining the health and integrity of the capillaries, veins and arteries.

But bear in mind that for maximum benefit, it's import to have all the bioflavonoids together instead of the individual compounds. This means that as much as possible you need to consume whole foods instead of relying on supplements. Again, supplements can sometimes be good concentrated sources of some of the compounds as well serve as stand-ins for some nutritional inequities.

Finally, remember that there are many other sources of bioflavonoids, including buckwheat, rose hips, apricots, black currants, plums and papayas. Broccoli, yams, cucumbers, green pepper, tomatoes, red and yellow onions and apples also contain a fair amount of these phytochemicals.

Broccoli. This dark green vegetable is a storehouse of many nutrients including, of course, phytochemicals. One of the most known anticancer vegetables, broccoli contains a well- studied, antitumor compound called sulforaphane. The power of this phytochemical comes from its ability to promote the formation and function of a group of enzymes called phase II enzymes. These enzymes are responsible for processing and removing carcinogenic substances from our cells.

In one study, rats were divided into two groups. Twenty-five of them were given a cancer-causing compound called DMBA, 29 of them were given both DMBA and high or low doses of sulforaphane. Of those that received just the DMBA, 68%

got breast cancer. However, of those that took the low dosage and the compound, only 35% got tumors. Of those that took higher doses along with the compound, only 26% got cancer. Although study has not been done on humans, the addition of sulforaphane to human cells grown in petri dishes showed an increased synthesis of the anticancer or phase II enzymes. Brussels sprouts, cauliflower, collard greens and kale are other vegetables that contain sulforaphane.

Cabbage. Like broccoli, this vegetable contains many nutrients and exciting phytochemicals that have been found to possess many benefits for the body. Some of these compounds are called isothiocyanates and indoles. Isothiocyanates function by inhibiting the production and activity of the "bad" group of proteins called phase I enzymes. These enzymes have a special knack of converting the benign, even beneficial compounds into carcinogens. Isothiocyanates simply snarl the enzyme, thereby minimizing the formation of cancer-causing compounds in the body. Isothiocyanates reportedly can also increase the activity of the phase II enzymes mentioned above, thus giving the compounds dual roles. In doing so, this crinkley cole slaw and sauerkraut maker can prevent esophageal, stomach, colon, liver and lung cancers. Also found in watercress, in one animal study, isothiocyanates reduced the risk of developing lung cancer by half when the animals were exposed to carcinogenic chemicals such as those found in cigarette smoke.

Breast and prostate cancers are believed to be a result of higher production of harmful versions of the estrogen and testosterone sex hormones. The indoles in cabbage and other cruciferous vegetables (such as broccoli, cauliflower, turnips, brussels sprouts) promote the activity of the enzymes that break down these harmful substances and thus minimize the incidence of the gender-related cancers.

Celery. This fibrous, riblike green has not attained the status or respect of the other vegetables like broccoli, cabbage and cauliflower. Yes, you have heard about its importance as a fiber source and as an ingredient in certain soups, chicken and other meat dishes, but celery contains phytochemicals that can be of a benefit to you. One of these phytonutrients is 3-n-butyl phthalid. This compound functions as a calming or sedative agent to the nervous system and also has a capacity to reduce blood pressure, through regulation of hormones that induce the condition.

For its healthful benefits, always consume fresh celery and avoid or discard any old or wilted celery that is more than 3 weeks old. This is because cancer-causing substances called furocumarins, found only in tiny amounts in the fresh celery, can significantly increase as the stored celery ages.

Onions, garlic and peppers. These three vegetables contain specific compounds or plant chemicals that make them such important dietary components. Onions, are rich in bioflavonoids and reportedly contain as many as 50 of these and other phytonutrients. Allylic sulfides (sulfur-containing compounds) are the predominant ones, and these compounds serve as cancer fighters in the body. For instance, researchers in China have shown that high onion consumption was attributable to a 40% reduction in the incidence of stomach cancer in one region of that country.

Garlic contains, among many compounds, a phytochemical known as diallylsulphide. It is this substance and others in this smelly, bulbous clove that block carcinogens from getting into the cells and inhibit those cells that have become malignant from growing further. The garlic compounds are also known to reduce cholesterol and blood pressure, improve circulation and strengthen the immune system.

Red pepper has similar benefits. The capsaicin compound, which gives peppers their hot characteristics, may help kill bacteria, neutralize the carcinogen chemicals such as nitrosamines and reduce the bad cholesterol and triglyceride levels in the body. This substance is also known to relieve muscular pain and elevate moods by releasing brain chemicals called endorphins.

Soybeans. For a long time, scientists couldn't figure out why there is less incidence of cancers including breast cancer, in Japan and other Oriental countries than in the West. Now the mystery seems to have been solved: it's because of the phytonutrients found in soy called genistein, daidzein and saponins. These compounds are effective in preventing the early development and spread of cancerous cells by blocking their food supply line.

When cancer cells grow and migrate to other parts of the body, they need new capillaries to bring them food. Genistein block the formation of the tiny blood vessels. For women, because genistein is similar to estradiol, one of the estrogen hormones, a known breast cancer promoter, the phytochemical blocks the formation of cancer by blocking the cell receptors in the mechanism of cancer initiation and formation. Saponins block cholesterol-absorbing sites in the intestine and hence help reduce cholesterol levels in the body. To obtain the beneficial effect of these compounds consume more soybeans and soy products such as tofu, soy milk, tempeh and tamari.

Teas. The most common active constituents of the humble green and black teas are tannins, catechins and theobromine. While theobromine acts as a central nervous system stimulant, the tannins and catechins primarily function as antioxidants in the body.

In terms of their overall effectiveness, the green teas, which are less processed than the black teas, may be more beneficial. In fact, this point has been postulated as the reason why there is a lower incidence of cancer and heart disease in a certain section of Japan where a large quantity of green tea is consumed than in those areas where less of it is consumed. In one animal study, catechins in green tea were shown to lower cholesterol and blood pressure and inhibit esophageal and gastrointestinal cancers. Catechins may also strengthen the immune system.

Besides serving as an antioxidant, tannic acid can help fight tooth decay. This phytochemical is lethal to the plaque-forming bacteria. In one experiment, when tannic extracts were added to saliva-coated tooth enamel, 85% of the cavity-forming bacteria were destroyed.

Tomatoes. Carotenoids are a group of related compounds that have remarkable benefits to the human body. Found in almost all the red, yellow, orange and green vegetables, carotenoids are associated with the reduction of all types of cancers.

There are thousands of these compounds, but the one of recent discovery and abundantly found in tomatoes is called lycopene. This compound and its relatives are fat soluble and hence are important protectors of the cell membrane and LDL cholesterol and triglycerides in the blood from free radical attack. This antioxidant protection hence can help reduce the risk of heart diseases, cancer, cataract formation and other degenerative conditions. For example, researchers in North Italy found that people who ate more servings of raw tomatoes every week had a 60% less chance of developing cancer of the stomach, colon and rectum than those who consumed fewer servings of the vegetable.

Unlike most vitamins, lycopene reportedly survives cooking and processing, so you are more likely to find lycopene in pasta sauce, ketchup, tomato juice and pizza. Other sources of lycopene are pink and red grape fruit, watermelon, guava and sweet red peppers.

P-coumaric and chlorogenic acids are some of the other compounds found in tomatoes. They too are effective in fighting the formation of cancer-causing substances in the body. Also found in pineapple, green pepper, strawberries and carrots, p-coumaric and chlorogenic acids are powerful in disabling the formation of carcinogenic substances called nitrosamines. These noxious compounds are formed when nitrates often used as food preservatives and the proteins from our diet interact in the digestive tract. By binding the precursor compound, nitric oxide, from forming, they prevent the formation of nitrosamine.

In summary, as you can see from the above examples, mothers were indeed right for demanding that we eat our vegetables when we were little. Daniel of the Bible and Hippocrates were astute observers about the benefit of foods, particularly those of plant or vegetable origin. To be the beneficiaries of their advice, we need to regularly consume our vegetables, fruits, grains and seeds. These foods may help fend off cancers, keep our blood vessels clean and our minds sharp, improve the appearance of our skin and provide us with a vibrant and dynamic health to the very end.

PART VIII
The World of Herbs

Herbal Samplers

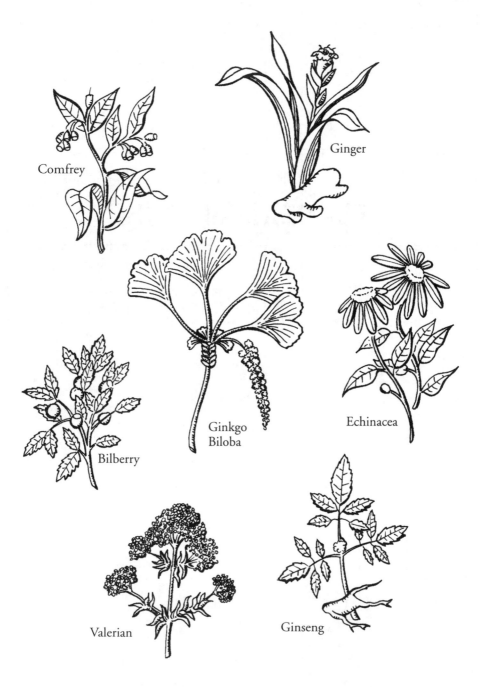

Comfrey

Ginger

Ginkgo Biloba

Echinacea

Bilberry

Valerian

Ginseng

Gifts from nature for the benefit of the human body.

CHAPTER 16
The World Of Herbs

AN INTRODUCTION

To most Americans, and for that matter to most people in the Western world, herbs or the use of herbs has been as alien as the use of vitamin and minerals supplements has been. In fact, if you randomly ask people in this country about the value of herbs to the human body most of them will probably draw a blank. Just as with vitamin and mineral supplements, though, the use and application of herbs in this country are now rapidly changing. This is so primarily because people are now finding that the best way to care for the body is not through drugs or synthetic chemicals but rather through proper nutrition and other natural means, such as homeopathy, herbs and chiropractic manipulation. Some or all of these practices, as John Lust, author of *The Herb Book,* puts it, are in "harmony with life" as opposed to being against it, which often can be the case with the synthetic drugs.

What Are Herbs?

The answer to this question can depend on how you perceive herbs. If you are a tea drinker, you may be thinking of the different herbal teas now available in grocery and health food stores. If you have a particular affinity for greens and spices, you may be thinking of the variety of fresh herbs or spices (parsley, sweet basil, etc.) that you can buy in the produce section of your supermarket. Gardeners and forest rangers may have their definition or perception of herbs. To them, herbs may mean those soft stalked plants or weeds that grow near the ground and die after they have flowered or completed their life cycle.

To herbalists, the term herb applies to those plants or parts of plants (such as roots, barks, leaves, flowers or seeds) that can be used to enhance, support and vitalize the human body. In this book only this last definition or interpretation will be used. Before, we discuss the many great attributes of herbs and their significance in our lives, let's first take a brief look at the historical background of these plants and their overall characteristics.

As you may well be aware, the use or application of herbs is not new. Herbs have been part of human societies for over 5,000 years. The oldest herbal book found in China dates back to 2700 B.C. This book documents some 365 plants and their beneficial properties. The Babylonians, ancient Egyptians, Romans and Greeks as well as American Indians depended on herbs for all kinds of home remedies and treatments. In Europe, herb gardens were common at monasteries and in private homes in earlier centuries.

According to the World Health Organization, some 80% of the world's population still relies on traditional medicines and remedies. Aside from uses in witchcraft, prayer, sorcery and psychic healing, herbs and plant extracts account for a very significant part of those remedies. Practically all the medicines of earlier eras were obtained or derived from plants. Even now, the active ingredients in a quarter of the pharmaceutical drugs come from plants.

Regarding their overall characteristics, herbs require you to remember a few rules of thumb. One, the quality and potency of the herb will depend on where the herb was grown, when it was harvested (seasonally speaking), what part of the plant was used (leaves, flowers, roots or bark) and how the herb was dried, processed and packaged.

As to regional or geographical variations, herbs grown in mountainous areas can have certain specific qualities or properties compared to those grown in the lowlands; those herbs grown near water or in warmer climates can still have other qualities or properties. Quantitatively speaking, plants grown in fertile or nutrient-rich soils can have a higher concentration of the active ingredients than those grown in poor soils or harsher climatic conditions. As mentioned above, seasons can also affect the distribution and concentration of the active ingredient in the plant. This to say that in spring the active constituent of the herb may be in the young leaves and buds, in the summer it may be in the fruits and flowers and in the fall and winter it may be in the roots and barks.

The quality of the herb can likewise vary depending on whether rootlets, twigs or leaves are used, or whether the herb has been adulterated with excipients of other plants. Sometimes age can be a factor, too; if the plant is old or too young, the quality and the quantity of the active ingredients may be low. As with vitamins and minerals, how the herbs are processed or extracted can determine the quality or potency of the herb. (For more information on this, see the reference given at the end of the book.) Bear in mind, however, that fresh herbs are often the most potent.

Two, with herbs you should not expect results on the first use or application. You have to give herbs time. Of course, there can always be an exception to this rule.

What Is the Specific Function of Herbs?

The list of herbs or plants to aid and strengthen the function of the body is long and growing. Of the some 250,000 plants discovered so far less than 1% are currently used for a variety of health and wellness-enhancing purposes. Those plants employed for such purposes range from the tonics—herbs that improve the overall function of the body—to those herbs that enhance the functions of individual organs and tissues. Thus, the tonics are generally for people who want or need energy and vitality. The herbs used for this purpose are seaweed (such as kelp), Irish moss, alfalfa, comfery, dandelion leaves, burdock, parsley, goldenseal root, ginseng, milk thistle and others. The herbs used for specific tissues, organs or body states (such as appetite, fluid balance, constipation) are equally varied.

Unfortunately, neither space nor point of emphasis permits us to list all these herbs and their benefits to the body. For more information on the different herbs and plants used for a variety of purposes, refer to some of the herb books listed in the bibliography. What you need to bear in mind, is that all herbs (including spices) and vegetables as well as other plants can have some benefits to the human body. Knowing the specific attributes of each herb, spice or plant can make you appreciate or value these wonderful natural gifts.

In summary, regardless of how you perceive or use herbs—as condiments you add to your favorite dishes or as substances you infuse to tea or as troublesome weeds in your yard or garden—from what we have said so far, herbs can have many important and healthful benefits indeed. You may also be one of those people who think of herbs as folklorish and therefore doubt their significance to the human body. Think again.

One, herbs have been used by many societies for thousands of years. This means, even though now we also have much scientific data that support their historical functions or benefits, even if we didn't, these plant extracts have been in experiment in many cultures much longer than drugs and vitamins and minerals have. They have a track record, a richer heritage than these substances.

Two, many of the drugs used today have their roots in plants, but from what we said earlier, the whole plant or herb can have greater benefit to the body than one or two components of the herb or plant. Most drugs contain just one active ingredient and can be tolerated by the body within limited ranges. Drugs are used to treat a disease or a symptom—as a quick fix or a mending device. Herbs, on the other hand, are used to support the function of an organ or the entire body.

Herbal Preparations and Methods of Application

Depending on their applications, herbs can be prepared in several ways. The traditional method has been to make any one of the following preparations using the end product for a given application.

Infusion. This method of extraction involves steeping the plant part (such as leaves or flowers) in hot water, just as you would steep tea, for a certain period of time (10 to 20 minutes is usually enough) to let the active ingredients and other substances such as vitamins and minerals release into the water. The amount of liquid and plant part used will depend on the concentration of the active ingredient you are trying to attain —usually 1/2 to 1 ounce of the plant part is used per pint of water. After the necessary allotted time, strain the fluid and drink or use for whatever external applications the herb is recommended. In the event the infused end product is bitter, you may add honey or sugar to make it palatable.

For whatever purpose you are using the herb, remember not to expect a result from one application. You may need to continue to use it for a certain period of time. Use a porcelain or nonmetallic pot or cup to make the infusion.

Decoction. This method of extraction is often for a plant's hard parts, such as the roots, bark or stems and in a situation where your goal is to remove the plant's active ingredients and mineral salts (instead of vitamins and volatile oils). Depending on the hardness of the raw material you work with, in this method of preparation, you simmer (not boil) the plant parts anywhere from 3 minutes to 30 minutes. The amount of water used can vary from a cup of water to a cup and a quarter, the latter amount being used when the herb is simmered for 30 minutes.

Tincture. For potent herbs and when the goal is to use a very concentrated form of the active ingredient, you use tincture as your technique of extraction. In this technique, you add 1 to 4 ounces of powdered herb into a 50% alcohol solution and let it sit for two weeks. You shake it once or twice a day for the duration of the extraction. After this time you strain or press out to yield the tincture. Tinctures are good for herbs that have a bad taste, for herbs you want to use as an ointment or when the herb is to be used for a long period of time. The alcohol solution serves to preserve the extract.

Extraction. Liquid extracts are a form of tincture but more concentrated than tinctures. They are usually obtained by removing some of the alcohol using low temperature and a vacuum distillation technique. When you remove the fluid completely, you're left with a thick pastelike residue known as solid extract. This residue can be dried and granulated or powdered to be used for a variety of applications. As you can imagine, a solid extraction method can give you a highly concentrated form of the active ingredient. If necessary, this extract can be made into a pill. Solid extraction can give you a much longer shelf life than any of the other forms of preparation.

Besides the methods of extraction described above, sometimes whole herbs can be dried and ground into a powder. At other times, honey or brown sugar can be added to a liquid containing the raw herb and boiled together until the right consistency is reached. Freshly cut herbs can also be pressed or processed through a juicer.

Freeze-drying is the other technique often used with herbs. In this process, you first freeze the whole herb and then under a very low pressure and high vacuum remove the water (or rather the ice) naturally found in the herb by sublimation——the transformation of ice into vapor. Freeze-drying is probably better than any of the other techniques because there maybe less degradation or loss of potency of the active constituents.

As indicated above, the extracted herb can be used for a variety of applications. You can make salve or poultice——a thick paste prepared by mixing the extract with carrier medium such as flour, corn meal, milk or water to be applied on a wound or a cut. Sometimes, you may also use herbal preparations as laxatives, ointments and liniments as well as emetics.

From the above brief introduction on herbs, you might by now wonder how can one be assured of potency of an herbal product——particularly given the potential difference in the quality of the herbs used as well as in the processing or manufacturing technique. In other words, knowing that herbs are not regulated the way drugs or medicines are, how can you be assured that you're getting what the manufactures says you're getting on its label of an herbal product?

Quantification and Standardization of Herbal Extracts

It's true that in the past, since the active ingredients were not known, it was difficult to precisely know what is contained in an herbal concoction. Now, besides the following common practices, we also have many sophisticated techniques to identify and quantify an herbal active ingredient.

The usual method of quantifying an herbal extract is using concentration ratios. For instance, a 4:1 concentration means 1 part of the solid extract is derived from 4 parts of the crude herb. A tincture is usually given in 1:10 or 1:5 concentration ratios, while liquid extract is expressed as a 1:1 ratio. These ratios can also be expressed in terms of grams or ounces. Hence, one gram of 3:1 extract is derived from 3 grams of the starting raw or crude herb.

If you're interested in the weight of the active ingredient, concentration ratios are not very useful because they can contain, besides the active ingredient, hundreds of other compounds, many of which may not be useful. But in some cases, these extraneous compounds may help the principal substance function better in the body. Nevertheless, in the past, accurately assessing or quantifying the active principle in an herbal extract was difficult.

Now, however, because of new tools and techniques of measurement, it's very easy to determine the active ingredients and measure their amounts. The most common techniques used are high pressure liquid chromatography (HPLC) and thin-layer chromatography (TLC).* By using these analytical tools, we can determine the amount of active ingredient in an herbal preparation and express this value in terms of grams or ounces. In other words, with these new techniques, we no longer have to talk about crude extract weights or concentration ratios. We'll have a more precise and standardized method of assessing herbal extracts. Thus, for instance, allicin is one of the many beneficial compounds found in garlic. Using the tools and techniques just mentioned, we now can give the amount of this compound in grams or ounces. This method of disclosure will enable us to know precisely how much of the useful ingredient we're ingesting.

---

* The analytical tools described above are commonly used in Europe, and there is no doubt they will be used here in the U.S. more frequently as the demand for herbs and herbal products increases.

CHAPTER 17
Herbal Samplers

As we indicated in the previous chapter, the kinds of plants or herbal extracts that can contribute to human health are many and cannot be covered in just two or three chapters. However, the following information on some of the most prominent herbs, widely used spices and herbal teas may be of benefit to you.

Astragulus. Steeped in Chinese tradition as an immune stimulant and for a number of other purposes, astragulus is finding similar uses in Western societies. Researchers here in the U.S. have confirmed these particular attributes of the herb. The active ingredients come from the root extract — usually prepared by decoction (simmering the root in water at low heat for a protracted period). Besides having a role as an immune stimulant (it helps increase the production of T-cells, the white blood cells of the body that attach foreign substances or invaders), astragulus may benefit the proper function of the heart and respiratory system. This herb also has adaptogen properties and thus helps prolong the function and life of the cells in the body by making them withstand extremes of physiological conditions.

The principal components of the herb include a polysaccharide known as astragalan B, a bioflavonoid and choline. Like most herbal products, the benefit of some of these active ingredients may not be immediate. For this reason, you may have to take the herb for several weeks before you see any significant effect. As we said earlier, there can always be an exception to this rule of thumb. Some people have reported seeing results within a few days of taking herbal products.

Baptisia Extract. This native American plant goes by various names, some of which are wild indigo, American indigo, horsefly weed and indigo broom. Baptisia is a multi-branched perennial plant that produces gray green leaves and yellow flowers.

The whole plant as well as the root bark can be used for many of this plant's beneficial properties. Although it has sometimes been used for a variety of external applications, it has been used for many internal purposes. These include its use as a stimulant, emetic or purgative as well as to enhance the function of the immune system.

Bilberry. Also called huckleberry or blueberry, bilberry is a shrubby perennial plant that is found wild in parts of Northern United States and in the woods and forests of Europe. For more information on other berries, see Chapter 15.

Now also cultivated, Bilberry has reddish bell-shaped flowers that turns into blue-black fruit on maturity.

The most important chemical components of bilberry are the bioflavonoids, particularly the anthocyanosides. As you can see below, anthocyanosides have been found to have beneficial properties in the body. These range from increasing the production of collagen and maintenance of its structural integrity to serving as antioxidants. Since collagen is the most abundant protein in the body and is the fabric that holds our skin, bones, blood vessels and other tissues and organs together, you can see that anything that helps with the health and function of collagen is also going to help with the overall health and structural integrity of the body.

More specifically, anthocyanosides maintain the health and function of arteries, veins and capillaries, fortify the brain from toxic substances by strengthening the blood-brain barrier and by serving as antioxidant. In the circulatory system they help disperse clot-forming platelets thus minimizing heart attack and stroke.

Because they function as an antioxidant and promote the health of protein fibers, anthocyanosides can help prevent or treat glaucoma, reduce peripheral vision loss and improve night time visual acuity. Anthocyanosides are also known to help reduce the effects of stress, improve memory, alleviate joint inflammation and enhance flexibility.

Because it helps lower blood sugar level and improve capillary fragility, the bilberry extract can also be important for those who suffer from diabetes. Reportedly, anthocyanosides are also effective in reducing cholesterol and triglycerides in the blood.

There are many other benefits of anthocyanosides, but just from the above description alone, you can see that blue-black fruit, of bilberry is an important food. To take advantage of this important fruit make sure you include it in your daily diet whenever you get a chance.

Burdock. This wide and long-leaved plant is used primarily as a blood purifier, but herbalists have also used it for a variety of applications, ranging from its use for coughs, colds and sore throats to help in healing stomach ailments to neutralization and removal of poisons and waste matter from the body. The herb does this by acting as a diuretic and diaphoretic (as a substance that increases perspiration). The herb can also restore the liver, kidneys and gallbladder to their normal operations during illness. This property of the herb is what classifies it as an "alterative," meaning that it helps alter or restore the body during illness.

In the literature, even antibiotic, antifungal and antitumor benefits have been mentioned of the herb. When applied externally, burdock can also be used to treat scrofuloderma (tuberculosis of the skin) and venereal eruptions, and other skin conditions, including those that are cancerous. The seeds, roots and leaves can be used for many of the herb's beneficial properties.

Chicory. This scruffy European native is often cultivated and found in the wild. Now it's also grown in the United States. Chicory has bright, iridescent flowers and yellow root bark with white stalk that contains milky juice.

Chicory is a tonic herb but also has specific functions to organs and tissues of the body. It helps stimulate the production of bile in the liver as well as serve as a cleanser to the liver and the spleen. It may also assist with nausea or stomach disorders and help heal skin that is affected by such things as insect bite, sunburn or rash. This interesting herb is also good for the kidneys as it decreases uric acid level (hence minimizing gallstones) from the body, increases urine flow and helps eliminate excessive mucus in the digestive tract. This herb is often recommended with people who have jaundice and for those with spleen disorder.

Comfrey. Comfrey is one of those herbs whose use by humans goes far back in time. Ancient Greeks, Native Americans as well as other societies used comfrey to treat many internal and external bodily problems.

Externally, comfrey's power comes from is ability to heal wounds, bruises, sores, fractures, broken bones and insect bites. Burns, ulcers, sprains swellings and pimples can also be treated with comfrey. Allantoin, a compound found in comfrey is responsible for rapid cell proliferation and healing of any of these maladies. For this purpose, a poultice of the root or fresh leaves is applied over the affected surface to help it heal.

Internally, comfrey can be used to stop bleeding of gums and hemorrhaging, relieve congestion in lungs and throat and alleviate irritation and inflammation of stomach, intestines, kidneys, urinary tract and the bladder. In short, any part of the body that is injured or bleeding can be helped by comfrey, so much so that comfrey is sometimes referred to as a *knitter* and *healer* herb.

Because of its high mucilage content (substances that swell without dissolving), comfrey root can also be an excellent demulcent—a liquid used to soothe inflamed surfaces and protect them from irritation. In the digestive tract, comfrey also promotes the production and secretion of pepsin, one of the enzymes that help digest protein.

For any of the above applications you can make a decoction, infusion or tencture of the herb. Although the root is used for many of the comfrey's benefits, the leaves can also be used for a number of external treatments.

To make a decoction, simmer 6 teaspoons of ground comfrey root in 3 cups of water for 30 minutes, cool, strain and put in the refrigerate. Heat and take 2-3 teacups a day from this batch for any of the internal benefits mentioned above. To enhance taste, you may want to add six to eight spoons of honey to the initial batch.

Dong Quai. Dong quai is one of the most popular herbs in China and Japan and has been in use there since ancient times. It has primarily been used to help with the function of the female reproductive system, including its ability to maintain the proper amounts of the female hormones and regulate menses after childbirth. Because it tends to cleanse and purify blood, dong quai is beneficial for the circulatory system. This herb also enhances the utilization of vitamin E by the body.

Dunaliella Salina. As mentioned elsewhere in the book, beta-carotene, a form of vitamin A is an important antioxidant that has many healthful properties. Beta-carotene is important for, among other things, healthy functioning of the immune system, the skin, the eyes and the mucous membranes. Dunaliella Salina happens to be one of the best sources of this important nutrient.

Echinacea. An indigene of North America, echinacea has been used by both Native Americans and health-care professionals for many purposes. These range from elevating the production of immune cells to stimulating the generation of new tissues, particularly when applied externally on burns or wounds. Echinacea also has overall tonic properties that it enhances the function of the body as a whole. This great herb has many wonderful qualities, some of which have been documented by researchers both here and in Europe.

For starters, echinacea can help boost the immune system, which is important for the health of the entire body. The herb does this by stimulating the production of T-cells (a type of white blood cell) and interferons (a group of protecting proteins) against viruses and bacteria. This amazing herb, which helps with the health of various tissues and glands, including the prostate gland is also an effective blood cleanser. Echinacea can help remove toxins from the body, enhance digestion and reduce the problem of gas in the digestive tract.

Echinacea has thick hairy leaves and large, pale purple flowers. It's the root, however, that has been used for a variety of its healthful benefits. A root extract usually contains a host of compounds, but the predominant ones are inulin,[*] glucose, fructose, betaine, echinacin, and echinacoside.

Whether you use it for a specific purpose or to aid in the overall function of the body, echinacea is one herb that you can appreciate having as part of your daily good nutritional program.

Fennel. Fennel is one of the common herbs you find in the produce aisle of your supermarket. It has a round light greenish bulb, stout stems and hairlike green leaves. A perennial plant, fennel can have very wide uses or applications in the body. It helps eliminate gas and aids with the proper function of the digestive tract. It helps remove congestion in the chest and throat and assists with the production and flow of milk in nursing mothers.

Fennel seeds contain a special type of oil that also can help with weight loss and weight management. In addition, this interesting herb can also be an effective liver and gallbladder cleanser. Because of its ability to dissolve uric acid crystals, fennel may also help eliminate gout. Its high vitamin A content can also help with nighttime vision and prevent snow blindness. Fiber, antioxidant phytochemicals and iron are fennel's other assets.

Garcinia Cambogia. Garcinia cambogia, also known as brindall berries or mangosteen, is a fruit that customarily grows in India and Thailand. Its primary function in the body is to suppress the appetite so that you have less craving for food. This interesting herb also tends to increase the oxidation of fat (through thermogenesis) while slowing or limiting the conversion of carbohydrate into fat. In this instance, the body converts more glucose into glycogen and stores it in the liver and muscles so that it can be used as fuel at times when you're low in energy. It's also reported that this herb may help with the health of the throat and the urinary tract.

The active ingredient in this herb is called hydroxycitric acid, and apparently it's this substance that blocks or inactivates the enzymes systems that are involved in fat synthesis and storage in the body. It is reported that 50% of the herb consists of hydroxycitric acid. This compound also blocks the formation of fatty tissues in the body, and with the proper exercise and nutritional program, such as the inclusion of metabolic enhancers such as chromium, L-carnitine and magnesium, one may be able to lose or maintain weight.

---

[*] a type of carbohydrate

Ginkgo Biloba. So far as we currently know, no other life from earth has witnessed and survived the climatic and other vagaries of the world for 200 million years in its present form as ginkgo biloba. The average life span of the ginkgo tree may, however, range from only 1,000 to 3,000 years. Considering its antiquity, it is quite possible to think that dinosaurs may have once plucked its leaves or scratched their shoulders against the trunks of this giant tree. This amazing, tall and hardy tree once grew in many parts of the world, but now it's found only in China. Although it bears fruit, only the leaves and the seeds are used by humans.

The ginkgo leaf extract has many chemical compounds, but the ones that have been extensively studied are the ginkgo-flavone glycosides, which you often see as 24% of the total compounds found in a ginkgo extract. The standardized ginkgo leaf extract (i.e., an extract that shows a 24% ginkgo-flavone glycosides content) has many important benefits to the human body. Some of these include their serving as antioxidant or free radical scavengers and in enhancing the utilization of oxygen and glucose by brain cells. The specific antioxidant activity involves the neutralization of free radicals that attack lipids (fats) of cell membrane and other fats elsewhere in the body.

The brain cells, for instance, are largely made from unsaturated fatty acids; hence, ginkgo biloba extract may serve as an antioxidant for these cells and the rest of the nervous system. Because the ginkgo extract may serve to facilitate entry of glucose and oxygen into the cells, brain cells may get sufficient quantities of these important nutrients and hence are allowed to function better.

A ginkgo extract has also been found to enhance nerve impulse transmission due to the brain's improved synthesis and turnover of brain chemicals (or so-called neurotransmitters.) It's reported that the circulatory system may also benefit by ginkgo extract, thus increasing blood flow to all tissues and organs of the body, which ultimately improve the health and nourishment of the body.

Like ginseng, ginkgo extracts have been used in China for thousands of years. And like ginseng, its use in Western societies is relatively new. In Europe and Mexico, ginkgo extract is fairly popular and is being sold under various trade names: Tebonin (Europe and Mexico), Tanakan (France) and Rokan (Germany). As mentioned earlier, although there can be many different concentrations of the plant extract, the extract that contains 24% of the active ingredient (ginkgo-flavone glycosides) is the one that's of greater benefit.

Ginseng. As you may be aware, there are generally three different ginsengs: American ginseng, Siberian ginseng and Korean/Chinese ginseng. The main difference among these different "nationalities" is their ginesnosides (the active chemical compounds in ginseng) content. Since there are may different ginesnoside compounds, certain ones are more predominant in one kind than in the other and the value of the ginseng will depend on the concentration of one or a few of those compounds. Bear in mind that ginesing contains besides ginesnosides, many other substances, including vitamins and minerals that can be of benefit to you.

The most frequent concentration of ginsenosides found in ginseng varies from 1% to 3%. A ginseng extract that contains higher than these percentages means that the extract is of the highest quality.

In terms of its benefits to the human body, ginseng is what is referred to as a "tonic" herb. Tonic herbs are those plants that enhance the overall performance and health of the human body. Be that as it may, in the Orient, ginseng has been used for many specific physiological or bodily functions. The following few examples illustrate some of those attributes of ginseng.

One, ginseng can help improve both mental and physical performance. This fact has been established with both human and animal studies. With this herb you're more likely to experience alertness, have enhanced memory and cope better under physically demanding situations such as exercise and athletic competition. Ginseng may give you these benefits because of its ability to improve energy metabolism and spare glycogen (your body's stored fuel), particularly during prolonged exercise. This wonder herb may also help you deal better with fatigue and everyday stress because it enhances the health of the adrenal gland, which is responsible for the production of anti-stress hormones. These effects of the herb are observed after its continuous and daily usage.

In the elderly, ginseng increases cellular enzyme activity and hence helps important organs, such as the heart and the brain, function better. Many people around the world also believe ginseng to be the world's greatest aphrodisiac. Some scientists in Japan have linked this to the herb's stimulatory action on the sex hormones.

Two, when the body is properly nourished, ginseng can stimulate protein synthesis and cell proliferation. Three, ginseng may help enhance the function of the immune system. This and all the other aspects of the herb may naturally help you build a strong and properly working body and mind. This great herb can also be good for the digestive and circulatory systems and, as mentioned, enhance the function of the male reproductive system. In addition, ginseng may function as an antioxidant, thus helping slow down the aging process. Ginseng has many other properties and benefits, the discussion of which are beyond the scope of this book.

Perhaps the best way to summarize ginseng's overall function in the body is to describe the herb in terms of its adaptogen properties. An adaptogen is a substance that maintains and normalizes the body function regardless of external or internal stresses. Adaptogens thus are substances that make the body adaptable in extreme situations by increasing its coping mechanisms.

Goldenseal. For a long time, some healthcare professionals in this country used goldenseal in an eye drop preparation, but now its use has been predominantly to help enhance the function of the immune system because of its antibiotic and anti-bacterial properties. This herb is particularly effective when used in combination with echinacea, the other immune system enhancing herb discussed earlier. Like echinacea, goldenseal has tonic properties and can be effective in treating wounds and infections. When used in combination with licorice, goldenseal can help lower blood sugar, which can be beneficial for those who suffer from diabetes. In addition, goldenseal may help stimulate appetite and improve digestion because it tends to sensitize or stimulate the function of the secretory cells along the digestive tract. Goldenseal also can be used to enhance the function of the nasal and throat mucous membranes.

The major active compounds in goldenseal are berberine, hydrazine and cana-dine. It's these compounds that have many beneficial properties. The extraction or preparation is usually made from the root or bark of the plant.

Marigold. Also called calendula by the ancient Romans, who observed that the plant bloomed on the first day or "calends" of the month, marigold is used exter-nally to treat skin conditions. These range from cuts, burns and bruises to wounds and skin irritations. Internally, marigold can be used to treat conditions of the stom-ach, colon and liver as well the gum. Because it has soothing properties, it can be a good gargle or mouthwash.

Milk Thistle. Milk thistle is one of those incredible herbs whose list of benefits never seems to end. Be that as it may, the primary function of the herb appears to center around the health of the liver.

For starters, milk thistle is important in removing toxins and in helping relieve liver-related chronic disorders such as hepatitis and cirrhosis. This herb also helps rejuvenate and revitalize liver function, particularly after a long and damaging pe-riod of alcohol consumption. Because it is rich in bioflavonoids, milk thistle is also an excellent antioxidant, protecting the liver and other organs of the body from free radical attacks.

The active ingredient in milk thistle is called silymarin. It's this compound that increases proteins synthesis in the liver and encourages the rejuvenation of this organ. Silymarin also has a blocking action against the absorption of toxins by the liver. Reportedly, toxic substances such as some wild mushrooms, cadmium and carbon tetrachloride (a dry-cleaning agent) can be safely processed and eliminated by silymarin.

Milk thistle also stimulates the production of super oxide dismutase (the body-born antioxidant enzyme) while preventing the depletion of glutathione (which is also an antioxidant) from the liver. Because of its antioxidant property, milk thistle helps boost the immune system by increasing the production of T-cells and interferons (soluble proteins involved in protection of the body against foreign invaders.) The kidneys, the heart, the brain and the rest of the nervous system also benefits from milk thistle.

Passion Flower. A hairy and climbing vine, passion flower is grown mainly in southern United States. Both the fruit and the leaves are used for their medicinal properties. Because they function as a calming, soothing or sedative agent, the leaves of a passion flower are used to treat nervous disorders such as hysteria, insomnia, nervousness and restlessness. Professionally prepared dosages, given for an extended duration reportedly can markedly improve epilepsy, Parkinson's disease, neuralgia, anxiety and hypertension.

Also, women whose hormones cause them to be irritable, the elderly who have muscular or motor control problems and hyperactive children can benefit from this plant.

Rich in bioflavonoids and many other compounds, passion flower can be used as a painkiller, an antiinflammatory and a germicide (particularly with bacteria that cause eye irritations).

St. John's Wort. According to one legend, this plant was so named because red spots that are metaphorical for St. John's blood appeared on the leaves of the *hypericum* plant on the anniversary of the saint's beheading. According to another legend, the saint had used the hypericum plant during the time of the crusades as balm to clean and heal battle wounds, and so the plant's name.

True to its legend, St. John's wort still can be used to heal wounds, ulcers, burns, bruises and other skin problems. The other important functions of the herb are its use as a sedative or relaxing agent for those who suffer from anxiety or nervous tension. Hypericin, the active ingredient in the herb, has also been used as an anti-

antidepressant.

St. John's wort has many benefits, including its use to treat insomnia, head-aches, anemia and bronchitis or congestion of the chest. This herb is also good for control of viral infection, tumors, boils, bladder problems and circulation difficul-ties.

Caution. When taken internally, hypericin ends up accumulating in the skin. This problem makes the skin of some animals, including humans, to be extremely sensitive to sunlight and can cause it to burn. Hence, when taking the herb, stay out of strong sun.

Schisandra. A native of China, schisandra is a thorny climbing vine that has been used for a variety of applications, including as a tonic and as an adaptogen to revitalize and enhance the overall function of the body. Many of this great herb's specific benefits are as follows.

Schisandra helps you cope with stress, improve your body's ability to forestall fatigue and increase the body's ability to function. Specific organs, such as the heart, liver and kidneys, the glands and nerves and the whole body can benefit from schisandra. The herb strengthens the cells in various organs and hence helps the body cope at wider ranges of physiological conditions, including fortifying it against stress.

Because it normalizes and calms the body, schisandra is very useful in situations where you may have stress, anxiety or a general below-par feeling. Schisandra also enhances circulation and digestion, and because it has antioxidant properties, it may boost the immune system, help with the health of the eyes and promote the well-being of other tissues in the body. In addition, schisandra help the body use calories more efficiently. Athletes and weight watchers may find this product a use-ful addition to their nutritional regimen. Women have used this herb in its native country to improve their sexual interest as well as promote youthfulness. Schisandra has pink flowers and red berries.

Spirulina. Also known as blue-green algae, spirulina has many important ben-efits to the human body.

One, this one-celled plant contains the highest concentration of beta-carotene and vitamin B12 (reportedly 250% more than liver, which is one of the best sources of the vitamin) and some of the best protein (with 80%-85% bioavailability) and holds 4 times the protein found in an equivalent amount of beef. This interesting algae also houses 26 times more calcium than milk, as well as a large quantity of phosphorus and niacin. Spirulina also contains a number of other key vitamins and minerals, including linolenic acid (or omega-3 fatty acid).

Two, blue-green algae, except for its lack of carbohydrates, is considered a complete food. To have a carbohydrate energy source, the body can still convert some of the amino acids from the protein it contains into glucose and use it as fuel. This plant of the sea is beneficial for the entire body, but the brain and the nervous system seem to thrive on it. Reportedly, the consumption of spirulina gives greater mental clarity and alertness. For some people though, the alertness could be too much, as it makes them feel wired.

Spirulina helps boost the immune system, normalize the cholesterol level in the body and suppress hunger or the desire to over indulge as well as helps the body eliminate toxins. Whenever you get a chance, include this herb as part of your meal. It's an incredible plant, indeed!

Valerian. This herb, which has been used for thousands of years has some great benefits. It can be used to calm or sedate nervous disorders such as anxiety or over-excitement, headaches, hysteria and insomnia and also works as a stimulant in cases of extreme fatigue or exhaustion. In addition, valerian enhances circulation and secretion of digestive juices and stimulates the muscular or peristaltic action of the digestive tract.

Witch Hazel. Witch hazel, whose name was derived from an Old English word that means "pliant or flexible" because the branches or twigs are highly flexible, is primarily used for external applications. Extracts of the bark, leaves or twigs can be used to alleviate pain or bruises and act as an astringent and a cleansing agent. It can also help heal wounds, bed sores, inflamed eyes, hemorrhoids and swellings. Extracts of the witch hazel plant seem to be particularly beneficial to the veins as they tent to strengthen and tone them, thus enhancing blood flow.

When prepared into a tea and taken internally, witch hazel can help stop or reduce internal bleeding, including hemorrhages and excessive menstrual flow. For women, witch hazel also helps in treating problems of the uterus, the cervix and the vagina.

A compress made of witch hazel can be used to treat irritated skin or eyes, burns, insect bites and infections. Because of its astringent properties to the skin, many cosmetic companies use witch hazel in their cleansers, hand and body lotions, message oils and aftershaves.

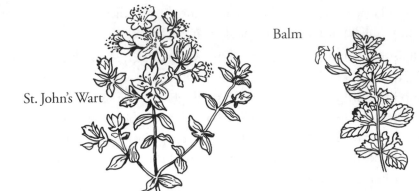

St. John's Wart

Balm

Feverfew

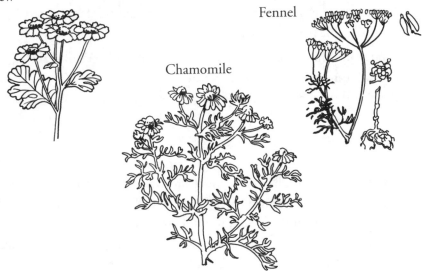

Fennel

Chamomile

Catnip

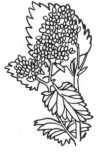

Mint

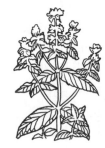

CHAPTER 18
Herb Tea Samplers

If you have browsed through the coffee and tea aisle of your supermarket or health food store, you are probably amazed at the variety of herbal teas now available to you. Not too long ago, when one thought of consuming tea, one may have considered the traditional commercial teas such as Lipton, Twining or Earl Grey. For most people, herb teas held no value or significance. Now our popular teas, such as Lipton have moved over on health food and grocery store shelves to make room for the dizzying array of herbal blends that pack these places like sardines.

Realizing the growing popularity and the many beneficial properties of herbal teas, enterprising individuals and corporations package and market an incredible assortment of such teas. These range from one or two herbs such as chamomile and peppermint to the ones whose ingredients list reads like those of multivitamin supplements.

Some of these herbs are formulated for specific conditions, and their names are as exotic as their blends: Throat Coat, Smooth Move, Gypsy Cold Care, Fast Lane and Emerald Gardens. Let's look at a sample of the different herbs you find in an herbal blend and the benefits they have to the body.

Cardamom. Cardamom is a seed herb that is also used to spice up certain dishes, particularly in India and the Orient. Often combined with other herbs, cardamom's primary function in a tea blend is to warm and stimulate the body. This herb is also good for indigestion, gas, colic and headaches.

Carob. In some tea formulations, you see roasted carob. Carob pods are found in a dome-shaped evergreen tree that is native to some parts of Europe and Asia. The tree is also grown in the Mediterranean region. Carob reportedly is very effective in treating kidney ailments and curing or preventing diarrhea. Naturally sweet, when present in a tea blend, it can help improve the taste of the tea while imparting its other benefits.

Catnip. This is another herb you are likely to see often in an herb tea. Before Lipton and other Asiatic herbs took over, catnip was the only herb tea drunk in Europe when people wanted a warm drink or a drink to treat bronchitis and diarrhea. American Indians used catnip as a sedative or calming agent. They also used it to treat colic, colds or flu in infants and children, as the herb tends to increase perspiration, which can lull a child to sleep. This herb also improves circulation, which is important for the proper function of the body. It may even be a benefit to those who have a swelling under the eyes. Its primary function in an herbal tea blend is probably to help calm, relax or ease the body.

Chamomile Flower. Chamomile has many external applications that make it such a useful plant. These range from enhancing the appearance of skin and hair (particularly blond hair) to treating dryness or flakiness of the skin to diminishing lines and wrinkles. This benefit of the herb does not involve much preparation at all. Simply steep the herb for 30 to 40 minutes and wash or treat the skin with the end product. Chamomile as a compress can also be used to alleviate stiffness and muscular inflammation.

Chamomile's popularity, however, is among tea drinkers, who view the herb as a calming or soothing one. It can also be very useful with hyperactive children. For either of these benefits, simply bring one pint of water to a boil, add two teaspoonfuls of the herb and steep for 30 to 40 minutes. If you are using herb tea bags, follow the instruction on the box. The vapor bath of the tea can be a good treatment for children and adults who have asthma or a cold.

The main constituents of Chamomile are essentials oils, flavonoids and tannic acid.

Chicory. A native of Europe and now widely grown here in the U.S., chicory has been used as a purgative of mucus from the stomach and other parts of the GI tract. It's important for the health and proper function of the spleen. It can also be used as an appetizer and to stimulate and enhance digestion.

Citrus Peels. The peel of an orange or a tangerine is believed to have a health-enhancing function in the digestive tract, including aid in minimizing the formation of mucus. It is also known to improve digestion as well as overall energy production of the body. Thus, as part of an herbal tea blend, it may help burn more calories, thus perhaps enhancing weight loss.

Hibiscus. This name is really a generic name for a whole class of plants that consist of 200 species and grow in many parts of the world. Many of these plants have important medicinal properties. Musk-mallow reportedly is one of the most commonly used hibiscus plants that has been used to relieve stomach problems, soothe or calm the nerves and freshen the breath. Those who have a high fever can also be treated with this herb, as it has cooling and detoxifying properties. As part of an herbal tea blend, it can help with these and other conditions.

Hops. The beer industry has long used hops as a preservative and flavoring agent. This important plant has also had a history of use as an easing or calming substance for those who are restless or wakeful at night. This relaxing and sedative action of the herb is good for those with muscle spasms, pain or fever. This plant is also good for the health of the gallbladder and liver, as it increases the production and secretion of bile. Because of its relaxing calming effect, hops reportedly can be effective as an enema.

Lemon Grass. Lemon grass, also known as oil grass or fever grass, can be excellent for colds, headaches and abdominal problems. A tea of lemon grass leaves can help ease dizziness, cold-related fever or stress. The presence of this herb in a tea blend can help the body ease with any of the aforementioned maladies.

Licorice. The major active phytochemical in licorice is glycyrrhizin or glycyrrhizic acid, which gives most of the herb's its sweet-tasting characteristics. There are, of course, also a whole variety of other compounds, including flavonoids, starch, sugars and amino acids. A native of Asia and Europe, licorice has many benefits, some of which include its ability to stimulate the adrenal glands so that they can help release the necessary hormones that help metabolize calories. This herb, among other things, has a calming effect on the nervous system. When taken along with other herbs, it is reported to have a balancing or harmonizing effect on the body.

Peppermint. Peppermint has been used since ancient times particularly in Chinese, Egyptian and Native American societies. This herb now grows widely in the United States, Europe and other parts of the world. Peppermint is a very commonly used herb because it has a soothing and calming effect on the body.

The herb has other functions that range from its ability to stimulate the functioning of the digestive tract to its ability to increase the supply of oxygen to the blood, which in turn facilitates the calorie-burning, or thermic, effect of the herb. Its overall function, however, is more for its tonic properties, because the herb enhances the proper functioning of the digestive tract as well as the rest of the body.

Spearmint. Spearmint is related to peppermint in terms of its function and benefits except that this herb tends to be milder, gentler and less stimulating than peppermint. Spearmint can be used for ailments involving digestion and circulation, for colds and fever and for cramps and muscle spasms. It also helps remove gas from the gastrointestinal tract and promotes sweating, which helps to reduce fever. Also, if you have a problem with nausea or vomiting, spearmint may help alleviate it. Because of its mild nature, it's often thought a better choice than peppermint for children. Women who suffer from morning sickness (as happens during pregnancy) may also find relief from this herb. Overall, spearmint is a soothing and calming herb that can be benefit you. Because its oils are volatile, it's recommended that you not boil it but steep it in a closed container.

Rose Hips. Rose hips refer to the fruitlike, fleshy hip that is left after the rose petals have fallen off. This hip is very rich in vitamin C, reportedly 60 times richer than any citrus fruit. Rose hips are also rich in bioflavonoids, a group of vitamin-like compounds that are often found along with vitamin C and that have many important roles including their benefit as an antioxidant. This group of substances is also important for the building and repair of tissues, particularly those of the circulatory system. Besides their independent roles, bioflavonoids are helpers of vitamin C. As discussed in Chapter 12, this vitamin provides tremendous benefits to the body. Perhaps the maximum benefit of vitamin C is attained when consumed along with its sister compounds (the bioflavonoids) and other compounds as in rose hips. The presence of these ingredients in an herbal tea preparation increases the nutritional value of the tea.

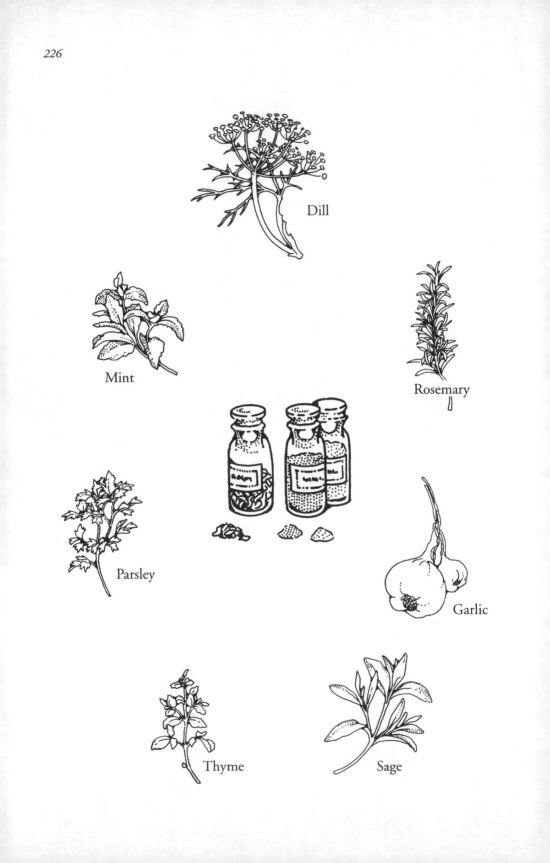

Dill

Mint

Rosemary

Parsley

Garlic

Thyme

Sage

CHAPTER 19
Spice Samplers

For most people, spices' importance ends with their use as food flavoring agents. But as you will see below, besides their culinary function, these mostly aromatic herbs have many benefits to the body. Although the number of spices used by various cultures is extensive, the following samples may help you appreciate the role spices play in your health.

Anis. This groove-stemmed, soft-stocked herb has had many uses since ancient times. In the digestive tract, anis when consumed as tea can help prevent the formation of as well as eliminate gas, alleviate nausea, cramps and colic (or severe abdominal pain), and for nursing mothers increase the production and flow of milk. Anis can also be a nice remedy for insomnia when taken with a glass of warm milk, and when taken as an infusion, help promote menstruation. A tea made from equal combination of fennel, caraway and anis reportedly is an excellent cleanser or purifier for the digestive tract. Because of its sweetness and pleasant flavor, you often find it in cough medicines.

Basil. Although grown worldwide and used to flavor foods, it's in India where basil is highly esteemed, almost considered sacred. Basil's healthful properties are many. When steeped into tea and drank, basil can help alleviate fevers, colds, indigestion, cramps, constipation, nausea and vomiting. This sweetly aromatic herb can also relieve gas and serve as a diuretic and a stimulant, particularly when you are tired or exhausted.

If you have a fever, simmer one ounce of the herb in a pint of water for 15-20 minutes and drink. Adding black peppercorns can enhance the herbs effectiveness.

Since basil increases milk production, a nursing mother can benefit by it. Because basil increases blood circulation, a pregnant woman taking it before and after a childbirth can also benefit from it. This herb can even benefit those with yeast infection of the mouth and throat as well as those who have headaches.

Bay. Bay leaves are excellent flavor enhancers when used with certain dishes. As you will see below, bay's function in the body is more impressive than its culinary uses. Also called laurel or sweet bay, this herb can be a great remedy for liver, pancreas, spleen, kidneys and lung problems. A tea of bayberries can be effective in treating sore throat and congestion of the nose, chest and lungs and help alleviate tonsillitis. The tea is also a very good remedy for colds, influenza and fever.

On the gastrointestinal and urinary tracts, the laurel herb can be an effective agent in eliminating gas and enhancing urine flow, respectively. Women who have menstrual and womb trouble can benefit from this herb by consuming it as tea.

When externally applied, the tea as well as the oil of bayberries can be handy in treating poisonous insect and snake bites, sunburns, itches, bruises and eczema. You may even use bay oil to improve the appearance of brown and black spots on your skin. In terms of usage, the bark, berries and leaves can be used for all kinds of treatments.

Black Pepper. Besides its culinary benefits, black pepper can be excellent as an expectorant for cold-related mucous of the throat. It is more effective when made into a tea and mixed with honey.

Black pepper can also be an effective insecticide, annihilating such household pests as roaches, ants, potato bugs and moths. Simply grind and sprinkle the spice where the insects are, and you should see them disappear.

Caraway. This common spice has many benefits beyond its use in the kitchen. It can help with digestion, in the prevention of fermentation in the stomach and elimination of gas from the bowel. For this purpose, crush an ounce of the seeds and add to boiling water and let it cool and steep for 20-30 minutes. Take two table-spoon of the infusion until relief is noted. This use of the herb can be very effective in treating digestive tract disorders of infants and children as well. For women, caraway helps promote menstrual flow, alleviate cramps in the uterus and increase the production and flow of milk.

Cayenne Pepper. Cayenne or red pepper is grown widely in warm climates through-out the world, particularly in Africa, Latin America, Asia and some parts of the U.S. This deceptively hot but harmless herb has been used to spice up foods in many cultures. In terms of its health merits, cayenne is one of the few herbs that stimulate the nervous and circulatory systems and serve as an overall tonic for the body. Some of the organs and tissues that benefit from cayenne are the spleen, kidneys, pancreas and digestive tract. Because of its stimulatory action, the glands along the digestive tract may produce more digestive juices in the presence of cayenne. So you can see the benefit of consuming red pepper along with your meals.

Capsicum is the active ingredient in whole red pepper, but the other substances include pectin, albumin, iron and phosphate compounds, magnesium and some oil. When taken whole, all these other substances can have healthful properties as well.

Because of its high vitamin A content, capsicum is also good for the eyes and can serve as an antioxidant for the rest of the body. This herb is also good for the heart, as it enhances circulation and improves the health of the veins, arteries and capillaries. In addition, it helps reduce the bad cholesterol while raising the good cholesterol. In the liver, cayenne increases fat-metabolizing enzymes and hence may help reduce fat production and deposition in the body, an important benefit for those who are struggling with their weight. Cayenne pepper has many other benefits, many of which are beyond the scope of this book.

Celery. This ancient plant has many benefits, some of which include its use as an antioxidant and calming and easing agent for the body. Because it tends to cause perspiration, some herbalists think celery may even help with weight loss. This herb has also been reported to help in balancing the acidity of the body. A combination of celery juice and carrot juice reportedly helps ease arthritic spurs. This interesting plant is also supposed to enhance sexual drive and serve as a stimulant to the kidneys to increase urine flow. Because it contains a fair amount of sodium, it helps enhance the function of the stomach lining and is good for the joints.

Cinnamon. The use of this herb goes back to the ancient Chinese, Roman and Egyptian cultures. Cinnamon's special attribute is that it helps with indigestion, heartburn and cramps. It's also an excellent antifungal and antibacterial agent. Hence, those who have yeast infection or athletes foot can benefit from this herb. Add 10 or so cinnamon sticks in four cups of boiling water, simmer for 5-7 minutes, remove from heat and let cool for 40-45 minutes. Apply the solution for either of the problems mentioned.

Cloves. When steeped into tea, cloves can be good in curing nausea and relieving gas in the digestive tract. This spice is also good for circulation, digestion and treating vomiting. Clove oils can help relieve toothaches. You may also chew cloves for this purpose. Because cloves have antibiotic properties, they can also be used as germicides.

Coriander. A small annual plant, coriander has been cultivated since ancient times. The seed is used both for its culinary and medicinal benefits. In the digestive tract, coriander can help eliminate gas, allay cramps or griping and other disorders and enhance the muscular tone of the stomach and the rest of the GI tract. Because of its pleasant taste, coriander is often used to enhance the flavor of foods and other medicinal preparations. It also has a diuretic and alterative (capable of favorably altering disease conditions) properties.

Cumin. Primarily used to make curries, it enhances the flavor of fried foods such as beans, rice and chicken. In terms of its health merits, cumin, can be good for the heart, the uterus and the mammary glands, as it increases the production and secretion of milk. You may use the tea or capsule of cumin powder for many of its internal benefits. Of course you can also use it with the appropriate dishes to derive the benefit of the herb. When externally applied in liniments (a thin substance rubbed onto the skin), it can stimulate circulation to the area.

Dill. Dill is an annual plant widely grown for its use as a spice; it is also found in the wild. It's a multipurpose spice that can be sprinkled on a variety of dishes. But beyond its role in enhancing the flavor of foods, dill has a number of healthful benefits. When used as tea, it can help alleviate upset stomach and prevent the formation of gas in the intestines and has calming or quieting effect on the nerves. It can reduce swelling and pain, stimulate appetite and fight off insomnia. When used in combination with other herbs such as anis, coriander, fennel and caraway, dill will help promote the flow of milk in nursing mothers. Chewing the seed of this herb is also supposed to relieve bad breath. If you have problems with hiccoughs, this herb may be the answer to the problem.

Fenugreek. The use of this spice/herb goes back to the ancient cultures of Egypt, Greek and Asia. Since ancient times, fenugreek has been hailed both for its medicinal and culinary uses. Medicinally, the seed of fenugreek can be used to remove congestion of the throat and chest, as an astringent, as a demulcent to relieve inflammation of mucous membranes and as an emollient to soothe and treat skin problems. The tea of fenugreek can be excellent in purging excessive mucus from the throat and gut that collects when one consumes large amount of milk and cheese.

This herb can be used to treat diabetes and gout, increase milk production in wet mothers and because of its spermicide properties, even prevent pregnancy. This funny sounding herb can also be used to treat boils and carbuncles and help with anemia and rickets.

Garlic. Garlic is the reigning king of all spices in that it has been used throughout history for a number of remedies—from warding off evil spirits to protecting against the plague and helping with wound healing to fighting cancer and a number of other diseases and maladies. This amazing spice is a true wonder of nature indeed and has been used to treat many internal and external infections and other diseases. Externally, garlic can be used to treat infections of the eye, throat, vagina and nose as well as burns and insect bites. It's also a great insect repellent. Internally, it can be used to treat parasites of the colon (when used as an enema), control fever, combat viruses and bacteria and alleviate hemorrhoids. This herb is also beneficial to the heart, stomach, lungs and spleen.

Garlic has many other benefits. These include improving blood circulation, lowering triglycerides and the bad serum cholesterol (while raising the good cholesterol), decreasing blood sugar (important for those with diabetes), reducing blood pressure and stimulating the immune system. Because it relaxes the nervous system, garlic may also help you keep insomnia at bay.

Ginger. We often use ginger as condiment to spice up or enhance the flavor of certain dishes. Ginger has, besides its culinary function, many healthful benefits. Some of these involve the elimination of gases from the intestinal tract, improved function of the liver, including its ability to increase the secretion of bile, and the processing of cholesterol. Because bile is involved in the digestion and absorption of fats and fat-soluble vitamins, it can be said that ginger may help enhance the processing of food in the body as well.

Ginger, like most plant extracts, contains several different substances. These substances include starch, protein, lecithin, fatty acids, triglycerides, protein-digesting enzymes, volatile oils (substance that give ginger its characteristic smell), vitamins and a variety of other compounds. All these compounds together help enhance the function of the body. Some of the specific functions of ginger are the ability to serve as an antioxidant, help with the digestion of protein and enhance circulation. Fresh ginger steeped in hot water (as tea) can be good for nasal and throat congestion.

Horseradish. This penetratingly pungent herb has many benefits. Some of these include serving as dilator of the nasal and bronchial channels (thus enabling the sinuses to open up and cleanse) and as an antibiotic or inhibitor of microbial and parasite growth in the body. Horseradish can also aid digestion by stimulating the cells of the gastrointestinal lining.

In addition, this root herb can be beneficial for the proper function of the kidneys and the intestines. When made into a poultice and applied externally, horseradish can stimulate blood flow to the area and help alleviate pain, such as in the case of rheumatoid arthritis.

Marjoram. In ancient Greece, marjoram was held as a symbol of love, so much so that people wore it as wreaths and garlands at weddings and called it "joy of the mountains." An ointment of the herb is supposed to enable the wearer to dream about his or her future mate. Marjoram, although native to Mediterranean countries and some parts of Asia, is now grown in the U.S. and other parts of the world.

In terms of its health merits, marjoram is used to calm the nerves, enhance digestion, treat rheumatism and sprains, relieve gas and stomach disorders and serve as tonic for the rest of the body. Marjoram can also be used to alleviate coughs and other respiratory disorders and as a mouth wash and gargle for sore throats. For women, marjoram can help relieve cramps and nausea associated with menstruation. In addition, a tea of the herb can be an excellent calming and sleep-inducing agent.

To make a tea of the herb, boil one pint of water, add one teaspoon each marjoram and oregano (an option) and let it steep for 30 minutes. After it cools, strain and refrigerate and use in an amount from this lot. You may want to reheat it before consuming it.

Also, you can add this herb to your bath water to help you unwind and relax if you have had a long and exhausting day. Lastly, the oil of marjoram can be used as a lotion for gout, rheumatism and varicose veins and to relieve stiff joints.

Mustard Seed. Mustard seeds, which can be either black or white, have many medicinal properties. It's the white variety that is combined with vinegar and turmeric (which gives mustard its yellow color) to make the pastelike spread that we use on sandwiches, hamburgers and hotdogs.

As medicine, mustard can be used both for internal and external applications. Internally, mustard is good in ease congestion of the chest as well as an emetic to remove poison or relieve discomfort in the stomach. It can also enhance appetite and stimulate the flow of digestive juices.

Externally, a paste of the herb (prepared by mixing black mustard and cold water) can help easing pain, sprain, spasm or rheumatism by encouraging blood flow to the particular area of the body. For this purpose, the poultice is spread over a thin cloth that overlays the wound or pain and is covered with a heavier cotton cloth and left until the skin begins to irritate or burn. Upon removal, the applied area is washed thoroughly to remove any remaining mustard. To complete the process and speed up recovery, apply grain flour such as rice or wheat on the treated area and wrap with dry cotton cloth. If you have sensitive or tender skin, this treatment may not work for you.

Nutmeg. Nutmeg is a seed herb from the great nutmeg tree, which is native to Indonesia but now is also widely grown throughout the world. However, it's only in Indonesia and Granada of the West Indies where the tree is cultivated commercially. The nutmeg tree has spreading branches and densely packed leaves.

Besides its use as spice for a variety of dishes, nutmeg and its sister herb, mace (from the dried shell of the fruit), have been used to treat gas, digestive disorders and stomach, heart, nervous system and kidney maladies. On the nervous system, nutmeg has a calming and soothing effect, producing a peaceful and almost euphoric state while dramatically increasing one's awareness and control. In addition, this herb reportedly heightens one's sensuality and sexual drive.

There can be some side effects with some people when taken in large quantities. These range from aching in bones and muscles to hurting eyes, sinus problems and diarrhea. For those who suffer from some mental disorders and need a treatment, these inconveniences may be minor compared to the herb's benefit.

Oregano. This wonderfully aromatic herb can be added to enhance the flavor of most dishes. As for its health benefits, oregano can improve the health and function of the stomach, increase appetite and help allay congestion of the chest and throat. As a carminative agent, it can help relieve gas from the stomach and bowel. Reportedly, oregano can alleviate deafness or pain and ringing in the ear and may even be used to get rid of a toothache. You can prepare tea, poultice or compress for many of it remedial applications. The whole plant is employed for oregano's many uses.

Parsley. This herb is the black sheep of the spice family. Although we are now finding that it contains a wide variety of excellent nutrients, in the past, parsley has been largely relegated to its use in garnishing and enhancing the appearance of foods. In terms of its nutritional and medicinal content, parsley is a rich source of iron, beta-carotene, calcium, potassium and phosphorus. This perennial plant can be an excellent treatment for diseases of the urinary tract, such as those inflicted by venereal diseases, for problems with the liver and spleen and for gallstones. It can also be an excellent diuretic and promoter of the health of the kidneys and of the circulatory system and can improve menstruation. This herb can be used to treat swollen glands and breasts as well as curtail the flow of milk (particularly important to mothers who are trying to wean a child.) The roots, leaves and seeds are used for a variety of the herb's benefits. To take advantage of parsley's benefits, use it liberally in your soup, salad and sandwiches.

Caution: Those who have a kidney infection should avoid using parsley.

Rosemary. Rosemary is a Mediterranean native that is now grown throughout the world. Besides its use in spicing up various dishes, rosemary has many healthful benefits. These range from enhancing digestion to promoting liver function, including the secretion of bile. In many cultures, this herb has been used to treat maladies such as stomach and headaches and to soothe and calm the nerves. Rosemary also promotes circulation in the capillaries (the tiniest of blood vessels), which thus helps bring more nutrients to all tissues of the body. In addition, this herb reportedly enhances memory and relieves tension and depression.

You may even see rosemary in shampoos and rinses. It's used in these products because of the herb's ability to darken and maintain a healthy scalp and youthful hair. To derive this benefit, you may make your own product by making an infusion of the herb and applying it after you shampoo your hair.

Rosemary tea can be prepared by adding a half teaspoon of the herb to a pint of boiling water and letting it steep for ten to fifteen minutes. Rosemary, which has antioxidant properties itself, can be an excellent source of vitamin E, an important antioxidant, particularly as a protector of cell membranes, fatty tissues and fat molecules in the circulating blood.

Caution: Excessive consumption of rosemary can be fatal.

Sage. Another use of this word in the English language means a wise man or a philosopher. As the name of an herb here it means "savior of mankind." It reportedly can function as a strengthener of memory and as a promoter of wisdom and longevity.

Among its many other benefits, sage helps reduce the secretion of bodily fluids such as sweat (beneficial to menopausal women who may be experiencing hot flashes and night sweats or those with tuberculosis), breast milk (useful to women who are trying to wean a child) and saliva and mucus (beneficial to those who have a cold or chest congestion).

A tea preparation of the herb can be used for depression, nervous disorder, vertigo and trembling. You can also gargle sage infusion to help heal sore throat, laryngitis and tonsillitis.

For these and other benefits of the herb first boil 1-1/4 cups of water. Remove from heat and add 2 tablespoons of the sage and steep for 30 to 35 minutes. Strain and add honey or sugar if necessary and drink half a cup of the infusion twice a day. For women who want to stop milk production, two cups a day of sage tea consumed over a week reportedly helps bring their milk secretion to a halt. For this purpose and to make a larger supply at a time, boil one quart of water, remove from heat add 8 tablespoons of the herb and steep for 45 minutes. Sweeten appropriately and drink two cups daily.

Sage has also been used to heal skin sores, to promote the health and regeneration of the liver and as a natural coloring agent for graying hair. In addition, sage can enhance circulation and serve as an antioxidant for the heart and the rest of the body.

Caution: Heavy and extended use of the herb may lead to poisoning.

Thyme. In ancient Greece, the name thyme conjured up power, strength and bravery. But the herb's beneficial properties lie in its ability to help ease congestion of the chest, throat and nasal cavity and alleviate gastrointestinal disorders such as stomach cramps, gastritis and gas buildup. It also serves to soothe the nerves and can be used as a disinfectant and germicide. When applied externally, thyme can help control athlete's foot, scabies, lice and crabs. The extract of the herb can also be used to heal wounds and bruises and alleviate rheumatism. Because of its antioxidant properties, thyme may keep cells from becoming cancerous.

It is reported that alcoholics can benefit from this herb because it causes vomiting, diarrhea, sweating and hunger along with a detestation for alcohol. For this to work, the herb has to be used repeatedly for a long period of time.

For this purpose, steep 1 to 2 teaspoon of the herb in one cup of water and drink this amount daily.

PART IX

Supplements: What You Should Know About Them

The myth of the balanced diet

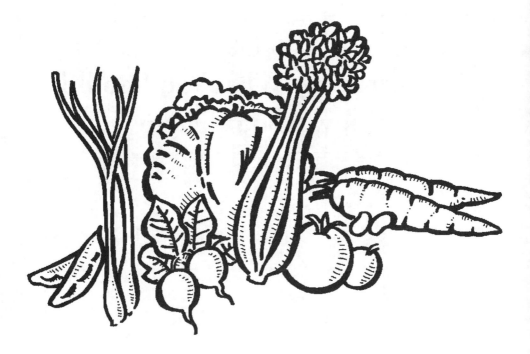

What you see is not necessarily what you get.

CHAPTER 20
The Significance of Supplements

If our food supplies were optimal, we would get every nutrient our body needs from the foods we eat. If our lives and the environment we live in were perfect, we would rely entirely on our daily rations for our good health and well-being. Unfortunately, neither of these cases is true, despite what some professionals and laypeople tell you.[1] These people often pipe up with their advice and say, "If you're eating a balanced diet, you do not need supplements."

This statement, as much as it is trite and meaningless, could also be dangerous. The fact is, as was discussed in Chapter 1, nationwide surveys, have shown that Americans get everything but balanced meals. In the 1978 survey, for example, only 3% of the nearly 21,000 people studied were found to be free of any nutritional deficiency.[2] The other 97% were found to be deficient in a number of minerals, vitamins, proteins and carbohydrates.

What is interesting in these findings is the fact that the deficiency problems were not limited to people of a certain class, race or economic status.[3] You would think the rich, who have the means, would be free of malnutrition. According to the survey, that was not the case.[4] There are many reasons why there is such widespread malnourishment. Nowadays, not only do the nutritional contents of vegetables vary depending on where they are grown (see Table 20.1 on page 240), but many fruits are picked before they have fully matured. Vitamin and protein synthesis, as well as mineral content, is the highest when fruits are allowed to ripen before being picked.[5,6,7]

Add to this the fact that a great percentage of the food you buy from your supermarket is processed, canned and filled with all kinds of additives (preservatives, artificial coloring and flavoring agents). Processing and canning strip off many nutrients in foods.[8,9] Additives can cause allergic side effects as well as other serious health problems.

Furthermore, the lifestyle of the baby boom generation is such that people would rather eat out than prepare the so-called well-balanced meal. Fast-food outlets have proliferated in the past few decades because they appeal to this eat-on-the-run generation. The foods from these outlets are far from being well-balanced. Preservatives, fat, salts and processed breads are often the predominant content of these meals. None of these is nourishing or healthy for you.

Table 20.1 Variation in the Mineral Content of Vegetables
Produced in the United States

		Percentage of Dry Weight			Millequivalents per 100 Grams Dry Weight			Trace Elements Parts per Million Dry Matter				
	Total Ash or Mineral Matter	Phosphorus	Calcium	Magnesium	Potassium	Sodium	Boron	Manganese	Iron	Copper	Cobalt	
SNAP BEANS												
Highest	10.45	0.36	40.5	60.0	99.7	8.6	73	60	227	69	0.26	
Lowest	4.04	0.22	15.5	14.8	29.1	0.0	10	2	10	3	0.00	
CABBAGE												
Highest	10.38	0.38	60.0	43.6	148.3	20.4	42	13	94	48	0.15	
Lowest	6.12	0.18	17.5	15.6	53.7	0.8	7	2	20	0.4	0.00	
LETTUCE												
Highest	24.48	0.43	71.5	49.3	176.5	12.2	37	169	516	60	0.19	
Lowest	7.01	0.22	6.0	13.1	53.7	0.0	6	1	9	3	0.00	
TOMATOES												
Highest	14.20	0.35	23.0	59.2	148.3	6.5	36	68	1938	53	0.63	
Lowest	6.07	0.16	4.5	4.5	58.8	0.0	5	1	1	0	0.00	
SPINACH												
Highest	28.56	0.52	96.0	203.9	257.0	69.5	88	117	1584	32	0.25	
Lowest	12.38	0.27	47.5	46.9	84.6	0.8	12	1	19	0.5	0.20	

Source: Firman E. Bear Report, Rutgers University.[1]

Our polluted air and water and the personal stresses we experience every day are some of the other influences that deplete our body's nutrient reserves. These elements are also some of the major causes of free radicals in our body's. It's important that to live a healthier and happier life, we need to supplement our diets.

One more piece of information that shows the progressive decline in the mineral content of farmlands in the United States is the data you see in Table 20.2. In a four-year study of crops grown in 11 states, researchers found that the mineral content of these crops progressively dropped from one year to the next. The total decline (the difference in the mineral content of crops between the beginning and the end of the study) is shown by the negative percentages in the first column.

As discussed in Appendix C, minerals are very crucial to the proper function of the body and mind. Because minerals are water soluble, they don't get stored in the body for too long (unless they are, of course, part of tissue structure like calcium in bones and teeth). Most get flushed out of the body within 24 hours. For this and the reasons given on pages 244-245, you should not only try to eat a balanced meal as often as possible but also include quality mineral and vitamin supplements with your meals.

Table 20.2 Decline of The Trace Elements in Corn

Element	% change	Beginning	Ending
Calcium	-41%	.047%	.025%
Phosphorous	-8%	.26%	.24%
Potassium	-28%	.34%	.245%
Sodium	-55%	.022%	.01%
Magnesium	-22%	.0128%	.10%
Iron	-26%	21.20 ppm	15.70 ppm
Copper	-68%	2.56 ppm	.82 ppm
Zinc	-10%	22.01 ppm	19.90 ppm
Manganese	-34%	4.88 ppm	3.23 ppm

Source: Dr. H. DeWayne Ashmead. Conversation on Chelation and Mineral Nutrition[2]

Something You Should Know About Supplements

The food industry has not been regulated by the federal government* in the way drugs are regulated.[1] As a result, what you see on food labels is not necessarily what you get. Until new food labeling reform took effect in May 1995, some food manufacture used to put such nonsensical labeling as "no cholesterol" on plant-extracted oils, cereals and other nonanimal-derived foods. Cholesterol is found only in animal products such as milk, eggs and meats. Labeling like this, besides being irrelevant, was misleading.

Even now, what you read on vitamin, mineral and other supplement labels may not truly reflect the content or quality of the nutrients. In other words, unless you buy your supplements from a highly reputable company, chances are you are wasting your money.

Let's see what could happen to some of these supplements. Refining minerals from ores and synthesizing or extracting vitamins from plant or other sources is a highly capital intensive (or costly) process. As a result, only giant companies, such as Eastman Kodak and Hoffmann-La Roche in this country and Takeda Chemical Industries and others in Japan manufacture the raw materials for the supplements you use.[3]

These giant companies serve as sources to the various vitamin companies, contract manufacturers and layers of middlemen. Although some of the reputable vitamin companies try to maintain their image by providing the best ingredient formulations they can, what happens to the vitamins that go through the middlemen and

---

* See "Food Labeling Reforms" on page 9 for changes that have taken place since 1990.

even contract manufacturers is often a matter of guesswork.

A contract manufacturer, for example, may put together products for any company that places an order with him. Since his name is often not on the labels, he may not adhere to the rigid quality control that a company with its reputation on the line might. To cut costs, he also may use inferior raw materials as well as cheap fillers in his formulations. This is often reflected in the wide price differences you see among various vitamin and mineral supplements in your local health food or drug store. Those that cost more are usually the better products.

Similarly, a middleman's concern is in getting the raw materials from the original manufacturer as cheaply as he can. Then he sells them to vitamin companies, contract manufacturers or other middlemen for a good profit. The original suppliers have no control over the quality of the raw materials once they have sold them. How these materials are handled, processed or formulated is up to the middlemen, contract manufacturers or vitamin companies.

Since most of the vitamins are very sensitive to oxygen, light, moisture and heat, they could get damaged during storage, processing or formulation. Therefore, to maintain the integrity of the raw materials, your vitamin and contract manufacturers will have to have a very high standard of inventory control. This can be done by purchasing only the quantities they are going to use immediately or by adhering to first-in, first-used inventory control methods. Storing and processing them away from damaging moisture, heat and light is also important.

In other areas, companies that pride themselves on providing the best products to the end user also make sure that they use the best binders. Equally important are the dispersion and uniformity of the ingredients in the carrier medium as well as the compression of the tablets or capsules formed from these products. If the end products, such as those you take in a pill, are too tightly compressed or are inaccessible to the digestive enzymes because of the type of fillers used, they will simply pass through your body without getting processed and absorbed. Some of them can also settle out on the digestive tract, causing local irritation and other complications.

Finally, companies that can stand behind their products try to ensure maximum shelf life in their products by making certain that they are packaged and sealed in containers that can affect neither the potency nor the longevity of the products.

This can ensure that what is being claimed on the labels is 100% accurate. All these precautions cost money, and you see them reflected in the prices of the products. So if you want the best products, you'll have to pay the price. Figure 20.1 offers a summary of what was just discussed regarding the various routes vitamins and

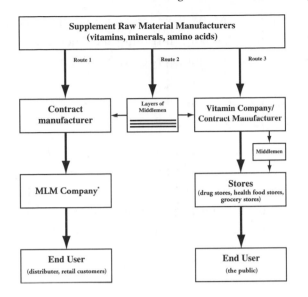

Figure 20.1 Various Routes Your Supplement and Ingredients Could Take
*Multi-level Marketing Company.

minerals as well as the finished supplement products could take before they reach the consumer.

Currently there are generally two major routes or distribution channels for nutritional products. The one marked Route 1 represents multi-level companies. These are companies that manufacture or have their products manufactured by contract manufacturers and sell them to independent distributors who in turn use as well as sell them directly to the public. Route 3 depicts the traditional distribution channel. Through this path, nutritional products go from the vitamin companies or contract manufacturers to stores (such as grocery, drug or health food stores) which in turn sell them to consumers. General Nutrition Center (GNC) is a franchise company that is similar to an MLM company. Instead of using independent distributors, GNC employs independently operating stores to sell its products.

The major difference between the two routes is that the nutrients that go through Route 3 not only could have been handled by a number of middlemen both before and after their formulations by manufacturers but also could stay longer in storage or on store shelves before they reach the end user. This practice could affect the potency or viability of the products.

On the other hand, those nutrients that go through Route 1 are not usually handled by middlemen; and once they are formulated as supplements, they are immediately shipped to the MLM company, which in turn ships them to the end consumers. With this route, both the distributor and retail customer can get quality products whose nutrient integrity and potency are still intact.

Do You Need To Supplement?
Here Are the Reasons Why You Should.

As mentioned earlier, we often run into people who seem to think that if they eat balanced meals they will not need supplements. Unfortunately, as much as we would like to believe in such a simplistic belief, there are many reasons, why we need to incorporate supplements as part of our daily meals. The following statements will help you deal better with people who seem to think that supplements are unimportant in their diet.

1. Americans get everything but a balanced meal. According to government surveys, people in this country are deficient in a number of key vitamins and minerals. There are many reasons for this problem, including a change in the lifestyle of people: eating on the run, consuming too many refined foods, more single people and unattended children, more working couples and absorption problems—particularly with the elderly.

2. The nutritional content of foods varies widely because

    a. minerals are not uniformly distributed throughout the United States. The mineral content in foods varies depending on where foods are grown. For instance, selenium is one of the most important nutrients, both to human and animal health. It has been found that this mineral is not uniformly distributed in this country or elsewhere in the world.[10,11] Thus, to take advantage of the health-giving properties of selenium, we should include supplements that contain this mineral.

    b. some of the agricultural lands in this country have long been depleted of their mineral content, and as a result, foods grown in these lands may be low in mineral content.[12,13,14] This is evidenced by the tremendous variation in the mineral content of vegetables shown in Table 20.1 and the decline in the mineral content of the soils as shown in Table 20.2.

    c. fruits and vegetables are picked before they have fully matured; consequently their vitamin and mineral as well as their carbohydrate content may not be as high it could be.

    d. shipping, storage, canning, cooking and processing can destroy or remove some of the nutrients in foods. This means that if you are one of those people who use canned and prepackaged foods frequently, you may not get all the nutrients that you normally obtain from fresh foods.

3. environmental pollution and mental and physical stress can deplete our tissue nutrient reserves. As a result, many of us may need more nutrients than what are ordinarily found in our daily meals.

4. as we age, our gastrointestinal tract's ability to break down and process food slows down, and consequently the minerals and vitamins that are naturally found in grains and other foods may be poorly processed. This means that we not only need to increase our intake of vitamins and minerals as we get older but also have a better way of delivering them into our system—like the chelation technology some companies use to formulate their products.

5. research indicates that when certain nutrients are taken in higher amounts, they have many health-giving properties. One way of ensuring this benefit is, of course, with quality supplements.

6. supplements are a good way of minimizing obesity. What this means is that to have higher amounts of vitamins and minerals, you would need to consume larger quantities of carbohydrates and protein-based foods—because vitamins and minerals are bound to these foods. This practice could bring with it many unwanted health problems, including obesity. Taking quality supplements decreases the risk of overeating to get all required nutrients.

7. as we age, the production of enzymes, hormones and other digestive chemicals is lowered. Quality supplements (vitamins, minerals and amino acids) may help sustain the production of these key body substances.

8. as we age, our bodies are more susceptible to free radical oxidation, which can lead to lowered immunity and other health-related conditions. The inclusion of quality antioxidant supplements (beta carotene, vitamins C and E, selenium, etc.) may help a person deal with these problems more effectively.

9. even if you are one of those rare people who eat well-balanced meals, supplements may act as a security blanket—a standby against a missed or insufficient meal.

10. finally, don't expect supplements to do what medicine does for you—make your headache go away or heal a wound. What supplements can do for you is create an environment in which your body can function better and look and feel healthier.

The Safety Issue of Vitamin and Mineral Overdose

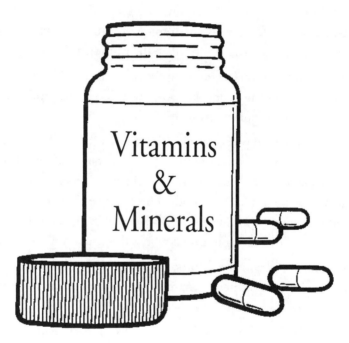

Know enough to allay your fears and exercise caution when necessary.

CHAPTER 21

Do You Have To Worry About
A Vitamin or Mineral Overdose?

Many distributors are concerned about the possibility of a vitamin or mineral overdose. They worry particularly if they take a large number of products on a daily basis. This concern, often associated with taking drugs, is a legitimate one. But as you'll see below, it's unlikely you would consume so much that your life would be threatened. We hope that this chapter will help alleviate your fears and make you aware of your limitations and any potential problems that may come about from taking too many vitamins and minerals. Before we get into the actual discussion of vitamin and mineral toxicity, however, let's talk about some basic guidelines.

One, remember that anything, including water, can be dangerous when taken in excess. So unless a dosage is prescribed by your physician, always stick to the amounts recommended on the labels. Try to eat healthful and wholesome foods as much as possible.

Two, unlike drugs, which can become toxic at higher intake levels, vitamins and minerals are tolerated over very wide dosage ranges. This is primarily the reason, as shown in Table 21.1, why there are such high mortality rates from drug overdoses, while there are none from vitamin supplement overdoses. Drugs don't become incorporated into tissues or have biochemical roles in the way vitamins and minerals do. These foreign substances, as soon as they have done their job, are broken down and, it is hoped, are removed from the system. To the organs (liver and kidneys) responsible for processing them, drugs can be burdensome.

Three, vitamins and minerals are nutrients. They are involved in a wide range of metabolic activities—from the conversion of food into energy to building tissue and other structures. So they are constantly used up, the rate of usage being higher if you have a stressful situation or other physiological conditions. Except perhaps for the fat-soluble vitamins, most of the other vitamins and minerals don't get stored in the body.

Four, as explained below, to develop a toxic level of vitamin or mineral overdose, you'd have to be taking the supplement for a long time. Not to say that you would do it, but if you're an adult, a onetime ingestion of a large amount of vitamins is very unlikely to cause harm to your body.[1] Before you take any higher doses than those recommended for each product, though, do consult your physician and use Tables 21.2 and 21.3 as your guide.

Having said all this, let's talk about the potential problems with some of the vitamins and minerals.

Common Vitamins and Minerals That Potentially Cause Problems When Taken at Considerably Higher Doses Than the RDA and for a Long Period of Time

In the literature, vitamins A, C and D and a few B vitamins are cited as causing problems when taken in large doses and for a protracted period. Among the minerals, iron, magnesium, selenium, iodine and zinc may cause some unwanted side effects. Let's look it each of these substances closely.

Vitamin A is normally found in dark green vegetables, dairy products, organ meats and fish oil. Vitamin A, an excellent antioxidant, is also very important for the healthy function of the body. The largest reserve of this vitamin is found in the liver, where up to 1,000,000 International Units (IUs) can be stored, evidently without side effects.[3] But as shown in Table 21.1, the minimum toxicity level is 25,000 to 50,000 IUs. The adult RDA is only 5,000 IUs.

According to a recent report released from Boston University School of Medicine, vitamin A dosage above 10,000 IU per day can cause birth defects. This study was based on a study of more than 22,000 pregnant women. If you are pregnant, keep your vitamin A intake below 10,000 IUs. Beta carotene has not been found to cause adverse effects. The body converts it into vitamin A as it needs it. Both vitamin A and beta carotene are fat soluble.

The symptoms of vitamin overdose when this occurs are chapped lips, headache, hypertension, dry skin, swollen liver and aches and pains. The symptoms go away once the person stops consuming the vitamin. According to Dr. Michael Rosenbaum, coauthor of *Super Supplements,* vitamin A overdose is extremely rare.[4] Nevertheless, use the figures in Table 21.2 as your reference to ensure that you're within a healthy dosage range.

Vitamin C is a water-soluble vitamin, and you should not be concerned about toxicity. However, reports have popped up about some side effects when the vitamin is taken at high doses. Some of these are related to gastrointestinal discomfort such as gas, bloating and diarrhea. Others pertain to the formation of kidney stones.

Table 21.1 Comparative Causes of Death—Annual Average in the United States.[2]

Adverse Drug Reactions	60,000 to 140,000
Automobile Accidents	39,325
Food Contamination	9,100
Boating Accidents	2,064
Household Cleaners	24
Acute Pesticide Poisoning	12
All Vitamins	0
Commercial Herbal Products	0

Oxalic acid is a by-product of vitamin C metabolism which, along with uric acid in those who are susceptible, may lead to the formation of stones in the kidneys. Large doses of vitamin C are reported to suppress the elimination of aspirin and other drugs.[5] There are also researchers who disagree with these assertions.[6,7]

Vitamin D is important for the formation and growth of strong bones because the absorption of calcium, key for bone development, is facilitated in part by this vitamin. However, being fat soluble, vitamin D can also accumulate in the body, particularly in the liver.

The problem associated with a high consumption of the vitamin is that your body could end up with more calcium than it needs, which incidentally happens very rarely. The concern is more in not getting enough of this important mineral. In any case, if and when it happens, the affected individual may experience confusion, kidney trouble, weakness or lethargy and an abnormal function of the heart.

The minimum toxicity dose is five times the RDA, or 2,000 IUs. Anything over 1,000 IUs, if taken for several weeks, may show some signs of toxicity in the body.[8] So, if you're concerned about this vitamin, you may want to add up all the vitamin D in the supplements you're taking and see whether it comes to anywhere near this amount.

Niacin, an important B vitamin, when taken at much higher doses than the RDA, can have many side effects, including redness and warm, tingling and itchy feelings in the skin, increased blood sugar levels and increased production and secretion of uric acid, which can lead to the formation of gout. Although doctors occasionally recommend as high as 1,000 mgs for heart patients to increase their HDL (the good) cholesterol, amounts as low as 100 mgs have resulted in the common niacin flush.[9,10]

Pyridoxine (vitamin B6) has had its own share of side effect stories when taken at super high levels. Side effects range from a tingling sensation in the body (also called "pins and needles" or "sensory neuropathy") to a loss of balance and coordi-

Table 21.2 Quantitative Evaluation of Vitamin Safety[13]

Vitamin	Recommended Adult Intake[a]	Estimated Adult Oral MTD*
Vitamin A	5,000 IU	25,000 to 50,000 IU[†]
Vitamin D	400 IU	1,000 to 2,000 IU[††]
Vitamin E	30 IU	1,200 IU
Vitamin C	60 mg	2,000 to 5,000 mgs[b]
Thiamin (B1)	1.5 mg	300 mgs
Riboflavin	1.7 mg	1,000 mgs
Niacin	20 mg	1,000 mgs
Pyridoxine (B6)	2.2 mg	2,000 mgs[c]
		200 mgs[c]
Folacin	0.4 mg	400 mgs[d]
		15 mgs
Biotin	0.3 mg	50 mgs
Pantothenic Acid	10 mg	10,000 mgs

*Minimum toxic dose—the smallest dose of a nutrient that has been shown to be harmful when taken over a period of time.

[†]If you are pregnant keep your intake of vitamin A below 10,000 IU.

[††]This figure is from Wardlaw and Insel's book, *Perspective in Nutrition*, 2d ed., St. Louis: Mosby, 1993, p. 363. John Hathcock in *The Nutrition Debate*, eds. Gussow, J. and Thomas, P., published by Bull Publishing, Palo Alto, Calif. (p. 303), on the other hand, puts the minimum toxicity dose for vitamin D for adults at 50,000 IUs. The conservative figure given by the previous authors is chosen here for greater safety.

[a] The highest of the individual RDA (except those for pregnancy and lactation) or the U.S. RDA, whichever is higher.

[b] To produce slightly altered mineral excretion patterns.

[c] For antagonism of some drugs; 2,000 mg for most adults.

[d] For antagonism of anticonvulsants in epileptics; 400 mg or more for most adults.

nation. For some of these conditions, the amount of pyridoxine consumed has to be upwards of 2,000 mgs or more per day. Although some scientists have reported doses as low as 50 mgs causing side effects, others have reported the absence of the problems even at doses as high as 200 mgs.

Iron is very important for our health because blood, the conveyor of oxygen, cannot form without this mineral. Women between the ages of 13 and 40 have to be watchful of their iron intake, as they tend to lose quite a bit of blood through menstruation. Large doses of this mineral, however, can also be toxic to blood vessels and a number of organs in the body. More than any other nutrient, iron has caused deaths from overdose in children. This happens mainly in unattended children who open and consume their mother's iron pills. Be careful how you store any iron supplements. In California from 1987 to 1993, there were 20 iron poisoning deaths of children who accidentally took large doses of iron pills.[11]

Table 21.3 Quantitative Evaluation of Mineral Safety[13]

Mineral	Recommended Adult Intake [a]	Estimated Adult Oral MTD*
Calcium	1,200 mg	12,000 mg
Phosphorus[b]	1,200 mg	12,000 mg
Magnesium	400 mg	6,000 mg
Iron	18 mg	100 mg
Zinc	15 mg	500 mg
Copper	3 mg	100 mg
		<3 mg[c]
Fluoride[d]	4 mg	20 mg
		4 mg[e]
Selenium	70 mcg	1,000 mcg
Iodine	0.15 mg	2 mg

*Minimum toxic dose—the smallest dose of a nutrient that has been shown to be harmful when taken over a period of time.

[a]The highest of the individual RDA (except those for pregnancy and lactation) or the U.S. RDA, whichever is higher

[b]As the orthophosphate ion.

[c]For people with Wilson's disease (because these people lack the enzyme that processes copper).

[d]As fluoride ion.

[e]Level producing slight fluorosis of dental enamel.

Finally, **selenium** over 1,000 mgs, **zinc** over 500 mgs and **iodine** in excess of 2,000 mgs may have a compromising effect on the body.[12] For all these minerals, as well as with the rest of the essential nutrients, try to stay within the recommended ranges. May you have good health and success in all your endeavors!

PART X
The Amino Acids

Protein Foods

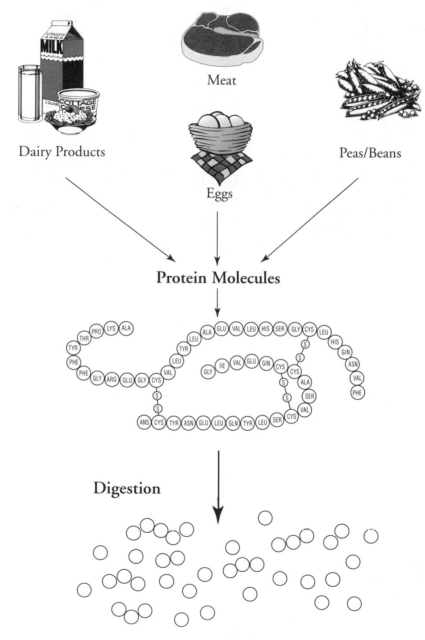

Dairy Products

Meat

Eggs

Peas/Beans

Protein Molecules

Digestion

Amino Acids

CHAPTER 22
The World of Amino Acids

Not too long ago, when people talked about food, they talked about carbohydrates (or starch), fats, vitamins, minerals and proteins. When they thought of protein, they thought of steak, milk, cheese, eggs and bacon. For a layperson, amino acids were never part of his/her every day dietary vocabulary.

Ten or fifteen years ago, if you were an iron-pumping athlete, you probably heard about protein powders. Perhaps you used one occasionally to supplement the mound of eggs, fruits and carbohydrates and the carton of milk you consumed every day. Ten or fifteen years ago, even as an athlete, you probably never heard of protein being classified as whole protein, partially digested protein (peptides) or free form amino acids.

Now, even if you are not an athlete, all you need to do is go to your local health food store and browse through the food supplement section. You'll find an incredible array of amino acids that come as powders, as individual tablets or capsules and as partially digested or part of a whole protein. You'll come home thinking you're amidst an amino acid revolution of which you have not been aware.

This seemingly sudden explosion of amino acids in our lives is a result of several years of research that sought to understand the function and chemistry of the brain. For instance, until a decade ago, there were no more than a dozen known brain chemicals (neurotransmitters). Now there are over 50. Not too long ago, scientists believed that the blood-brain barrier (a membranous "foolproof" tissue of cells that protects the brain from poisons that may come along with blood) would allow only oxygen and selective nutrients into the brain. Recently it has been found that besides these nutrients, it will allow others to pass through as well.

Some of these are amino acids that serve as parent substances to many neurotransmitters. These chemicals are responsible for such things as your mood changes, your ability to fall asleep and your sex drive. If you have become a victim of depression or some psychiatric disorder, you may not have to take prescription drugs or chemicals to deal with these problems. Instead, you may need to take amino acids. This is just the tip of the amino acid iceberg. As researchers make more inroads in this area, your treatment of or immunity from diseases will be primarily through proper nutrition. Before we discuss this important new area further, let's first understand how the body breaks down proteins from the food you eat and utilizes the resulting amino acids.

The Making and Distribution of Amino Acids in the Body

No matter what their sources, all protein foods will have to be disassembled into their components (amino acids) before they become usable by the body. That job of disassembly, or breakdown, is left to the enzymes (proteins themselves) found at various stages in your digestive tract—mainly the stomach and the small intestine. Once the proteins are broken down, the resulting amino acids are small enough to slip through the intestinal wall and be swept up by the bloodstream that brings them to the liver.

The liver is a master distribution center in which all the nutrients are temporarily stored and from which they are rerouted to various parts of the body later. The liver can sometimes be filled to capacity, in which case the nutrients just stay in the blood going around and around until they are picked up by various tissue cells (skin, muscles or brain tissues) that need them. In the case of amino acids, once they enter the cells, they have to be reassembled into the protein that fits that particular tissue.

For example, skin cells have to sift through the hundreds of amino acid molecules that are there and construct a protein specifically designed to meet their needs: a collagen fiber, a hair or a new skin cell. The same thing is true for muscle cells that make muscle fibers and the bone marrow that makes the hemoglobin in the red blood cells. The amazing thing about all this is that although there are only 20 amino acids that the body utilizes, the order in which these amino acids are fitted, the frequency with which one or more amino acids are used and the length of amino acid chains determines the character of a tissue. For instance, in hair, nails and, to some extent, skin, the sulfur-containing amino acids cysteine and methionine predominate.

All these are dictated by the master substance, DNA. How DNA decodes or transcribes such tangible entities as hair, nails and skin from its over 100,000 microscopic library of genes is a fascinating and somewhat complicated process. For now, however, just remember that fundamentally you are a blonde or a brunette, brown or blue eyed, dark or fair skinned because of your genes. The health and appearance of these respective features depend on the amount and quality of foods (particularly the amino acids) you have in your diet.

The words *amount* and *quality* are very important when it comes to proteins. As you know, there are many different sources of protein. There are meat (like beef, poultry, fish, pork), dairy product (milk, cheese), egg, legume, and cereal sources. The amino acid amounts (particularly the essential ones, discussed in Chapter 23 on page 265) in each one of these products differ widely.

Regarding quality, whey (a cow's milk by-product) has the highest biological value*—95% (eggs, 94%; red meat, 80%). Although eggs as a protein source are excellent and red meat is good, they are fraught with danger. With eggs, you have to worry about cholesterol. With red meat, you find saturated fats, preservatives and sluggish digestibility, which have bad health ramifications, including constipation and possibly colon cancer.

Without supplements, along with steak or eggs you will have to eat vitamin- and mineral-rich foods and hope that all the necessary nutrients will be extracted from these various foods, get absorbed and end up in the cells at the same time so that the synthesis of the appropriate protein will take place. This may or may not happen. If it doesn't happen, all the amino acids that got into the cells may not be utilized. The body uses whatever necessary nutrients are available to meet some critical needs, such as synthesizing an important enzyme, and just skips the less essential processes.

Once they are in the cells, the amino acids will have to be utilized immediately, or else they get eliminated. They don't hang around waiting for many minerals and vitamins to come blasting through a cell membrane and help them get metabolized, which, incidentally, brings us to the quality of protein you need to consume.

Quality, in this regard, pertains to the number of essential amino acids (those nine or so amino acids your body is not capable of producing) a particular food source provides you. For example, most legumes and cereals are not a great source of protein because they contain fewer of the essential amino acids. On the other hand, soybeans, dairy products and meat are a great source because they are rich in the essential amino acids. The more essential amino acids you have, the greater the freedom the body has to make all kinds of important health-providing tissue or blood proteins.

To illustrate the significance of this, let's say you have a recipe for a particular size cake. The recipe calls for 5 measuring cups of sugar, 12 cups of flour, 10 eggs and 2 cups of butter. Say you have, instead, only 3 cups of sugar, 15 cups of flour

---

*Refers to the percentage of protein available to the body.

and more eggs and butter than you need. You can never make this cake exactly as the recipe calls for because you don't have enough sugar. The fact that you have an extra amount of flour is irrelevant. You either have to throw out all the ingredients or reduce the size of the cake.

When you don't have all the essential amino acids in your diet the same thing can happen in your body. If the cells don't have all the amino acids that call for a strong, lustrous hair recipe, they simply abandon that "project" (or make a weak, tired looking one from what they have at hand). Or, they may use these ingredients to make some simpler, but just as important, molecule like an enzyme or a hormone. In either case, the hair still suffers because of a shortage of the ingredients necessary to make it.

Incidentally, the simple example above also illustrates why doctors first look for telltale signs in the skin and hair when studying a disease or nutritional deficiency that is not expressed elsewhere in the body. Because having beautiful skin or hair is low in the order of importance as far as your body goes, they are the first to suffer when you have a disease or nutritional deficiency. Other critical needs such as the synthesis of hemoglobin, a digestive enzyme or some other protein, for instance, takes precedence over other less essential needs. This is how the body manages life in its propensity to sustain it.

Metabolic Pathways

Another way of looking at how the body allocates food when there is a limited amount of it is to look at the metabolic pathways. Amino acids are perhaps the most versatile of all the nutrients. Besides serving as structural (building blocks) and functional (enzymes and hormones) components in our body, they are used as precursors to many other biological molecules that contribute to your health, well-being and longevity.

How well all these other end products are met is to a large degree determined by how well your body is supplied with raw materials (amino acids). For instance, norepinephrine (NE) is a neurotransmitter synthesized by the brain (and by the adrenal gland), and it serves to increase blood flow in the arteries. It also serves as a relaxant of certain muscles and in enhancing mental keenness and long-term memory. NE is produced by the brain from two amino acids known as phenylalanine and tyrosine, where the former acts as the precursor to the latter. Any significant drop in the production of NE can affect a person's behavior as well as performance. A severely low level of NE can lead to depression and anxiety. Similarly, tryptophan serves as a precursor to niacin (vitamin B3) and the sleep-inducing brain chemical called serotonin. In the event that your diet is short of niacin, your body can naturally make this important vitamin from tryptophan. Now suppose you don't have enough of the amino acid (and vitamin B3) in your diet. The end result can be insomnia, depression and other mental and physical disorders we covered under niacin.

The point of these two examples is to show that amino acids, besides having a role as building blocks of proteins, have many metabolic functions. Your having sufficient amounts of these substances, along with the necessary cofactors (vitamins and minerals), is very important to achieving optimal health. In the above two metabolic processes, vitamins C and B6 are the cofactors. Any condition (such as alcohol, cigarettes, antibiotics, stress, coffee, contraceptives) that destroys or interferes with the absorption of these vitamins can also curtail the production of serotonin, niacin or norepinephrine.

In biochemistry, the various routes one or more substances can take are referred to as "metabolic pathways." The object of a good nutrition program is to avail the body of sufficient amounts of nutrients to attain all the metabolic activities. This means that you have to have not only sufficient quality proteins to meet all your critical needs but also enough to meet other biologically less important ones such as your skin, hair and nails. In the absence of good nutrition, these tissues suffer the most.

CHAPTER 23
The Essential Amino Acids

Amino acids are the basis of life. From your oxygen-carrying hemoglobin to the thousands of enzymes that catalyze the multitude of metabolic processes to the various tissues and chemicals that make up your body, amino acids play a crucial role. In addition, current research in medicine and biochemistry is showing the importance of amino acids in areas of health that were never considered before. These range from the use of amino acids in fighting jet lag, curbing appetite and relieving arthritis to fighting free radicals, soothing pain and a number of other health-related problems. (See Chapters 24 and 25).

There are 20 amino acids in all living things. Of these, about 11 are synthesized by the human body. The other nine or so have to be imported from outside. Since your body cannot make these internally from other foods, they are called *essential amino acids*. These amino acids must be obtained from the foods you eat. Let's see what each of these nutrients can do for you.

Arginine

Although arginine is not considered an essential amino acid for adults, growing children and certain athletes need it because it's believed to be involved in the activation and release of growth hormones (GHs) from the pituitary gland. GHs are important agents for increasing body size and muscle mass, as well as for metabolizing body fat. Both in humans and laboratory animals, arginine was found to have stimulatory effects on the immune system, making the subjects studied less susceptible to infectious diseases and cancer.

In addition, arginine is the parent molecule to spermine and spermidine, important substances that enhance male fertility. Reportedly as much as 80% of arginine in males is found in the seminal fluids. Because arginine is an important component of collagen, supplements of the amino acid were found to increase wound healing. In other areas, arginine has been found to have uses in relieving kidney disorders, in weight reduction and in the detoxification of ammonia. Arginine is not recommended for growing children or pregnant or lactating women.

Histidine

One of the benefits of this essential amino acid is its use in the treatment of rheumatoid arthritis, ulcers, excessive acidity and anemia. It can also help you in the production and flow of digestive juices, the production of blood cells and the repair and growth of tissues. In addition, histidine has been known to reduce tension and anxiety, thus bringing calm and peacefulness to your life. Pregnant women who suffer from nausea and heartburn can benefit from this amino acid.

Whenever your histidine level is low, mental disorders such as paranoia, loss of appetite and lethargy, excitability and irritability can take place in your life. This apparently is due to histidine's ability to suppress some of the stress or anxiety-inducing electrical activities (called beta waves) of the brain.

In the immune system, histidine acts as a precursor to histamine, a chemical that is secreted by the mast cells of the skin and the respiratory canals in response to allergens. (See Chapter 25 for more information on this.) This same substance "tames" the immune cells and keeps them from becoming overreactive to harmless substances, which is usually the case with allergic reactions. Women who suffered from an inability to achieve orgasm (or frigidity) have benefited from this amino acid. Histidine is also an important detoxifier of metals from the body because of its chelating ability.

Isoleucine

This essential amino acid is one of the three branched chain amino acids. The others are leucine and valine, discussed below. Aside from its role in energy production and regulation of blood sugar, isoleucine is involved in the synthesis of hemoglobin—the important life-supporting protein.

Leucine

For those athletes who train intensely, the essential amino acid leucine can be an important supplement because it's one of the few amino acids that contribute to the production of energy. When your blood glucose level is low, this amino acid and others are used as an alternative energy source. Contrary as it may sound, however, excessive use of leucine can lead to hypoglycemia. This is particularly a problem with infants who suffer from a disease called leucine-induced hypoglycemia. Other than this, leucine is important in the synthesis of proteins and in healing wounds, skin and muscle tissues.

Lysine

As an important part of bone and skin tissues, the essential amino acid lysine is necessary for proper growth and development in children. In adults, lysine is especially useful to those who are recovering from surgery, healing a wound or mending an injured tissue. Part of its role in bone formation comes from the fact that lysine serves as a transporter of calcium across the intestinal wall. It is also known to aid in mental acuity and the production of energy from fatty acids.

In other areas, lysine is useful in minimizing herpes breakouts and in boosting the immune system. Any significantly low level of lysine in the body can lead to a number of disorders, including loss of energy and concentration, growth retardation, thinning of hair, anemia and complications of the reproductive system.

Methionine

This essential amino acid is one of the few sulfur-containing amino acids that is useful in suppressing free radical activity in the body. This helps slow down the aging process and fights the onset of certain cancers. As an important component of skin, hair and nails, methionine can enhance the strength, appearance and quality of these body parts as well. As a metal chelator, methionine is useful in purging heavy metals like cadmium, aluminum, lead and mercury out of the body. These metals, besides their free radical-generating potential, can cause tension and hyperactivity, skin problems and other complications.

Another important area methionine is involved in is the metabolism of fat. In the liver, this important amino acid increases the production of lecithin, which plays a role in the mobilization of fat from arterial, liver, heart and brain tissues. Indirectly, methionine can also help increase the level of choline—one of the important precursor brain chemicals involved in the synthesis of acetylcholine. Bear in mind, that excessive consumption of alcohol can destroy this important amino acid.

Phenylalanine

Besides its use in lowering the effect of jet lag, discussed in Chapter 24, this essential amino acid has been found helpful in treating depression and in boosting one's energy level. It does this by increasing the activity of the thyroid gland and the secretion of thyroxine—the hormone involved in the metabolism of carbohydrates and fats. The production of insulin and a variety of enzymes is also influenced by this amino acid. The significance of these two pieces of information is that those who wish to lose weight can benefit from a supplement of phenylalanine. Phenylalanine also plays a role in one's sex drive, improved memory and mental disposition.

Dopamine and norepinephrine, two brain chemicals known to heighten one's mental acuity, memory and learning ability, are synthesized from phenylalanine. A corollary to all these is also phenylalanine's role in relieving pain associated with overworked muscles, headache, lower back problems and arthritis.

There's a disease called phenylketonuria (PKU), which affects people who lack the enzyme that catalyzes the conversion of phenylalanine into tyrosine—a precursor of the hormone thyroxine. Those people who have PKU should not take phenylalanine supplements, as it can lead to an excessive accumulation of the amino acid in the body, which can have very serious side effects. Those who take prescription drugs that are MAO (monoamine oxidase) inhibitors should also not take phenylalanine or tyrosine supplements, since these two can lead to very high blood pressure.

Both vitamin C and vitamin B6 are important cofactors for the conversion of phenylalanine to the succeeding brain chemicals. Any consumption of phenylalanine without these vitamins and minerals will not have beneficial results. Instead, that person can have side effects like irritability, headaches and other related symptoms.[1]

Threonine

Although there is not a whole lot known about this amino acid, what we know so far is very important to the health of the skin and teeth and for protein synthesis. All the connective tissue proteins, like collagen, elastin, cartilage and enamel, contain a fair amount of threonine. The nervous system, as well as the heart and the skeletal muscles, also contain this amino acid. In conjunction with aspartic acid and methionine, threonine can help in controlling fat buildup in the liver, heart and arterial walls.

Tryptophan

Tryptophan has many important benefits in our body. One of these is in treating a sleep disorder known as insomnia. Serotonin, the primary brain chemical that induces sleep and influences moods, is derived from tryptophan. A sufficient production of serotonin can also help you release tension and stress that may have accumulated throughout the day. Because migraine headache is sometimes triggered by anxiety, anger or overexcitement, those who suffer from this malady sometimes find relief from tryptophan.

Tryptophan also functions as an antidepressant and a precursor of niacin, a key B vitamin involved in a number of metabolic processes. For those who suffer from eating disorders, tryptophan has sometimes been found to curb appetite, thus enabling them to control their weight.

Unfortunately, as much as tryptophan has been found to have many benefits, in recent years it has (wrongly) been linked to a disease outbreak called eosinophilia myalgia syndrome (EMS). This disease, characterized by an unusually high white blood cell count, can lead to respiratory disorder, rashes, swelling, fatigue and muscle pain. This happened in late 1989, and in this particular incident, there were also a few deaths. Because of this incident, the FDA issued a recall of all tryptophan supplements.

After months of investigation by the Centers for Disease Control (CDC), the real culprit was found to be not tryptophan itself but a contaminated batch of tryptophan manufactured by a Japanese company. There were 21 deaths that resulted from taking this tainted amino acid. Although the mystery now has been solved, the FDA has not given the green light for manufacturers to supply tryptophan.

Valine

This essential amino acid is the third member of the branched chain amino acids (BCAAs). Leucine and isoleucine are the others, discussed above. These three amino acids are important components of muscle tissue and constitute about 35% of the amino acids found in these proteins.[2] This trio also contributes an important source of energy during intensive exercise. They also help speed up wound healing from burns or surgery. Because of their role in protein synthesis and energy production, the BCAAs contribute to the physical development of children in the formative years. In foods, whey has the highest level of BCAAs.

Words of Caution

Theoretically, you should not have to worry about supplements, because they are food and food-based products. Occasionally there arises a situation in which people are prohibited from taking certain foods and food supplements for specific medical reasons. For this reason, we recommend that you consult your physician before you start any new nutrition or weight loss program.

Regarding amino acids, particularly if you plan to take individually formulated ones, there are certain health warnings or medical conditions that you should be aware of. The following is a summary of information given by Dr. Robert Erdmann in his book *The Amino Revolution,* published by Simon and Schuster, 1987, pp. 50-55.

1. People who take antidepressants containing MAO (monoamine oxidase) inhibitors should not take phenylalanine, tyrosine or tryptophan.

2. Arginine is believed to stimulate herpes breakout and therefore promote its ability to spread. Ornithine does the reverse. Histidine is thought to induce premature menstruation. A high level of this amino acid also tends to increase the intensity of schizophrenia. If you suspect or observe any of these problems, reduce intake or stop altogether.

3. High blood pressure can be lowered with phenylalanine and tyrosine supplements, but do consult your physician before taking these supplements.

4. When in doubt, always talk to an expert.

CHAPTER 24
The Many Roles of Amino Acids in Your Health

Simply speaking, your body is nothing but a well-ordered package of chemicals and fluids. It's these chemicals that influence your emotions, thought processes and mechanical and metabolic functions, as well as your protection level against illness. When you realize that all these are dependent on your diet, you'll come to appreciate and respect the food you eat. Of the many food-derived chemicals found in the body, those made from amino acids are the most prevalent.

Perhaps the most crucial area where amino acids play vital functions is the nervous system. The network of nerves in your brain and in the rest of your body depends on neurotransmitters and electrolytes to transfer information from one cell to the next. This can be processing a thought, recalling stored information or responding to outside stimuli.

The nervous system is built from discrete units of cells called neurons. Each neuron contains a cell body, dendrites (branchlike fibers) and an axon (a long sheathed fiber). Information, or a stimulus, enters a neuron through the dendrites, passes through the cell body and finally is carried away by an axon, which transmits it to the next neuron. At each point where the stimulus enters and leaves a neuron, there exists a gap called a synapse. Under excitation in the form of electrical impulses, this gap is temporarily bridged by a release of neurotransmitters, which are usually stored in tiny sacs at the tip of axon branches.

That, simply speaking, is how your entire body functions as a whole, integrated system and how the brain processes and responds to the hundreds of requests it receives each second. Nearly all the neurotransmitters found in your brain are made from amino acids. You can imagine how terribly paralyzing it could be if you had a severe deficiency of these vital nutrients in your body. Even small deviations from optimum levels can lead to headaches, confusion, depression and other symptoms, such as overexcitement and feelings of euphoria, which we sometimes experience for some unknown reason. Each neurotransmitter is responsible for arousing or inducing a specific mental state—from feeling sleepy to being angry, depressed or happy.

Many of the chemicals that help you manage stress, as well as enhance your sexual functions (discussed later), are also manufactured from amino acids.

Several researchers have found a direct correlation between the quantity and quality of amino acids eaten and the level and activity of the neurochemicals produced by the brain. Thus, having a rich source of quality amino acids, along with the necessary cofactors (minerals and vitamins), can help you maintain a healthy and properly working brain.

Some of the specific areas where amino acids are found to have great benefits are in managing stress, coping with jet lag, alleviating depression and enhancing memory and mental acuity. Let's briefly discuss how each is influenced by the presence of sufficient amino acids in the body.

Amino Acids for Stress Management

To the human body, stress is anything that upsets or interferes with its internal steady state or condition, called homeostasis. Examples of homeostasis vary, from your body temperature (98.6 degrees) to blood contents (water, electrolytes, glucose, proteins, fats and many other components), all of which have to be maintained within rigidly controlled limits. Anything that disrupts these conditions threatens the health and well-being of the individual.

In life, there are many adverse factors that throw the human body off balance. These range from environmental (pollution in air and water, irradiation, food additives) to psychological (worries, internal conflicts, loss of a job or a loved one) and physiological factors (eating excessive amounts of sugar, fats, proteins or salts). Hot and cold weather and bodily injuries such as burns, wounds and surgery are some of the other conditions scientists often lump together and refer to as stress-inducing factors.

Getting stranded in a traffic jam, facing financial pressures, having a bad relationship with a boss or one's significant other and preparing for an event are some of the other factors we often associate with stress. Incidentally, any strong emotional experience, such as love or hate or any negative emotion, can also be stressful to the body. Thus, the expression "hate hurts the hater, not the hated" has a scientific basis as well.

One thing health-disrupting factors have in common is their tendency to interfere with the digestion and absorption of nutrients as well as to speed their depletion from the tissue and blood reserves. When you are under stress, the production and release of many of the gastric juices and intestinal enzymes are curtailed. Under such conditions, people frequently lose their appetite, and when they do eat, the food stays longer in the stomach, causing cramps, diarrhea and gas.

Elsewhere, the body not only is getting insufficient nutrients from the intestinal tract but also begins to mobilize many of its reserves to deal with the stress. Vitamins A, C and E, biotin, inositol, the B-complex group and the minerals calcium, zinc, magnesium, potassium and others become quickly depleted. During this time, the synthesis of proteins slows down while the dismantling of tissues begins as the body needs fats and amino acids for fuel and to meet some critical life-sustaining functions.

Some of the life-sustaining chemicals that are produced by the body during stress are the adrenal hormones. These hormones prepare you to physically flee from danger by increasing your heart rate and raising your blood pressure and metabolism. Thyroxine is one of those essential hormones metabolized in higher concentrations during a stressful situation. This hormone, along with enzymes and other mineral and vitamin cofactors, facilitates the conversion of glucose and fatty acids into energy. With a sufficient amount of thyroxine, cells are able to use oxygen more efficiently, which is so important in a "fight or flight" situation.

The adrenal hormones are synthesized from two amino acids (phenylalanine and methionine) with the help of a number of minerals and vitamins. In a shortage of these amino acids, any of the cofactors or enzymes can limit the production of the adrenal hormones. The result is often a weakened immune system that leaves you open to infections and diseases. Prolonged exposure to stress can also manifest itself as depression, anxiety, insomnia, premature aging, muscular pains and a digestive disorder known as dyspepsia.

During this time your body needs, more than anything else, foods that are rich in amino acids (particularly phenylalanine, tyrosine, methionine and glutamine),* vitamins A, C and E, and all the B-complex vitamins, and the minerals calcium, iodine, magnesium, manganese and potassium. In addition, getting plenty of rest and exercise can help your body ride out the accumulated stress. Serotonin is a sleep hormone synthesized from tryptophan. Having a sufficient amount of this amino acid in your diet can help you sleep well at night.

Since stress is one of the conditions that generates free radicals, you should also not forget to include the supplements or foods in your diet that contain high levels of vitamins A, C and E, selenium and the amino acids cysteine, lysine, methionine and glutathione.

---

* See the section Words of Caution, on page 265.

Amino Acids for Minimizing Jet Lag

Along with being simply tiresome and boring, long-distance air travel can literally and figuratively make you feel out of place. The time differences can throw your biological clock out of whack and make you feel lethargic, irritable, disoriented and foggy headed. This temporary mental and physiological condition is referred to as "jet lag."

In a time when people hop from one time zone to another with such frequency and ease, finding a way to minimize or shorten the effect of jet lag becomes a very important health and business matter.

At the moment, conscientious travelers use a variety of sleep-inducing drugs and opiates to help them have a restful night and be alert and clearheaded the next day. These drugs, in addition to being addictive, could cause a number of side effects. It seems that the best alternatives to these drugs are amino acids and their derivatives. Both glutamine (a derivative of glutamic acid) and phenylalanine are frequently used to fight jet lag. These nutrients stimulate the brain enough to make you alert and less tired after a long flight, a much healthier alternative than drugs.

Amino Acids and Depression

Medically speaking, depression is a feeling characterized by sadness, despondency and a negative outlook on oneself and one's surroundings. Depression can be temporary, lasting only a few hours, or of a long-term nature, in which case it can be very serious and dangerous to one's health. In either situation, the expressed symptoms may vary from anxiety and mood changes to fatigue, sleeplessness, loss of appetite and lack of interest in one's surroundings or activities. In the extreme situation, even hallucination and delusions can occur.

Depression may have some definite causes, such as loss of a loved one, being out of a job or failing an exam. It may also arise from illnesses such as stroke or cancer, hormonal changes (especially in women), excessive use of drugs or heredity. Sometimes, depression may also have a psychological basis—stemming, for example, from poor mental and emotional childhood development.

Many nutritionists and other health professionals, seem to believe, that a deficiency in the proper nutrients and the inability of the brain to use nutrients properly are some of the fundamental causes of depression. Considering the type of organ we are talking about, this seems to be a very valid interpretation.

First, as we said in the previous pages, anything that upsets the homeostasis of the body or any agent that places stress on a person tends to deplete nutrients from the body. The resulting symptoms in the brain tend to be emotional (as in depression) or physical (as in headaches). Because the brain is such an important organ that governs our entire body, any deleterious effect on it also tends to have a paralyzing effect on the rest of the human organism.

Second, it's important to understand that the brain is a very sensitive, most complex, highly nutrient-dependent and yet finicky organ. For example, while most of your other organs and tissues can use fats, proteins and sometimes even alcohol for fuel, the brain is one of the few organs that depends almost exclusively on glucose as its energy source. The brain is only 2% to 5% of your body's weight, yet it consumes 20% to 25% of the fuel in your body.

The various electrolytes (sodium, calcium, potassium, magnesium, chloride, water, etc.) are also essential for the health and proper functioning of the brain. Information between the minute gaps of your brain's 14 billion cells is transmitted via neurotransmitters that are made from the nutrients you eat.

It's self-evident that any major imbalance to these nutrients as a result of stress, alcohol or other drugs, can lead to temporary or long-term brain health problems. For instance, a low level of glucose in the blood can often result in headaches, fatigue, depression, nausea and shaky muscles, while higher levels can lead to hyperactivity, nervousness or jitters. When you are low in electrolytes, you may become light-headed, confused or moody or experience some other behavioral changes. Even some of the degenerative brain diseases such as schizophrenia and Parkinson's disease are believed to be linked to abnormalities in certain brain nutrients.

Depression, whether of long or short duration, is perhaps one of the most common mental ailments, affecting roughly 20 million Americans. Biochemically speaking, it's strongly believed that depression is caused by an insufficient synthesis of the stress-relieving brain chemicals called catecholamines from their amino acid precursors. Adrenaline and noradrenaline are two such chemicals. These hormones influence brain activity and how we mentally react to things around us.

Both of these are synthesized in the brain from tyrosine and L-phenylalanine. Low levels of these amino acids can limit the production of the two brain chemicals. This, in turn, increases the chance of succumbing to depression. Other amino acids, such as DL-phenylalanine, methionine and tryptophan, are also important antidepressants.

Amino Acids for Memory and Keenness of Mind

How the brain stores and retrieves information is not exactly known. Several theories have been advanced to explain how it might work. One of these theories involves messenger RNA* (one of the key molecules found in our cells), which is involved in protein synthesis, cell growth and replication. It is believed that RNA somehow influences the brain cells' ability to store and retrieve information.

Since the formation of RNA is dependent on enzymes and their cofactors, and since enzymes are made up of amino acid precursors, having an adequate amount of these food nutrients should have beneficial results in improving memory. RNA polymerase, the enzyme that makes RNA, is dependent on a substance called spermine, which is produced from the amino acid arginine. Vitamins C and B6 and the minerals magnesium and manganese are important for the formation of spermine from arginine.

The other aspect of memory is not only storage but also transportation of information. That beautiful piece of music you heard, a face you saw, food you tasted or the softest substance you touched all have to be communicated to your brain cells in order for them to be recorded and to be retrieved later. The transportation of these pieces of information is accomplished by means of tiny electrical and chemical currents.

While the electrolytes do the electrical aspect, the neurotransmitters do the chemical part. One of the most important neurochemicals involved in information transfer and storage is acetylcholine. This brain chemical is made from choline—one of the B vitamins derived from lecithin (also called phosphatidyl choline). The enzyme that synthesizes acetylcholine is also dependent on the presence of sufficient amounts of amino acids. It is believed that one of the reasons we lose our memory as we age may have to do with an inadequate formation or loss of activity in this enzyme.

Sharpness of mind is also dependent on the food you eat. The brain as a center of the highest metabolic activities is also an area of your body where there are going to be large amounts of metabolic waste. One of these waste products is ammonia, produced from a metabolic breakdown of protein. Unless ammonia is removed regularly, it can build up in the brain, causing confusion, depression and the inability to concentrate or think clearly. If excess amounts of it are retained, it can lead to irritability, convulsions, nausea and even death.

---

* Short for ribonucleic acid.

Glutamic acid combines with ammonia to produce a harmless end product, glutamine. The latter ultimately converts into urea, which ultimately gets eliminated from the body through the urine. However, because the brain-blood barrier doesn't allow glutamic acid to pass through, nutritionists often recommended glutamine supplements that can get past the barrier. Once in the brain, glutamine converts into glutamic acid and begins its mopping up operation on ammonia.

Amino Acids—The Fountain of Youth

Fundamentally, it's what you put on your skin through metabolic processes that will determine the appearance of your skin and how you feel internally. Yes, nowadays, there are some skin care products that contain remarkable ingredients, which can give you a youthful appearance by retaining the moisture in your skin. This moisture-holding ability of the ingredients can keep your skin appearing soft and supple. What will benefit you even more is the strengthening of the structural aspect (the collagen and elastin matrix) of your skin by consuming the right nutrients in your diet. (See Chapter 5 for more information.)

Amino acids play crucial roles. They are the stuff your skin is made of, and as such, they can serve as the legendary fountain of youth. As we said earlier in the book, one of the causes of aging is the formation of free radicals in our bodies. These free radicals speed the process of aging—for example, the breakdown of collagen and elastin matrices. This condition leaves us susceptible to many health hazards, including cancer and other degenerative diseases.

Not only do amino acids help repair damaged tissues, but also some amino acids can even serve as free radical quenchers and heavy metal detoxifiers. Both free radicals and heavy metals such as cadmium, aluminum, mercury and lead are aging elements. When you supply your body with a rich source of key amino acids like methionine, cysteine, taurine and cystine (the four known amino acid antioxidants) you help it purge itself of these toxic substances.

Cysteine also seems to be the predominant amino acid found in collagen, and this amino acid is very important for the health and appearance of your skin. Zinc is very important for the health of your skin as well. This mineral is critically involved in the synthesis of collagen and in keeping skin soft and flexible. Speaking of flexibility, glycine is another important amino acid that gives the collagen its spring-like properties. Both cysteine and glycine, as well as zinc, help minimize the appearance of stretch marks, which pregnant women often acquire.

The other benefit of amino acids is keeping the digestive system young. It's been said that some of the problems that come with aging may be associated not with not eating the right foods but rather with having a poor digestive system, which slows down with age. Thus, as you get older, one of the best things you can do for yourself is boost the function of your digestive tract. In this regard, amino acids will serve you well. Since the multitudes of enzymes that help you digest your food are made up of amino acids, having adequate amounts of these nutrients will help improve the digestion and absorption of foods.

Furthermore, amino acids are involved in the production of various hormones. Some of these hormones are directly involved in keeping you young. Arginine, for example, is one amino acid that stimulates the pituitary and thymus glands to produce growth hormones, which are important substances that keep muscles and skin youthful. Tyrosine is the precursor of thyroxine, a hormone that helps keep muscle tone and aids development.

CHAPTER 25
Amino Acids and the Immune System

The immune system is perhaps one of the most abused and least understood systems of the human body. Both internally and externally, it's being constantly challenged by thousands of agents such as cancer, bacteria, fungi, viruses, parasites, protozoans and a variety of toxic chemicals. Some of these can be pretty harmless, even beneficial to the body (e.g., those bacteria found in the intestine that help us digest our food), while others can be detrimental to our health, even life threatening.

These potentially harmful agents vary from the common cold, flu and influenza viruses or allergic substances that can make your life miserable to the AIDS (HIV), hepatitis, rabies or polio viruses that are severely life and health threatening. Others, such as the cocci bacteria that lead to meningitis, tonsillitis or pneumonia, or the bacilli that produce leprosy, tuberculosis and many other viruses and bacteria can be equally deleterious to your health and life. Various chemicals (food additives, pesticides, herbicides, etc.) and heavy metals (lead, mercury and cadmium) are some of the recent additions that are also found to cause or lead to health problems.

Some of these agents make their assault on your body via air, water and the food you consume, while others may enter the body through direct physical contact. Regardless of their means of entry or point of contact, your body uses its immune system to a large degree to stave off most of the above intruders. This defensive mechanism can be your skin—a tough oil- and sweat-secreting organ that contains chemicals that have an antiseptic or neutralizing effect on antigens. The tiny hairs and the mucus in the nasal and respiratory tract also help trap and sweep away some of the aforementioned microorganisms. The various chemicals and digestive enzymes in the intestine and gastric juices can also help destroy or deactivate many of the bacteria and viruses that get past the nose and throat.

As we all know, some of these health hazards get not only to our stomach and intestines but also into the cells and fluids in our tissues and organs. They may manage to get through a nick or fissure in your skin or through the soft tissues in the mucous membranes of the nasal and digestive tract. Here is where most of the antigens (foreign matters) suffer a serious blow.

For example, when you cut your skin with a dirty blade you're likely to introduce germs or microbes into the damaged skin. The first response is the production of histamines. This leads to inflammation, swelling and heat. This is followed by the arrival of white blood cells that engulf and destroy the intruders.

As more blood is pumped into the area, some of the phagocytes (white blood cells) and other substances called complement proteins, which have the capacity to dissolve (lyse) the foreign organisms, leak out of the blood vessels and pervade the inflamed tissue.

These above mechanisms are your first line of defense and are sometimes called *innate* or *natural* immunity. The next, perhaps more sophisticated, line of protection is the *adaptive* or *acquired immunity* system. The cells responsible for this line of fortification are a rather prolific and highly specific bunch. The cells of the acquired immune system are divided into *B-lymphocytes* and *T- lymphocytes.* Although both are "born" in the bone marrow, the way they function and come to maturity differs widely. After birth, the B-cells migrate to intestinal tissues and the liver, spleen and thymus glands for full development. The T-cells populate and mature mainly in the thymus gland. Functionally, the B-cells specialize in the manufacture of great quantities of differentiated protein substances called antibodies.

Upon sensitization by antigens (virus, bacteria, etc.), the B-cells multiply and enter the bloodstream to become what are known as plasma cells. It is these cells that produce weapons of mass destruction (antibodies), which have the ability to bind to the surfaces of the antigens and trigger a series of reactions that eventually destroy and remove the invading substance from the body. When you have a cold, the stomach flu or any other infection, a fantastic quantity of antibodies can be released in a matter of seconds.

After a given species of microbes is destroyed, some of the B-cells remain in your body for the rest of your life as memory cells. If you have two or more encounters with the same substance, they can quickly multiply to produce antibodies and destroy it, in some cases before you are even aware of its existence in your body.

The T-cells, on the other hand, simply multiply and directly attack any intruders with their "bare hands," so to speak. They have no ammunition of their own. The T-cells are divided into three groups. The *killer* (cytotoxic) T-cells exist primarily to recognize and destroy foreign substances, including your own cells that may become cancerous. They are the search-and-destroy team of the immune system. Many of them survive their first attack and go on to cause more damage to other existing antigens.

The *helper* T-cells coordinate and facilitate the functions of many of your immune cells, including the B-cells, white blood cells and the killer T-cells. For example, the killer T-cells can function and multiply with great force. The B-cells can gear up their production of antibodies with the assistance of the helper T-cells. Incidentally, HIV (the virus that causes AIDS) thrives by destroying the helper T-cells and thus incapacitating the multiplying and protective ability of the killer T-cells. Under such circumstances, many infectious diseases, including tumor cells, become rampant, posing serious health and life threats.

The third group of the T-lymphocytes is known as the suppressor T-cells. Their function, as their name implies, is to end the production of B-lymphocytes and killer T-cells after an infection or a disease is over. Without this group of cells, the body could go on producing the two cells, wasting unnecessary nutrients and their immune protective forces.

Furthermore, an unchecked proliferation of the killer T-cells in the body could potentially lead to a condition in which it destroys itself (autoimmune disease). These T-cells could begin to indiscriminately attack everything they come in contact with, including your normal tissue cells. For example, rheumatoid arthritis—a crippling disease affecting the joints (wrists, fingers, toes, etc.)—is believed to result from an autoimmune disorder. The production of relative numbers of the helper and suppressor cells is monitored by the prostaglandins, organic molecules that are synthesized from the omega-3 fatty acids we discussed in Chapter 7.

Along with the two main lines of defense (the natural and acquired immune systems), your body is buttressed with a number of antiviral chemical secretions from certain immune cells and with a variety of toxin-mopping vitamins and amino acids acquired from your diet.

Interferons, for example, are protein molecules released by virus-infected cells to coat and protect neighboring cells from further infection by the same or other viruses. There is a strong indication that these protein molecules may also be involved in curtailing the proliferation of cancer cells. As another example, many of the complement proteins mentioned earlier are produced by the macrophages of the white blood cells.

What's interesting in all this is that given the fact that nature has presented us with countless microorganisms as our enemies, it has also endowed us with an almost fail-proof defense system that enables us to face and defeat most of the challenges placed upon us daily. The various lines of defense discussed above, including those memory cells that are put in place so that you won't be sick again from a second exposure to the same strain of microbes, and the many nutrients available to help fortify your immune system can ordinarily assist you in maintaining good health and well-being.

Although the different lines of defense may often be good enough to help us cope with most of the microorganisms and certain cellular errors within our bodies, our modern stressful lifestyle, bad eating habits, the hundreds of toxic chemicals we get from our food, water and air, as well as cigarettes, alcohol and other drugs, can erode the strength and endurance of our immune system. This often seems to be the case when certain individuals catch a cold or the flu more easily and frequently than others and when some HIV-infected individuals die of AIDS sooner than others.

Once the immune system is weakened through abuse and poor dietary practices, the body is more susceptible to infections by any number of microbes, as well as predisposed to the development of cancer. As you might know, cancer is currently the number two cause of death.

It seems that although we have very little control of the polluted city air we breathe and some of the toxic chemicals we get through food and water, we can, through a proper diet, exercise and rest, shield our immune system and ensure our health. According to one nutritionist, cancer and many of the degenerative diseases we have today are preventable by as much as 90%. A good nutrition program and abstinence from many health-threatening habits (such as excessive alcohol, other drugs, cigarettes and stress) will enable us to lessen the onset of many of those diseases.

In short, you can think of your immune forces as a well-fed army. When you have a well-trained and well-fed army, it fights with all its might and strength at the time of an invasion by an aggressor. The same thing is true of your immune system. Wholesome and well-balanced nutrition is the key to your being healthy, feeling strong and staying young.

The Role of Amino Acids and Other Nutrients in the Immune System

It's evident that the quality of your health and well-being will very much depend on the health and integrity of the individual parts that comprise the immune system. These include the health and proper functioning of your skin, nasal and respiratory mucous membranes, the adequate secretion of gastric juices and intestinal enzymes, as well as the strength and sufficient production of the white blood cells, the many complement proteins and the B- and T-lymphocytes. The ability of these individual members to fight diseases or to enable your body to recover quickly from disease, will, in turn, depend on the variety, quality and sufficiency of the food you eat.

In this regard, amino acids along with other essential nutrients (vitamins, minerals, essential fatty acids and carbohydrates) will be of primary importance in keeping your immune system strong and healthy. All the tissues that cover the major entry points (skin, throat, lungs, the nasal cavity), all the immune cells, the antibodies and the various secretions (hormones, interferons, enzymes, complement proteins) depend on amino acids for their development and function. These tissues and chemicals help preserve your health and well- being.

Besides the various microbes that pose threats to our health every day, we also have free radicals, heavy metals (lead, mercury, cadmium, etc.) and other toxins to contend with. Amino acids, both as integral parts of enzyme systems and as individual molecules, have neutralizing and health-preserving functions as well. As mentioned at various points in this book, free radicals not only accelerate the aging process and promote the incidence of cancer in our body, but also disrupt the normal operation of the immune system.

The problem of free radicals with respect to our health ranges from their attacking the various immune cells and deactivating or destroying certain enzymes to heightening our allergic response to different substances in our environment. To use the previous analogy, just as the once strong army of a nation can be weakened (thus making the country vulnerable), when there are forces internally that disrupt its unity, your immune system, too, can become fragile and weak when you have free radicals and other toxins that go around your body and attack the very forces that were meant to defend you.

Amino acids, particularly those that contain sulfur such as methionine, cysteine, taurine, the branched chain aminos like leucine, isoleucine and valine and others, can function both as free-radical quenchers and as heavy metal chelators (molecular traps that grab hold of these toxins and remove them from the body). Glutathione (a three-member amino acid molecule containing cysteine, glutamic acid and glycine) is also a very powerful chelator and free radical scavenger. Glutathione helps boost your immune forces and fight cancer, allergies and premature aging. Glutathione was shown to be directly absorbed into the bloodstream when administered orally.[1] This is in contradiction to the theory that it may get metabolized by digestive enzymes.

When glutathione combines with selenium, you have the enzyme glutathione peroxidase, which is one of the most potent destroyers of superoxide free radicals. These are the most vicious free radicals in the body, and they tend to destroy just about anything they encounter, including the various immune cells. When this happens, not only do you make your body an easy target for various infectious diseases, but you also increase the incidence of cancer and other degenerative conditions with it.

Selenium and amino acids are indeed some of the best known anticancer and immune-boosting agents in our bodys. In the presence of sufficient amounts of these nutrients, our bodies can go on producing immunity-fortifying cells and antibodies while minimizing the occurrence of the degenerative diseases. That is why in areas of the world where there is a low level of selenium in the soil, cancer, heart and other diseases predominate.

Other Nutrients and the Immune System

Besides selenium and amino acids, there are many nutrients that are very important to a healthy functioning of our immune system. For example, vitamin A is very important in cell growth and cell division. We mentioned earlier that the immune cells, including those of the skin and mucous membrane, are some of the most prolific in our body. An adequate amount of vitamin A can therefore be critical to the proper development and multiplication of these health-preserving cells. If you are sick, healing a wound or recovering from surgery, higher doses of this vitamin (preferably the beta carotene version) can be of great benefit to you. Retinol, the pure form of vitamin A, can be toxic when taken in large doses.

Similarly, vitamins C, D and E and all the energy-producing B-complex group are crucial to the health and disease-fighting abilities of the body. For instance, vitamin C is the key nutrient that helps us develop and maintain strong collagen—the fibrous, durable tissue, often referred to as the "glue" that holds everything in us together. In addition, this vitamin is involved in the production and deployment of the various immune cells to wound or infection sites in our bodies.

Vitamin E is another crucial nutrient that helps us maintain a strong immune system. In animal studies, this vitamin was found to increase the antibody-producing ability of immune cells. In humans, it seems, the vitamin's benefit lies in its capacity to neutralize free radicals and therefore help the immune system maintain normal production of the necessary disease-fighting forces in the body. Vitamin D facilitates the formation of healthy bones and therefore the production of precursor immune cells from the bone marrow (white blood cells and B- and T-lymphocytes).

An adequate amount of energy is important for the growth and proper functioning of the immune cells. These cells require energy to move around the body and fight infection or heal a wound. The B vitamins, such as vitamin B6 (pyridoxine), folacin and pantothenic acid, are directly involved in energy production, cell growth and antibody formation.

In addition, minerals such as zinc, copper and iron are also important in the maintenance of a healthy immune system. Zinc is a very versatile mineral that is also involved in the synthesis of RNA and DNA—two important substances in cell growth and division. It goes without saying that high amounts of zinc in your diet will help your body speedily produce the required disease-fighting cells and antibodies. Furthermore, zinc, manganese and copper are the three minerals that function as structural components to an important enzyme system called superoxide dismutase (SOD). These enzymes neutralize the dangerous oxygen free radicals that form during metabolism. Any significantly low level of these minerals can lead to an increased destruction of immune cells as well as body tissues.

Clearly, from the above discussion, a good nutrition program can help create a very strong and formidable barrier between the delicate, highly vulnerable and sensitive tissues of your body and the harsh, dangerous and often life-threatening microorganism world out there.

A good nutrition program can also help minimize the occurrence of cancer and other degenerative diseases such as Alzheimer's, arteriosclerosis and arthritis. Unfortunately, for many of us, a good nutrition habit is a rarity, because convenience and practicality seem to take precedence over living a long, healthy and disease-free life. In our stressful and fast-paced lifestyle, we would rather grab our meals from a fast-food outlet or a sit-down restaurant than prepare a healthy and nutritionally balanced meal.

Every day, the environment (air, water and noise pollution) and our pressured job or work situation put a tremendous amount of stress on our body and health. As if this is not enough, some of us smoke, drink excessively and do other drugs. When you combine these with our fat-rich, processed-and-additive-filled foods, you have one terribly abused and nutritionally deprived body on your hands. For all the above reasons, perhaps now, more than in our ancestors' time, we need a very nutritious and well-balanced diet.

Amino Acids for Your Allergies

Allergic reactions are some of the most common irritating problems for some, a downright misery for others and fatal for a few. Often these problematic physiological expressions happen when one is unaware or unsuspecting. You may be out working in the garden on a beautiful spring day when all of a sudden you realize your nose is itching, your eyes are watering and your throat is gasping for air.

In a different scenario, you may have just returned from hiking in the neighboring woods when you find blistering red rashes covering your arms, legs or wherever your skin has encountered the offending agent. In yet another scenario, for some unknown reason, you may find yourself feeling depressed, moody or experiencing vomiting, diarrhea or a throbbing headache.

All or some of these are examples of your body's overly defensive reaction to allergens (foreign substances, such as pollen, ragweed, cat hair, house dust mites, food, bee stings, etc.). Your immune system has no way of telling a harmful organism, such as a virus or bacteria, from a benign substance, such as a pollen, a speck of hair or the feces of a dust mite. It simply prepares and springs to action whenever it detects foreign protein substances that come in contact with the body. In this regard, you might compare your immune system to an overzealous watchdog that bolts and barks at every moving object within the periphery of your home.

Just as this dog can become terribly obnoxious, irritating or a downright problem to you, so will an immune system that reacts to many harmless substances. For reasons that are still unknown, some people are more susceptible to allergens than others, but the series of events that take place when one has an allergic reaction are invariably the same—similar to what happens when you have an infection by a harmful organism like a virus or bacteria.

Upon entry, the allergens are recognized by the body's defense systems, such as the B-cells, which after a few days produce antibodies and release them to the bloodstream. The newly made antibodies find their way to the mast cells—a special group of cells found throughout the body but highly concentrated in the skin. At the next exposure to the allergen, the antibodies attach themselves to the mast cells and, in conjunction with specialized tissue hormones called kinins, activate the release of histamine contained in them. Histamine is an amino acid-derived compound that produces the characteristic reddening of the skin, watery eyes and sneezing when you are exposed to poison oak or ivy or a pollen.

Some allergic reactions, however, are not as harmless or benign as these. In sensitive individuals, they can be quite a nightmare. The problem with these people is that their bodies "panic" at the slightest exposure to the offending allergen and start producing far too many immune forces (B- and T-cells and antibodies). The production and mobilization of such a great number of forces by the body can result in an almost self-destructive reaction called autoimmune response. In this case, the immune cells begin to attack body tissues. When this happens, the suffering individual can experience headache, depression, irritability, fatigue, diarrhea and sometimes a lung-constricting and chest-tightening, asthma-like symptom. On the skin, conditions such as eczema, hives and inflammatory lesions may develop. Food-related allergens can cause havoc on the intestinal wall, including the insulin and digestive enzyme-producing pancreas.

Because the immune cells tend to concentrate at the points of contact with the allergens—such as the skin, the respiratory channels and the intestinal wall—several remedial measures can be taken. Some of these involve antihistamine drugs. Since histamine secretion in the surrounding tissues is what causes the itch and redness in the skin, watery eyes, sniffling and coughing, as well as diarrhea and vomiting, the use of antihistamine drugs has a relieving and blocking effect. These drugs are merely a quick fix, however, with many possible side effects (such as drowsiness, nausea, loss of appetite and blurred vision).

Through proper nutrition involving amino acids and antioxidants, you can help contain the problems encountered with allergic reactions. In those cases where partially digested proteins may manage to get past the intestinal wall (resulting in a food allergic reaction), having sufficient, quality digestive enzyme-building amino acids will be of great benefit. For example, glutamic acid and histidine can stimulate the production and release of stomach acids as well as the digestive enzymes. Histidine can reverse some of the effects of an allergic response. Ironically, this amino acid, which serves as a precursor to histamines, works by suppressing the production of helper T-cells, one of whose functions is to stimulate the B-cells to produce antibodies. When you have fewer antibodies, you also have fewer of the many problematic symptoms associated with allergic reactions.[2]

Another associated culprit that is believed to heighten a person's sensitivity to allergens is a high level of free radical generation in the body. These substances can not only speed up your aging process and cause degenerative and other health-threatening diseases but also apparently make those predisposed individuals more sensitive to allergic reactions.

Prostaglandins, those rather intriguing and fleeting hormonelike chemicals we discussed in the section Essential Fatty Acids (EFAs) on page 78, have been found to play an important role in the production and activity of the immune cells. One of these substances, called prostaglandin E1 (PGE1), for example, controls the formation of suppressor T-cells. As we have mentioned earlier, the suppressor T-cells control the production of the helper T-cells, which in turn monitor the synthesis of antibodies.

This biochemical chain of events can be thwarted by free radicals that can block the synthesis of PGE1. This means that to have a stronger immune system you need to have many antioxidants. All the free radical-quenching vitamins (A, C, E), minerals (selenium, copper, iron, zinc, manganese), amino acids (cysteine, methionine, lysine) and amino-acid-formulated compounds like glutathione can be very helpful in keeping these biochemical pirates at bay. In addition, the inclusion of phytoantioxidants, discussed in Chapter 15, can be of great benefit.

Glutathione peroxidase, the enzyme produced from glutathione and the mineral selenium, is actually the one that acts as a neutralizer of the free radicals. According to the literature, impressive results have been obtained by using glutathione to reduce the allergic responses experienced by certain individuals.[3]

CHAPTER 26
Amino Acids for Your Heart and Digestive System

Amino Acids for Your Heart

In Chapter 7, we talked about how the accumulation of fats in our blood vessels can lead to heart attacks and other heart disease. We also talked about how certain substances known as HDLs are good because they tend to dredge any accumulating fats from the circulatory system and that LDLs are bad because they encourage the reverse. In our discussion of fats in that chapter, however, we made an important, but not stated, assumption. We presumed that those fats that were moved by the HDLs were either burned, converted into body fat or removed from the body via the liver and the gastrointestinal system.

An amino acid-derived substance called L-carnitine is a key compound that helps us metabolize fats. In the body, L-carnitine is synthesized in small amounts with the help of vitamins B6 and C and iron. It functions by literally towing fat across the mitochondrial membrane so that it can be burned as fuel.

The significance of this nutrient is manifold. One, when you have a sufficient level of L-carnitine and fat is continuously brought into the cells by the HDLs and you're using up energy, you will be able to keep the blood vessels relatively clear of plaque-forming fats. You can imagine what would happen in a reverse scenario. It can be analogous to a traffic jam or a blocked water pipe. When you have a high L-carnitine level in the body, cholesterol and saturated fats will be continuously mobilized and burned.

Atherosclerosis is a degenerative disease that results from the deposition of fat in the arterial walls, impeding the normal flow of blood and nutrients. This condition can lead to the deprivation of sufficient oxygen to various tissues, including those of the heart and the brain. This can result in confusion, weakness, shortness of breath, chest pain (angina), in its mildest form, and a heart attack or stroke, in the worst case.

Atherosclerosis develops gradually. It results partly from your body's inefficient utilization of fat, as when you are deficient in L-carnitine or the enzyme that facilitates the synthesis of L-carnitine.[1] Other risk factors such as smoking, high blood pressure, gender and genetics are also contributors to this debilitating disease.

Early on, besides occasional muscle cramps and pains that you might be experiencing (particularly when you exercise, fast or eat a high-fat diet),* there are generally no outright symptoms to indicate something ominous might be lurking in your blood vessels.

Nonetheless, over time, what seems to be critical is what you do or don't eat on a daily basis. This will determine whether you're going to have clear blood vessels or clogged ones. This includes eating less fat and supplying your body with enough amino acids so that it can make its own L-carnitine or having L-carnitine supplements in your diet.

Since L-carnitine functions primarily as a mobilizer of fat, certain individuals, such as diabetics, alcoholics and overweight people, can benefit from a sufficient quantity of this nutrient in the diet. Diabetes is a disease arising from your body's inability to process glucose—your body's primary source of energy. This often results from a deficiency of insulin (juvenile diabetes), a reduced secretion of insulin or the body's resistance to the action of insulin (adult-onset diabetes) or excessive loss of dilute urine (diabetes insipidus) caused by the failure of a malfunctioning pituitary gland to secret the antidiuretic hormone.

When any one of these conditions occurs, your body mobilizes fat from the tissues to use as fuel. The end result is not only the accumulation of fat in the blood vessels but also the production of incompletely burned (oxidized) fat products, known as ketone bodies, in the cells. The condition is called ketosis. An abnormally high level of ketones in the tissues can be fatal. Fasting or starvation are two of the other situations in which ketosis may develop. L-carnitine can therefore help those who suffer from diabetes to burn fat more efficiently and completely.

Alcohol tends to deplete the body's sugar reserve (which lowers a person's energy level) as well as the amount of fat buildup in the body. Alcoholics and overweight people can thus benefit by L-carnitine's ability to induce the usage of fat as fuel, which at the same time helps them maintain a steady glucose level. These people can not only lose their fat but also have a supply of energy. Several experiments, both here and elsewhere in the world, have shown the beneficial effects of L-carnitine in such cases.

---

* These tend to increase the use of fats as fuel.

Amino Acids for Your Digestive System

The importance of amino acids in your digestion lies in their function as precursors to the many enzymes, hormones and the fast-dividing epithelial cells involved in the processing of food in your gastrointestinal tract. All the enzymes that are secreted by the cells in the lining of the stomach and the pancreas depend on the sufficient availability of amino acids for their synthesis.

One of the few blood-related diseases is one that results from the unavailability of vitamin B12. This disease is called pernicious anemia, and it's caused as much by the lack of vitamin B12 as by the absence of a protein complex called the "intrinsic factor." This substance literally wraps the vitamin and transports it across the intestinal wall. Without sufficient amino acids and the necessary mineral cofactors, the synthesis of this important protein substance can be severely compromised.

CHAPTER 27
Amino Acids and Your Sex Life

The reproductive system is a truly remarkable part of the human body. Think of it. When it works properly, it's the basis of procreation (the seat of life). It's also one of the most fundamental sources of pleasure, the foundation of a good couple relationship, and perhaps the main factor that brings two individuals intensely close, emotionally and physically, to each another. When it doesn't work, it can also be the provenance of one's silent anguish, frustration and pain.

Regarding the above, there's perhaps nothing that undermines a man's masculine self-esteem more than his inability to have sex. It's said that a man prefers to be shot or have any number of other diseases rather than become impotent. Somehow it seems as though a man's entire ego and male identity are wrapped up in his ability to have an erection and to reach an orgasm. A woman, similarly, can suffer from a sexually desolate condition known as frigidity. This problem (an inability to reach orgasm) is reportedly widespread among women. A man may also suffer from a frustrating sexual problem known as premature ejaculation.

For a long time, scientists have attributed these sexual disorders to deep-seated psychological problems. Although this may be the case in certain instances, current research into these and other similar sexual dysfunctions seems to indicate that poor nutrition often may have more to do with it than any mental block or disorder these people may be experiencing. For example, according to one nutritionist, certain amino acids (such as histidine, lysine and arginine) can help reduce or even eliminate the lack of orgasm associated with women. Similarly, men can deal with the problem of impotency, as well as premature ejaculation, by using the right amino acids. Another expert, Dr. Carl Pfeiffer, was able to effectively treat men who suffered from premature ejaculation by using methionine.[1]

Another major problem involving the human reproductive system is infertility. Women, as well as men, can suffer from this condition. To couples who want to have children, it can be one of the most frustrating and financially costly situations—as these individuals often end up spending much money trying to find a cure for their predicament. Perhaps, not surprisingly, some of the infertility problems, too, seem to arise from nutritional deficiencies.

A shortage of amino acids and vitamins as well as many key minerals can often lead to some of the characteristic preconditions that lead to infertility. In men, for instance, infertility is a result of low sperm count or sperm clumping. In one, you have fewer sperm cells, in the other, the sperm cells are knotted together, making them less motile. This means they cannot travel the distance required in the female reproductive canal to reach an egg and fertilize it. Both these conditions were found to have been caused largely by a lack of the necessary nutrients.

Like many of the body chemicals and organic fluids, semen* and sperm cells are made mainly from amino acids, with the help of vitamins and minerals. In this case, the key amino acid was found to be arginine, which serves as a precursor to two key chemicals called spermine and spermidine. These substances were found to have a direct effect on the sperm count, as well as the unclumping (and therefore greater motility) of the sperm cells.[2] Zinc and vitamin C, as well as L-carnitine, were also found to be of great benefit, both in increasing sperm count and in improving the motility of sperm cells.[3] The end result, of course, is improved fertility in the man.

Fructose and prostaglandins are believed to help activate the womb muscles. Fructose, which gives sperm cells energy, and prostaglandins (those hormonelike substances discussed previously) are important constituents of semen. The normal production of both these chemicals is facilitated by testosterone—the male sex hormone. (Testosterone is the substance responsible for the production of secondary sex characteristics, such as the growth of beard and pubic hair and the development of the testes and the penis, as well as for the sex drive.)

In either case, these and the previous situations presuppose that you have to have the necessary precursor nutrients in order for the body to be able to produce healthy and properly functioning sperm cells. All the nutrients (amino acids, fructose, minerals and vitamins) found in the seminal fluid that enable the sperm to move more effectively are dependent on the quality and completeness of the food you give your body. When you have a healthy and properly functioning sexual system, you will be able to have a prolonged and satisfying sex life as well.

Besides poor nutrition, infertility in men can come about from testicular tissue damage, radiation, removal of the prostate gland and sexually transmitted diseases (such as gonorrhea and syphilis) that can render the male reproductive organ ineffective.

---

* Semen—the fluid emitted during ejaculation containing sperm cells and other organic substances. 95% of the semen is produced by the prostate gland, 4% by the seminal vesicles—a pair of glands found above the prostate gland but below the bladder. The other 1% is sperm from the testicles.

Regarding women, infertility can result from a number of physically limiting situations—the inaccessibility of the egg to sperm, for example. These include a blocked ovarian tube due to the growth of a cyst or tumor, a misshapen uterus or a highly acidic and hostile environment in the uterus. All these, and other similar situations, can either impede sperm cells from reaching the ovary or kill them altogether.

In other instances, the egg may not ovulate, or be released from the ovary to be available for fertilization. This problem is often a result of an insufficient production of the hormones that are responsible for both the development of the ovaries and their activation or stimulation to release the egg. These hormones are called the follicle-stimulating hormone and luteinizing hormone, and both are synthesized in the body from amino acids.

In addition to the amino acids, a number of the vitamins—including vitamins C and E and a few of the B-complex team (such as B6, folic acid, B3)—can be of a great benefit to women. With these nutrients, one expert recommends the inclusion of the amino acids cysteine, methionine, histidine, arginine and phenylalanine and the minerals selenium, magnesium and zinc.[4]

CHAPTER 28

The Importance of Amino Acids and Other Nutrients During Pregnancy

Pregnancy is one of the major events that takes place in a couple's life. First, by conceiving and carrying a baby to term, these individuals bring a new life into the world. This new life is a manifestation of the couple's healthy and properly functioning reproductive systems. Second, from conception to delivery, the mother goes through many biological and physiological changes. Since nearly all of these changes are nutritionally dependent, understanding the significance of quality food to you and your fetus will enable you to cope better during those months and have a healthy child.

Third, since increasing research in prenatal nutrition is finding a good correlation between the quality of food the mother eats during pregnancy and the proper physical and mental development of her baby, eating well-balanced meals during those months will aid you in making a lifetime investment in your child's health. If you are pregnant now or plan to be in the future, the discussion below should help you become more astute in your choice of nutrients.

The Physiological Changes That Take Place During Pregnancy

There are many changes that take place in a woman's body during pregnancy. Some of these are the following:

Blood Volume

It is reported that by the time of delivery, a pregnant woman will have increased her blood volume by roughly 25%. All this new blood is made from the food the mother eats—mainly the amino acids and iron, which make up the hemoglobin portion of red blood cells. As you must realize, this new additional blood is important to transport nutrients and oxygen to the fetus as well as to serve as backup in case of a sudden loss through hemorrhaging or other similar accident.

Having a rich source of iron and amino acids will therefore be important to a pregnant woman during this important time. Equally important are foods that are rich in electrolytes as well as carbohydrates. Beginning around the end of the first quarter until about the beginning of the last trimester, the woman's cardiac output (amount of blood pumped out of the heart each minute) is increased by 25% to 30%.

This is a lot of work for your heart, and you need a good source of fuel as well as electrolytes (minerals like calcium and magnesium) that help the heart maintain its rhythm. Vitamin C is important in protecting and strengthening the supporting blood vessels. Vitamin B complex and the amino acid L-carnitine are very important in the metabolism of carbohydrates and artery-clogging fats. From these examples, you can see you need a good mix of nutrients during those crucial months to accommodate the changes taking place in your body and to support the growing fetus.

The Liver

During pregnancy, your liver also will have an added responsibility in maintaining and supplying your expanding body and your fetus. The liver has many important functions. Just to name a few, the liver serves as a storage and metabolism site for many nutrients, as one of the places where proteins and many other organic molecules are synthesized and as a purging organ for many toxic metabolic by-products as well as for those that filter from the digestive tract. Like the heart, it has to work harder to accommodate the increased blood volume. As a response to the added demand placed upon it, the liver also increases in size. All these changes require good nutrition.

The Digestive Tract

The digestive tract is one of those organs that is immediately affected by the erratic behavior toward food by pregnant women. First, during the early period of pregnancy, women often have an aversion to the smell, taste and even sight of foods that they ordinarily eat. This sometimes leads to their eating little and depriving their bodies of important nutrients. Second, pregnancy tends to make women want to eat unconventional foods and nonfood items (pica). Often, the digestive system will have to make adjustments to these new tastes.

The above condition and other reasons lead to disturbances in the digestive tract. Some of these are chemical—such as the secretion of fewer digestive enzymes and less hydrochloric acid. Others can be physical—such as a reduced peristaltic action due to temporary loss of muscle tone and strength in the digestive tube. As a result of all these problems, food does not get digested, staying longer in this dark, moist environment, which leads to constipation and putrefaction. These are not very healthy for anybody, let alone for a pregnant woman, who needs sufficient nutrients for her growing fetus and herself.

Skin Condition

We discussed elsewhere in this book that the first places doctors look for signs of malnutrition are the skin, hair and nails of a person. These tissues are sacrificed first whenever there are nutritional deficiencies. Because of hormonal changes and finicky eating habits, many pregnant women tend to have problems with their skin, hair and nails. The solution: force yourself to eat and make sure you get the right nutrients.

There are many more changes that come with pregnancy, but the most important thing is to make good nutrition your ally as much as you can. You have a responsibility to give that growing fetus a good start in life. After all, it will be constructed entirely from the food and water you give it during its formative months in the womb.

The Importance of Optimal Nutrition During Pregnancy

From the brief discussion above, you can see that the quality of nutrients you take in during pregnancy will determine how well your body will cope during these major physiological changes as well as help you to have a healthy and properly developing baby.

If we go by the national surveys, most of us don't get adequate nutrition. Most of us also have many life and environmental challenges (such as pollution, stress and food additives) that threaten our health and deplete our bodies' nutrient reserves. Because of these challenges, pregnant women, more than anybody else, should be concerned about the quality and diversity of their nutrient intake.

When we talk about quality products, we are talking about those that are rich sources of the amino acids, carbohydrates, vitamins and minerals one needs to take together to take full advantage of the nutritional value of foods. During the developmental or construction stages (through mitosis or cell division), the fetus is entirely dependent on the mother for its supply of nutrients.

Thus, having optimal nutrients during this construction period is very important for the developing fetus. For example, a shortage of sufficient amino acids during this time could lead to poor brain development, which has many consequences, including poor learning ability and emotional imbalances.[1] The raw materials for many of the increases (blood volume, breast and uterine expansion as well as the fetal and placental protein synthesis) come from proteins in the form of amino acids. Together with these, you need carbohydrates and key vitamins and minerals to help process the protein.

The Importance of Vitamins and Minerals During Pregnancy

A large percentage of the vitamins and minerals you consume function as metabolic partners to the thousands of enzymes in your body. In the body of a pregnant woman, the availability of greater concentrations of vitamins, minerals and other nutrients is crucial to the developing fetus. An insufficiency in any one of these nutrients can lead to a number of unwanted consequences.

Zinc, for example, is one of the minerals that is intimately involved in cell division and tissue repair. Having adequate levels of this mineral in your diet will, therefore, help the fetus to develop to normal size and be delivered at full term. On the other hand, it has been found that a significantly low level of zinc in a pregnant woman's body can increase the likelihood of spontaneous abortion or the baby's being born with birth defects.[2]

As another example, calcium helps lower blood pressure and minimize the incidence of toxemia (blood poisoning resulting from toxins) and eclampsia (conditions of late pregnancy characterized by hypertension, excessive protein secretion in the urine and accumulation of fluid in body tissues). Because the fetus uses up a fair amount of calcium for its own developing tissues, extra amounts of calcium in the diet of the expectant mother will help minimize the above problems and the loss of the mineral from her own bones (a precondition to osteoporosis).

Magnesium is calcium's partner in that one facilitates the absorption of the other when they are found in the right amounts (magnesium to calcium ratio of 1:2). Because magnesium is involved in muscle relaxation, an abnormally low level of it can apparently lead to spasms in the placenta and umbilical cord.[3] To prevent spontaneous abortion as a result of this problem, doctors often give magnesium-deficient pregnant women intravenous injections of the mineral.

Another mineral, iron, is intimately involved in the synthesis of hemoglobin and other proteins that are produced in greater quantity during pregnancy. Any significantly low level of this nutrient can lead to anemia. According to one report, nearly 55% of the infants born to low-income families are either anemic or borderline anemic. This condition negatively influences the child's intellectual development and behavior.[4]

Another mineral that you don't see commonly mentioned but which is equally important is iodine. This mineral, as discussed under the "trace elements" section earlier, is important in the synthesis of thyroxine, the thyroid hormone involved in the production of energy. If a pregnant woman is deficient in iodine, she is more likely to give birth to a mentally retarded and diminutive child, or a cretin. Some of the complications associated with cretinism are coarse skin, poor muscular coordination and hearing problems.

In addition to minerals and amino acids, there are key vitamins that are equally important for the health of a pregnant woman and her fetus. For example, vitamin C is very important for the formation of tissues in the fetus and for strengthening the circulatory system of the mother. Vitamin B6 is another nutrient that is crucial for the health of the mother and the fetus. The conversion of carbohydrates into energy and proteins into tissues cannot be accomplished adequately without this important vitamin.

Folacin or folic acid is another B-complex vitamin that is intimately involved in tissue formation and development. Vitamins A, D and E and the essential fatty acids (discussed in Chapter 7) are also very important. As you know, vitamins A, C and E are great antioxidants, and pregnant women can benefit from these vitamins during the stressful times of pregnancy. These vitamins can help neutralize many free radicals that may form during such a dynamic period.

Note: It's considered medically expedient to consult your physician before you include any supplements into your daily nutrient regimen. If needed, bring your supplements and show your doctor what you are taking, or plan to take in addition to your normal meals. Give this person literature, if you have any, on the supplements.

CHAPTER 29
Nutrition and Breast-Feeding

Alternatives to breast-feeding have been available for the rich and well-to-do for thousands of years. In earlier centuries, rich and aristocratic women of Europe and Russia who wanted to preserve their figures hired wet nurses to feed their babies for them. In this century, and here in the U.S., infant formulas have sold in record numbers—reaching their peak with the baby boom in the '50s and early '60s. In those two decades, nearly 90% of the mothers in this country reached for bottles of formula instead of their breasts to feed their infants.[1] Contrary to this great popularity of infant formulas, however, several researchers around the country have discovered that for the health and proper development of an infant, presuming the mother is well nourished, breast milk is far superior to infant formulas, which are made mainly from cow's milk. As a result, women are increasingly nursing their babies instead of relying on infant formulas. According to some studies, although their numbers have also dropped, a greater number of poor and minority women still use infant formulas to feed their babies.

When a nursing mother is properly nourished, her breast milk has many health and nutritional benefits for her infant. When a child comes from the semisterile environment of the womb to a world full of health- and life-threatening viruses and germs, it needs some level of extra fortification against these microbes.

The baby is usually born with its own antibodies (called immunoglobulin G), but it also needs added protection. For this reason, nature, in its wisdom, has made the first batch of breast milk (known as colostrum) rich in antibodies. Colostrum not only serves as a protection against infections but also has laxative and cleansing effects on the brand-new digestive tract of the baby.

In addition, it's believed this first milk protects the child from allergies, now and in the future,[2] by speeding up the closure of the rather porous intestinal wall of the infant. Allergies usually develop when whole proteins, such as those from cow's milk or eggs, get past the digestive tract. So, the importance of making the intestine foolproof immediately after birth is apparent.

In terms of nutrition, breast milk is rich in vitamins, minerals and large quantities of quality proteins and lactose (milk sugar). These have greater advantages over cow's milk both in digestibility and absorbability of the nutrients.

Whey is known to contain the best proteins. The contents of human milk are very similar to whey. Cow's milk, on the other hand, also contains casein, the predominant protein. Because its molecules are bulkier, it's hard for the delicate and soft digestive system of an infant to digest.

Lactose, which you find in larger quantities (about 50% more) in human milk than in cow's milk, is a very important fuel for the infant. The fast-developing brain cells depend entirely on this sugar (after it's converted into glucose, of course, by the liver). Infant formulas, in addition to being low in lactose, often contain sucrose, which can negatively affect one's moods.

Breast milk is also a rich source of cholesterol. Although this may sound unhealthy to you, cholesterol is crucial to the growing nervous system. The sheath that covers the nerve axons and the cell membranes is in part made up of cholesterol. This otherwise important substance is also the precursor of vitamin D, an essential vitamin for the absorption of calcium. For the developing bones and teeth of a baby, the availability of sufficient vitamin D in the body is very crucial.

There are many more advantages to breast feeding, from both the mother's and the infant's points of view. These include financial as well as emotional rewards. Breast-feeding, on the whole, costs about $500 less per year than infant formulas. Moreover, this early bonding of infant and mother is believed to be very important for the psychological and emotional development of the child.

To make all the above worthwhile, for both the mother and infant, a woman needs to eat well-balanced and nutritionally dense foods. The best way for a nursing mother to ensure that she and her infant are getting quality nutrients is by including the best supplements she can find on the market.

CHAPTER 30
Nutrition, Menopause and Premenstrual Syndrome (PMS)

Nutrition and Premenstrual Syndrome (PMS)

Premenstrual syndrome, or PMS as it's often called, is one of the mysteries of nature that is yet to be fully understood. At one point or another, PMS affects over 90% of child-bearing-age women, and for some it can be so severe that it creates major havoc in their lives. The most common symptoms of PMS are irritability, depression, lethargy, loss of sleep and sometimes wild mood swings. Often, less apparent symptoms can include fluid accumulation in body tissues, an abnormal craving for sweets and breast tenderness.

Because some of these symptoms are almost identical to those in people who are hypoglycemic, PMS is often associated with an abnormal sugar metabolism. Although eating too many sweets could heighten or aggravate the problem, the occurrence of PMS is believed to be more hormonal—such as an imbalance of estrogen and progesterone levels in the blood.

Unfortunately, there is no one single cure for PMS. What a woman can try to do, however, is minimize the symptoms by eating the right nutrients. Doctors often find that women who are well nourished have fewer of the PMS-associated problems. When symptoms do occur, they are not as severe as in those PMS sufferers who are poorly nourished.

Those nutrients that have shown significant results are vitamin B6, vitamin E, magnesium, chromium and calcium. The omega-3 and omega-6 fatty acids were also found to be helpful. These nutrients are precursors to prostaglandins—those hormonelike substances that do many wonderful things in your body. The minerals magnesium and zinc and vitamin C and niacin are the necessary cofactors that can help transform the essential fatty acids into prostaglandins.

Some of the minerals, particularly magnesium and the amino acid tyrosine, are very important for the synthesis of dopamine and noradrenaline—key hormones that control our emotions and moods. Since PMS causes wild mood swings, having these nutrients in your diet can help minimize this problem.

Nutrition and Menopause

One of the other major concerns baby boomer women should have is menopause. Like other physiological changes that take place in the body over time, the female reproductive organs will gradually cease their job of producing hormones and eggs, and a woman will stop menstruating. Derived from the Greek, menopause literally means "month stop" from *men,* month, and *pausis,* stop. Sometime between the ages of 45 and 55, the menstrual cycle slowly comes to a halt. The symptoms of menopause too, like those of PMS, are caused by hormonal changes—in this case from a reduced production of the hormone estrogen.

When this happens, the associated symptoms are "hot flashes," night sweats and backaches. Also thin, dry skin and scalp result from a stoppage or lowered production of oil from the sebaceous glands. During this time, the appearance of the hair and skin suffers. The skin can become rough and ashen, while the hair becomes weak, dry and brittle and falls out more readily. Secretions of vaginal fluids also become scarce, causing sexual intercourse to be difficult and even painful for some women.

Equally difficult and stressful is what happens psychologically and emotionally. As a result of the hormonal changes, the menopausal woman can often become teary, irritable, depressed and anxiety-ridden. In addition, partial loss of memory and concentration can be equally disruptive. This is also the time when the woman begins to lose bone mass rapidly, which leads to osteoporosis (thinning of the bones). Menopausal women can also experience inefficient metabolism of food that leads to a buildup of fat in the tissues and blood vessels. This, of course, can be a major concern not only because of weight gain but also because of the problems associated with stroke and heart attack.

Until recent times, women did not experience these problems because they usually died before their ovaries stopped producing hormones. Today, women live long past menopause, and thus it is important to seriously consider, together with one's gynecologist, whether to take hormone replacement therapy. This can alleviate hot flashes, prevent bone loss and address the other symptoms of menopause. Recent studies have shown hormone replacement therapy to be quite safe, especially when compared to the high probability of a hip fracture and its related complications occurring in many women if hormone replacement therapy is not instituted at menopause.

A woman can also naturally help herself by eating foods that are rich sources of amino acids, vitamins and minerals. As discussed earlier, amino acids are the parent molecules to a number of brain chemicals, including those that give a person a sense of euphoria and well-being. In addition, exercise, meditation and relaxation can help to metabolize food more efficiently and bring a sense of well-being into one's life.

CHAPTER 31
The Disadvantages of Excessive Protein Intake

Having said so much about the importance of amino acids to our health, it's also important that we talk about the disadvantages of taking too much of them, particularly as bulk protein.

It is reported that the average American consumes as much as 100 grams of protein a day. This is far too much, as you will see below. Depending on your age, body size and level of physical activity, your protein need should not exceed 40 to 80 grams. Consumption of excess protein has a number of disadvantages.

One, if you depend on ordinary dairy and meat products as your protein source, as we said before, the fat these foods contain can place your health at risk.

Two, when you encumber your body with a lot of protein beyond its need for building and repair, what is left is often converted into and stored as fat. The body can use protein as fuel, but only if your body is depleted of its carbohydrates. In ordinary circumstances, carbohydrates are the fuel of choice, followed by fats. Proteins are the least in order of preference. Moreover, only a few of the amino acids really get into the Krebs cycle.

The use of proteins as fuel, besides requiring several steps of conversion, is also wasteful. First, in order for the protein to be used as a fuel, it has to be converted into glucose. Before any conversion takes place, however, the nitrogen portion of an amino acid will have to be stripped from the parent molecule. The by-products of this process are urea, uric acid, creatine and others. These extraneous products can be toxic if accumulated, and the body quickly eliminates them via the urine and other excretory organs.

Three, protein-rich foods can often be a burden on your liver and kidneys, which are the organs responsible for processing and removing nitrogenous waste from your body. This elimination process can lead to an excessive water and mineral loss, as well as to overworked and malfunctioning organs. Particularly wasteful are those you get from legumes. The protein in these foods is of inferior quality, and as a result, your body tends to convert them to fuel or simply eliminate them.

The consumption of too much protein can lead to other complications as well. Many adult males and relatively fewer postmenopausal women suffer from gout—

an extremely painful joint inflammation that occurs from the accumulation and formation of uric acid crystals in the joints. This often results from the excessive consumption of protein-rich foods and, ultimately, from the buildup of uric acid in the blood.

Osteoporosis is a progressive thinning or hollowing of the skeletal system, resulting from the erosion or depletion of calcium from the bones. Osteoporosis affects women more than men.* Among other things, the consumption of excessive protein is believed to be the cause of osteoporosis. The body keeps a certain amount of calcium in the blood to meet many electrolytic demands (for contraction of muscles, for transmission of nerve impulses, etc.).

When there is a continuous water loss by urination or sweating, you also deplete the level of calcium in the blood. The contraction of muscles and the transmission of information between nerve cells are more critical than maintenance of sturdy bones. Therefore, when the calcium level is low in the blood, more of it is released from the bones to meet those needs. The frequent elimination of urine caused by the existence of excessive protein in the system can thus threaten the structural integrity of your skeletal system.

Four, the consumption of too much protein itself can cause much wear and tear on your body. As an analogy, you can think of a milling machine that is loaded with too much grain that squeaks and grunts from the weight. Your body is no different. To process the excess bulk that sits in your stomach, the body will work extra hard, gearing up the synthesis and secretion of extra enzymes and hormones necessary to digest the food.

In doing so, you also abuse the various glands along the digestive tract that produce those enzymes. Some of these enzymes play an important role in preventing diseases such as cancer, diabetes and other degenerative diseases. Thus, if you continue to abuse these glands, after a point they begin to function improperly. Read Chapter 33 for more information.

Five, as you get older your metabolism rate slows down. That means that anything that you don't burn as fuel or use to repair and build tissues is converted into fat and stored. That's why it seems amazingly easy for an older person to gain weight

---

* Women are afflicted with osteoporosis nearly 4 times as often as men. By age 65, the average woman loses 25% of her bone mass. As a woman ages, particularly past menopause, estrogen (the female hormone), which helps calcium to remain in the bones, dwindles. Anything that interferes with the absorption and circulation of calcium in the blood (e.g., excessive fat, fiber, stress, alcohol, smoking, coffee and other drugs) can increase the loss of calcium from the bones.

faster than a healthy, young person. With age should come knowledge and wisdom. Not only should you eat less protein as you get older, but also the protein you eat should be of the highest quality, free of saturated fats, cholesterol and a number of other dubious chemicals.

How Much Protein Does a Person Need?

The RDA for protein varies from .8 gm/kg per day for those who are 19 and over to 1 gm/lb per day for infants six months and under. These values are considered sufficient to meet the protein requirements for building and maintenance of body tissues. For instance, the RDA for a 165-lb adult who is not overweight is a little over 56 grams per day. Pregnant women, on the other hand, need an extra 10 grams of protein per day. Lactating women require 15 and 12 grams per day for the first and second six months of lactation, respectively.

PART XI
Digestion

The Digestive System

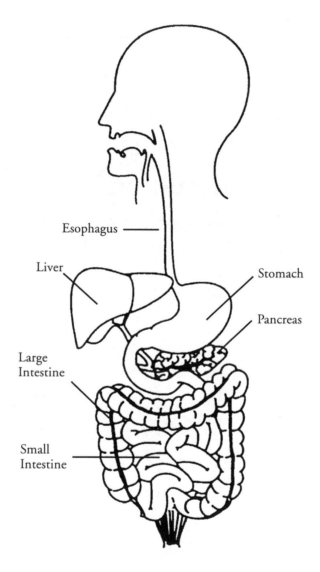

Esophagus

Liver

Stomach

Pancreas

Large
Intestine

Small
Intestine

The tireless, living food-processing machine.

CHAPTER 32
Proper Digestion: The First Step to Good Health

Someone once said that one of the greatest pleasures in life comes from filling and emptying an organ. Regarding this notion, eating is perhaps one of the most pleasurable activities we all engage in every day. It is also a crucial activity because our health and well-being are dependent on the food we eat. Yet most of us have little clue as to what happens to the food we eat once it gets past our lips and into our digestive tract. Like a sunrise or the change of seasons, we take this important, life-giving daily activity of ours for granted. This lack of interest or understanding is perhaps one of the reasons why we have such an unprecedented proportion of food-related degenerative diseases in this country.

As you will see below, much of our day-to-day mental well-being, as well as our long-term health or demise, is dependent not only on the type of foods we put in our bodies but also on how well these foods are digested or processed once they enter our digestive tract.

First, as was mentioned elsewhere in the book, for food to be of any benefit to us, it has to be reduced or broken down to its basic components—proteins to amino acids, fats into glycol and fatty acids and carbohydrates into glucose and other simple sugars. At a microscopic or molecular level, it is these simple molecules that are capable of being transported across the gastrointestinal wall and into the bloodstream. The nutrients are then carried by the blood to the cells where they can be used to fuel, repair and build tissues.

Second, in order for the above nutrients as well as vitamins and minerals to be picked up and transported across the digestive tract, there have to be as few interfering factors as possible. These factors could be substances that trap nutrients and make them unavailable for absorption or those that suppress their transportation across the intestinal wall. Some of these suppressors could be alcohol, cigarettes, coffee and certain medications.

Third, the nutrients that enter the circulatory system should be of the kind that won't upset or disturb the homeostasis ("steady state" conditions) of the body. This means that the foods we ingest should not only have the right balance of nutrients but also be of the kind that won't upset the body's rigidly controlled conditions. It also means that we should eat little or no sugar, sugar-based foods or saturated fats and that we should limit our intake of various foods to the level at which our bodies can process them without too much effort or encumbrance. In this regard, eating small but frequent meals is often considered the best approach.

Here are some of the specific problems that could arise from eating the wrong kind of food. Too much sugar may upset the body's glucose level, which also creates wild mood swings. Saturated fats are bad for the circulatory system. Too much food can strain gastrointestinal walls as well as the various glands that produce the digestive enzymes and juices. In the tissues, excess amounts of these substances must either be converted into fat and stored or be burned or eliminated from the body. If some of these substances are allowed to build up in the circulatory system, they can lead to many unwanted complications.

In order for us to be intimately involved in our health and well-being, we should have a good understanding of the food we eat and how it is processed by the digestive system and the rest of the body. It is amazing how easy it is for us to spend time and money on things that may have no inherent value to our health or long-term survival and do so little for the physical and biochemical self.

Every aspect of our physical, emotional and intellectual well-being is as much a reflection of a properly working digestive system as the variety and diversity of nutrients that enter our bodies. It is with the digestive system that our health's glory or failure begins. This complex and differentiated system functions by reducing long chain and branched food molecules (also known as polymers) into their individual components so that they are small enough to be absorbed by cells that line the gastrointestinal wall.

Let's see how the digestive system breaks down long chain and branched food molecules and readies them for absorption.

The Digestion and Absorption of Nutrients

The first stage of digestion begins in the mouth. Here, the tongue whips the food into a moist mass while the teeth pummel, knead and masticate it. Certain enzymes in the saliva (lipase, amylase and others) begin the initial chemical breakdown of starch and some fat molecules. After the chewing or mastication is complete, the food is turned into a spherical mass known as the bolus, which, with a squeeze and wavelike motion of the throat, is pushed down the esophagus.

The bolus arrives in the stomach. Here a strong acid (called hydrochloric acid) and a medley of enzymes that specialize in snipping and splitting protein, fat and carbohydrate molecules takes action. The stomach, a J-shaped, potlike organ, is also good at agitating and churning the food as the acid and enzymes untangle and rupture every morsel of food they come in contact with. From here, the food passes down to the small intestine, where, upon its entrance into the upper portion (the duodenum), it is drenched by another medley of digestive juices that come from the gallbladder and the pancreas.

The enzymes trypsin and chymotrypsin function as splitters or reducers of intact or partially digested protein chains. Their job is to reduce them to a size (as amino acids or short peptic chains—as two or three amino acid fragments) that will make it possible for the individual molecules to easily slip across the intestinal wall. The pancreatic amylase goes about finishing up all the partially digested carbohydrate molecules and maybe even chopping up those that managed to come down untouched by the previous enzymes. Another enzyme, called lipase, goes after fat molecules. The bile from the gallbladder is a handy fluid that helps emulsify or reduce fats to small droplets so that the lipase gets to the individual molecules.

As the food goes down the small intestine, more enzymes are added from the glands that line the wall. These enzymes tend to be those that cleave the last food fragments into individual units: amino acids, glucose and other small sugar molecules. It is these that finally get picked up by a layer of fingerlike projections of the small intestine called villi and microvilli. Because of these tiny microscopic outgrowths, the surface area of the small intestine is increased by over 600 times, which is actually equivalent to the size of a real tennis court. Its length may be only 12 to 15 feet.

It is on the intestinal surface that most of the food gets absorbed. The absorption process can be either by simple diffusion, by active transport (also called facilitated diffusion) or by engulfing. As you will see below, there can be many factors that interfere with this process. It depends largely on the kind of food you eat, the health of the digestive tract and the existence of interfering factors.

The large intestine serves as the place where large quantities of water get removed from waste matter. It also serves as a temporary repository of waste matter.

That, in a nutshell, is how the digestive system works as one whole and integrated unit and serves as a watershed to the cascade of metabolic events that take place later within the billions of cells in your body. When you think that very little solid food gets past our digestive tract without being broken down by the digestive processes and that life cannot exist without food, you can appreciate the tremendous importance of this living food processor, which we undignifiedly call our "gut." It is the digestive system that gives food meaning and purpose in our lives. There can also be many disruptive factors that interfere with this process, so let's look at them closely.

Digestion Disrupters

The process of digestion we described above may not be smooth or consistent from day to day or person to person. There are many factors that can disrupt the physiological and chemical processes involved in the digestion of food. Let's start with you. Without being aware of them, there are many things you do just before ingesting food that inhibit the production and secretion of digestive juices as well as interfere with the absorption of nutrients.

One of these could simply be not having sufficient time to sit, relax and enjoy your meal. The process of digestion requires the engaging of all those organs involved in the mobilization and breakdown of food that is placed in the digestive tract. This often entails the activation of key organs along the digestive tract through hormonal stimuli. Sight, smell, taste or even the thought of food can start a whole series of events, which are all concerned in the reception and proper digestion of food that arrives in the digestive system.

Unfortunately, when you eat in a hurry, your focus and energy are not concentrated on your food. This means that not only are all those key digestive organs not activated properly but also the food you consume will be underutilized by your body. The food consumed under such circumstances often stays longer than usual in the digestive tract and causes cramps, distention, constipation or diarrhea.

Similarly, depression, anxiety, overexcitement or stress can cause you to temporarily lose interest in food. Even if you have no physical or emotional disturbances, such simple practices as eating sweets, drinking too many caffeine-based beverages or alcohol or smoking cigarettes and other stimulants can have an equally disruptive effect on your digestive system. They could lead to a whole range of temporary or permanent problems involving the health of the digestive tract, including infections, ulcers, food poisoning and chronic diseases.

Another important concern you may have is what happens to the digestive organs and processes as you age. Unfortunately, like everything else in your body that atrophies with age, the digestive tract and all the organs that contribute to its function reduce their output of digestive juices. This in itself can be a limiting factor in the absorption and utilization of nutrients by the body. Add to this the fact that because most of the food in this country is processed, canned and prematurely harvested, there is a low nutrient content in foods.

Thus, not only do you have many of the disruptive factors mentioned above, but also you are dealing with a situation in which you might not be getting enough nutrients even if you have a healthy lifestyle. Although the health-eroding aspects of all the above factors are not apparent to you now, as the years pass, you may start to feel their impact.

Your Solution

The best thing that you can do to deal with some of the problems is to treat the whole activity of eating like an event, a celebration of something important in your life. Treat it with respect. Enjoy the anticipation as well as the act of consuming your meals. Take your time or slow down when you sit down to eat your meals. Nothing in life should be more important than your health and well-being. After a meal, relax for 15 to 30 minutes before you engage in any activity. By doing so, you can help your body concentrate its energy in processing the meal. This may enhance the digestion as well as the absorption of nutrients. If you are hungry but don't have time to sit down and have a relaxed meal, have something simple instead, like an apple or water. This option can help kill your hunger and sustain your body until you have time to sit down and enjoy your meal.

You may want to avoid or minimize your intake of the absorption-disruptive foods and drinks mentioned above before your meals. Although you may have no control over certain infections or chronic digestive disorders, you should have control over such everyday problems as stress, depression, anxiety or overexcitement. Even a chronic condition and infection can be dealt with effectively if you have the right kinds and sufficient amounts of nutrients in your body.

Digestion Disturbances

One of the by-products of digestion is what we often euphemistically refer to as gas. It's largely produced when bacteria in the stomach work on an improperly digested food. This happens, for example, if you eat your food too fast—without thoroughly chewing it and allowing the hydrochloric acid (HCl) and enzymes to break it down in the stomach. This means that before you're ready to eat, think about food. Think of some of the succulent foods you have eaten in the past. These thought processes stimulate the secretions of all the digestive enzymes in the saliva, the stomach lining and the pancreas gland. HCI, the strongest chemical in your stomach, kills bacteria and viruses and helps break down many of the foods. It is also produced in greater quantities when you mentally stimulate the secreting glands along the stomach wall.

A food that is not properly digested can become food for the bacteria in your intestines instead of for your body. The bacteria can start to break down this food and use it, creating gas as a waste product. Often, you may have noticed that when you eat your food in hurry, you end up with cramps and discomfort in your stomach. This food tends to stay longer in your system, causing pain and constipation. It's believed that one of the causes of colon cancer is when such food putrefies and the bacteria convert it into carcinogenic chemicals. High-protein and lower-fiber foods tend to linger longer and, as a result, putrefy and produce carcinogenic chemicals.

Some foods are more gas generating than others. Most protein foods, especially those rich in sulfur like eggs, cauliflower, beans and broccoli, can be converted into hydrogen-sulfide gas (the most offensive kind) by the intestinal bacteria. Most of the legume family (beans, peas, soybeans, etc.) have two soluble sugars called raffinose and stachyose that are equally gas forming and distending. Most grains, fibers and other plant foods convert into methane gas, which is not as penetrating and jarring to the nostrils.

Fibers can sometimes be a double-edged sword. They have many healthful properties in the digestive tract, but to some people, they can also be a nuisance because the bacteria in their intestines digest them and produce gas. There are some remedies to this problem, however. When you eat fiber-rich foods or supplements for the first time, try to take them in small quantities. The key is not to overwhelm your intestinal bacteria with too much fiber for the first time, in which case they begin to proliferate and start a feeding frenzy and produce large quantities of gas. Just start slowly and build up to the normal serving level.

There are also drugs you can take. The easiest and the safest remedy is activated charcoal, which you can buy from your local drug store or health-food outlet. It comes as a tablet or powder, and it's a powerful absorbent of stomach gases. Just take two to three tablets of this harmless substance with your meal and you should see an improvement.

You may also be one of those people who cannot properly metabolize milk, or rather, the milk sugar (lactose). The milk-processing enzyme, lactase, may be lacking in your digestive system, leaving the milk to be processed by the bacteria into gas. In this case, the easiest remedy is, of course, to avoid milk and milk products.

In summary, just remember that your overall health and well-being and even longevity are dependent on the nutrients that are processed and provided by your gastrointestinal tract. Without the proper functioning of this system, there is no beautiful hair or skin or healthy and properly working body or mind.

CHAPTER 33
Enzymes

We have now come to what is perhaps the most important and fundamental component of good health, wellness and longevity: enzymes. Unlike vitamins, minerals and herbs, which directly or indirectly affect the function of the body, enzymes (as discussed in the previous chapter), control the very fundamental processes or operations of the body. These range from the breakdown of foods in the digestive tract to their assembly or synthesis in the tissues and organs to their conversion into energy. In short, enzymes are the key that unlocks the essence of food in the body to give it strength, wellness, and vitality. This means that without enzymes, life would not exist and food would have no meaning or purpose.

What exactly are enzymes, and where are they made, you may ask. Enzymes are a special group of protein molecules that somehow behave as if they had a soul and a life of their own. They do what they do (break down food, synthesize or assemble food molecules, etc.) without instruction (at least as far as we know) from anywhere. They are the architects and the laborers as well as the housekeepers of our body. Everything that we are and do is controlled or facilitated by enzymes. This can range from thinking to blinking our eyes to engaging in physical tasks as well as to building and repairing tissues.

The body contains two major classes of enzymes: digestive enzymes and metabolic enzymes. The digestive enzymes are synthesized in the pancreas and in the cell along the gastrointestinal tract[1] as well as in other cells in the body. These enzymes are responsible for the breakdown or digestion of food. The metabolic enzymes are produced by every cell in the body and are involved in the conversion of food into energy or in using food to build and repair tissues.

Enzymes also can get involved in processing or converting toxins and pollutants into harmless substances. This is their scavenging function. Considering that many of us live in a polluted environment and consume food and water that may have been exposed to dubious chemicals, this housekeeping function of enzymes can be very important indeed.

Outside the body is a third class of enzymes, called food enzymes. As their name implies, these enzymes are responsible for all the activities that take place in plants, from germinating a seed to its growing and maturing into a plant to its blossoming and bearing fruit. Just as an organism decomposes after death with the help of its own enzymes, the enzymes in plants are responsible for making plants biodegradable. Most of the food enzymes are similar to the enzymes found in our bodies.

The Importance of Enzyme Supplements for Our Health

Before we discuss the significance of enzyme supplements to our health and well-being, let's talk about the specific functions of the different digestive enzymes found in our bodies. As you can see in the discussion on digestion in previous chapter, there are specific enzymes for the different classes of foods we consume every day. Hence, protease specializes in processing proteins; lipase, in breaking down fats; and amylase, lactase, and cellulose in snipping and splitting starch, lactose and cellulose molecules, respectively. (Starch, lactose and cellulose are all carbohydrates.) It can be said that nearly every single food molecule (or, for that matter, every chemical reaction) has its own specific enzyme that helps catalyze the conversion or breakdown of that food (or chemical substance).

It may be self-evident that without sufficient quantities of all the above enzymes, foods cannot be properly processed, and consequently our health and wellness could suffer. Does this mean that we need to be concerned about our supply of enzymes? Can there be a shortage or depletion of our enzyme supply? If so, could we benefit from an enzyme supplement? Let's answer each of these questions separately.

Our body's production of enzymes will depend on our age, the type of food we have been consuming throughout life and the stress and pollution levels we have subjected our bodies to.

 Like everything else that happens in our body's as we get older, our bodies' ability to secrete sufficient quantities of enzymes declines. For instance, in one study, the concentration of the enzyme amylase in the saliva of young adults was found to be 30 times stronger than in individuals over 69 years old.[2] In another experiment, the concentration and strength of the same enzyme taken from the pancreas of a group of older men were found to be many times weaker than that taken from the pancreas of younger men.[3]

Besides the normal aging process, extended consumption of processed, cooked and irradiated foods can deplete the body's reserve of both metabolic and digestive enzymes. As mentioned above, when consuming foods that have been processed and altered (i.e., foods whose enzymes have been destroyed), the body has to produce a large quantity of its own to digest and utilize such food. Interestingly, like muscles that increase in mass from the challenge of physical exertion, glands and organs responsible for the secretion of digestive juices and enzymes enlarge when repeatedly burdened with a large quantity of processed and cooked foods.[4] This fact has been demonstrated by comparing the pancreas of wild mice (mice that feed on raw food) with the pancreas of laboratory mice that were fed processed and cooked food.

Likewise, when our body is exposed to pollution or extraneous chemicals such as pesticides and food additives (preservatives, coloring and flavoring agents), it will use (and therefore waste) a large quantity of its own enzymes. This happens because, our liver, kidneys and other organs and tissues use enzymes to process or turn some of these chemicals (as well as viruses) into harmless substances. As these organs and tissues are stressed or burdened with the production of a large quantity of enzymes, they naturally enlarge to increase production and meet the demand placed upon them.

When we eat whole, uncooked foods, the enzymes that are naturally found in them can help break down those foods in the digestive tract. Cooking or microwaving foods destroys enzymes. This habitual practice will lead to our being dependent on our own enzymes to process the food and consequently may lead to the depletion of our bodies' reserve of enzymes. The long-term consequence of this reckless usage of our bodies' labor force can be a decline in the bodies' function, a greater susceptibility to degenerative diseases and in general a higher compromise of our health and wellness.

What is the solution to the above problem? The first solution to this challenge would be to consume whole and uncooked foods as much as possible. Because the enzymes that are naturally found in uncooked foods can help digest such foods, the body will produce fewer of its own enzymes in the presence of these foods. In other words, to quote Dr. Edward Howell, author of *Enzyme Nutrition,* "If we depend solely upon the enzymes we inherit, they will be used just like inherited money that is not supplemented with a steady income."[5] The uncooked, whole food may serve as a good source of that supplemental, steady supply of enzyme income.

The second solution to enzyme depletion can be the use of prepackaged enzyme supplements. When you think about it, this actually is a great idea. Because processed, cooked and chemically adulterated foods are omnipresent and that eating raw food is neither easy nor practicable, augmenting your diet with quality enzyme supplement may be an excellent alternative. Thus, a supplement may help you conserve your body's reserve of enzymes as well as help you process your food efficiently.

Use a supplement that has multiple enzymes, or enzymes that can help you process protein, carbohydrates and fat. Hence, for example, while protease, peptidase, help you to digest proteins, amylase, invertase, glucoamylase and lactase can help your body break down carbohydrates. Similarly, a lipase enzyme can help you process fat. As we said above, enzymes can very specific in their function. Thus, the above different protein and carbohydrate enzymes can help you digest some of the most common carbohydrates and proteins found in ordinary foods, when taken as part of a supplement.

PART XII
Water

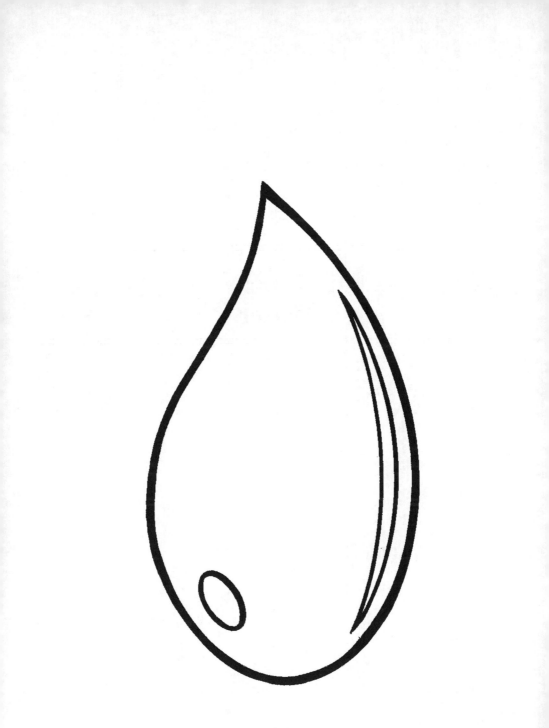

The Fluid of Life

CHAPTER 34

The Importance of Good, Clean Water to Your Health and Longevity

Throughout this book, we have talked about how good nutrition is the basis of good health, well-being and longevity. Good, clean water is an integral part of good health and nutrition. In fact, considering that about two-thirds of your body consists of water and that water is the medium in which nearly all the metabolic processes take place, the quality or integrity of this medium is very important indeed.

Some of the degenerative diseases such as cancer, arthritis, atherosclerosis (hardening of the arteries), kidney stones, cataracts, hearing loss, diabetes and a number of others that come with age could be caused by a lifelong consumption of bad water[1,2] as much as by bad nutrition. Unfortunately, as long as the water we use or drink every day satisfies our thirst, tastes reasonably OK and is readily available, many of us don't think twice about it.

In reality, as you can see below, the water you use from your tap, well or river can be the harbinger of many health hazards. These health problems are not cholera, typhoid, dysentery or any number of other water-borne diseases that have caused devastations in various parts of the world throughout history. The modern versions of these once fatal diseases are subtle, and in most cases, causes and symptoms may not be directly correlated. This is because many of the maladies that can be attributed to pollutants in water can also come from other sources.

From a number of disease-causing chemicals that are often found in our drinking waters and from the continuous rise in many degenerative diseases, as well as from specific correlational findings,* our drinking water has indeed come to be a growing threat to our health. For example, radioactive minerals such as strontium 90, radium 226 and 228 and common chemicals such as chlorides and nitrates are known to be carcinogens. Yet all these and many other substances can commonly be found in our drinking water—albeit some in tolerable amounts.

---

* For example, people who live in New Orleans near the delta of the Mississippi River are found to have a higher incidence of kidney and bladder cancer, as well as other urinary tract disorders.[3] Nitrates from farmland runoffs that often contaminate the water supply in the Midwest, are probable culprits, and are known to be a major health hazard to babies and adults alike.[4]

The Environmental Protection Agency (EPA) has called the water pollution problem "the most grievous error in judgement we as a nation have ever made."[5] Dr. Patrick Quillin, in his book *Healing Nutrients* writes that those who still drink normal tap water are either "uniquely blessed with an isolated pocket of clean water" or "very cavalier about (their) health."

What Could Be Wrong With Your Drinking Water

Besides the inorganic minerals that naturally abound in most ground and river waters, there can be countless chemicals, bacteria, viruses and even radioactive substances contained in the water you use every day. Some of these pollutants can come from agricultural runoffs. These can be pesticides, herbicides and fungicides, and fertilizers such as nitrates, sulfates and chlorides. Industrial and power plants also emit a lot of waste (which includes radioactive substances) into the atmosphere and the water supply above or under the ground. Similarly, hydrocarbons and other pollutants from auto exhaust fumes can find their way into the lakes, rivers and reservoirs from which your city draws your drinking water.

Moreover, because water is highly mobile and interactive (many organic and inorganic chemicals can dissolve in it), the pollutants that may exist in your drinking water may have come from far away. Because of this and the above reasons, the quality of the water you use for consumption should be of paramount importance.* Unfortunately, most of us are indeed cavalier about our drinking water. The sad thing about it is that our water pollution problem is not getting better. One writer refers to this worsening situation as a "scourge of major proportion (that could become) our legacy."

Here is a list of some of the substances that can be found in your drinking water:

EDBs	Zinc	Viruses
Strontium 90	Bacteria	Sodium
Algae	Silver	Lithium
Thorium	Aluminum	Radium 226 & 228
Tannins	Mercury	Herbicides
Magnesium	Pesticides	Lead

---

* Even in a situation in which the quality of the water is closely monitored, the allowable level for each contaminant has been determined without the availability of studies of their long-term, chronic ingestion even at these "low" levels.

Petroleum solvents	Iron	PCBs
Copper	THMs	Chromium
Benzene	Calcium	Sulfides
Cadmium	Sulfates	Barium
Nitrates	Arsenic	Fluorides
Rust particles	Chlorine	Silt
Chlorides	Sand	Cesium 137
Nickel	Carbon 14	Radon

Because of these and many other inorganic and organic substances, your water can sometimes look unappetizingly murky, taste heavy and muddy and smell stale and swampy.

The heavy metals—cadmium, lead, mercury and others from the list above—are known to generate free radicals, those chemical renegades that create havoc in your body. Nitrates, chlorine and chlorinated substances can be equally deadly. For instance, chlorine and chlorinated chemicals can generate free radicals on their own when they are acted upon by the enzymes in your body or can combine with the salt, water, hydrogen peroxide and hypochlorite (a compound found in most drinking waters) to make the dangerous singlet oxygen free radicals.[6] These chemical species, as mentioned elsewhere in this book, are believed to be one of the causes of cancer.

Similarly, nitrates are a problem because when they combine with the amino acids in your diet, they create nitrosamines—also well-known carcinogens. Then you have the radioactive elements such as carbon 14, strontium 90, radon and thorium that can collect in the bones to become a health threat. As you probably know, radioactive materials are carcinogenic as well.

Contrary to popular belief, the inorganic minerals such as calcium and magnesium that you find in most drinking waters may actually have a negative impact on your health.[7] Some of these minerals, for example calcium, can settle out in the arterial walls, causing them to harden, collect cholesterol and impede the normal blood flow. The technical term for this is atherosclerosis, which is one of the causes of heart attacks and stroke. The reason why they can be bad when found in water but good when found in food or nutritional supplements is discussed further on in this section.

Minerals can also collect in the joints, kidneys, pancreas and inner ears, as well as eyes and other tissues, leading to arthritis, kidney failure, diabetes, hearing loss and cataracts. According to Dr. Allen Banik, because of the impact they have on many vital functions of the body, too many minerals in your drinking water can "destroy every fond hope you have by striking you down ... and will draw your activities from the great out-of-doors, into creaking rocking chairs and finally into bedridden old people's homes."[8]

Considering how important minerals are to our health, the above statements may come as a total surprise to you. Minerals are very, very important indeed, because your muscles, heart, brain and many other body processes depend on minerals for their proper functioning. You need, however, only the minerals you get from organic sources, from the food you eat or from supplements.

Studies have shown that the amount of minerals the body metabolizes from drinking water (whether it be mineral, tap or well water) is less than 5%. And according to the *American Medical Journal,* "the body's need for minerals is largely met through foods, not drinking water." Similarly the National Water Quality Association has remarked: "The amounts of minerals found in water are insignificant when compared to those found in the food we eat."

To understand how waterborne minerals behave in your body, you can think of a river that carries sand, silt and many other organic and inorganic matters in it. This river, as it flows from higher grounds to the lower, flat lands, leaves behind much of what it carries along its course, banks and delta. Over a period of time, much of the material could collect so high and wide that it could cause the river to divert its course.

The blood in your arteries is similar to such a river in that it, too, tends to deposit any excess material along its path until, after some point, the sludge of minerals and fat harden and begin to interfere with the normal flow of blood. In your body, excess cholesterol, fat and mineral sedimentation are some of the major causes of circulatory disorders.

Amazingly, the average person could consume roughly 450 pounds of inorganic minerals from tap and well water in his/her lifetime.[9] Where do you think some of this gunk ends up? Your kidneys try to get rid of as much as they can. What is left may slowly accumulate in the blood vessels, joints, lungs and other tissues in your body, leading to some of the diseases that come with age.

The Solution

Your best solution is to drink pure water, free of any of these substances. This means distilled water. Distillation, in combination with pre-carbon filtration, can give you water that is 99.9% pure. Despite popular belief, this is the kind of water that is ideal for drinking. Your food and supplements, not your drinking water, can provide you with the minerals your .

Reverse osmosis (RO) is perhaps the next best method of water purification. Manufacturers of RO systems claim that their devices can remove anywhere from 85% to 93% of substances found in water, but these percentages go down over time. Some critics have put the figures as low as 50% to 70% after a few operations. In either case, RO filters seem to have more problems than the manufacturer or a door-to-door RO water filter salesperson would be willing to admit to.

Such problems include quality variability in the filtered water, short service span of the membrane, carbon and sediment filters (lasting only 1 to 2 years) and water wasting. With steam distillers, you have none of these problems. Although a good quality in-home steam distiller costs about $200 more than a similar size RO, which cost $500 to $600, steam distillers can last as long as 20 years. The replacement cost for the heating element in the steam distiller is $20, while the RO's may cost about $75.

Let's now see how the city purifies the water you drink every day. The most common methods of water purification (carbon filtration and sediment filtration) remove only 20% and 5%, respectively, of matter contained in water. These two methods, are used by most cities and towns to bring you filtered drinking water.

Depending on where you live and the type of water (soft or hard, lake or river or groundwater) that exists there, your city may use different treatments and filtration processes. Most of these treatments are designed to make the water safe (free of disease-causing bacteria and viruses) and to reduce unwanted smell, taste and appearance.

In typical filtration, a combination of several processes may be used. For starters, long-term storage is used to settle much of the suspended matter and bacteria. This may be followed by aeration to reduce taste and odor and by coagulation and sedimentation to enhance the color and lower the material content. Because coagulation often entails the addition of several chemicals, such as ferrous sulfate, lime, sodium aluminate and ferric chloride, the resulting water can become hard and corrosive.

The last three steps of purification involve softening, filtration and disinfection. The softening process uses ion-exchange resins to remove most of the calcium and magnesium. The filtration process can be accomplished using either fine sand, underlaid with gravel or just large grains of sand. Both of these processes are used to improve the appearance as well as to reduce the mineral and bacterial content of the water. The final stage of the purification involves disinfection. This step most commonly uses chlorine, but ozone and ultraviolet radiation are also used to kill bacteria and to disable viruses. In addition, copper sulfate, to control algae growth, and activated charcoal, to trap odor and organic chemicals, may be used.

After all these steps, the maximum your town's filtration systems can do is to remove only up to 25% of the substances contained in your drinking water. This means that from the list of substances you saw earlier, the sediment filtration stage removes mainly sand, silt and rust particles, while the others and the activated carbon filter help remove bacteria and organic substances such as benzene, THMs, PCBs, petroleum solvents and some of the pesticides and herbicides. The activated carbon filtration can also remove bad taste, odors and chlorine. Otherwise, nearly 75% of what you see on the list, *if* they already exist in the water being processed, can end up in your tap water.

The other problem, often not apparent to the average consumer, is old, corroding water pipes. In fact, your city's water purification centers may have done the best they could in filtering your water supply. What they often don't have control over are the leaching metals such as copper, lead, nickel, cadmium and others that may be found in the network of underground water pipes.

Depending on the condition of the water itself (acidic or basic), the duration of contact it has had with the pipes since it left its source and the age of the pipes, you could have various levels of leaching and contaminations as a result of the above metals. For instance, a significant level of leached copper can change the appearance of your water to blue. A high level of lead in drinking water can cause a number of physical and neurological disorders, particularly in children, that affect a child's mental development and learning abilities. The heavy metals listed also are known to be free radical generators, as we said in earlier chapters, and can initiate a number of diseases and speed up aging. To deal with these problems, you have a few choices.

The first option is to purchase distilled water for drinking and cooking. It may cost you considerably less than what you ordinarily pay for bottled water.

The second option is to buy and install your own steam distillation or reverse osmosis system. A distillation system, as we said earlier, is the best. You consistently get top quality water, and the system can last you a long time compared to an RO system. If this is too expensive, find a water company that at least uses reverse osmosis and purchase your water from it. In the long run, though, you might be better off owning a purification system.

The third option is to use tap water cautiously. If your piped water has not been in use for some time, such as overnight or when you've been on vacation, turn the faucet on and let the water run for at least 3 to 5 minutes. This will help flush any accumulated leached-out minerals in the water. If you depend exclusively on your tap or even bottled and spring water for your drinking and cooking, eat foods that are a good source of antioxidants. Vitamin A, for instance, as retinol or beta carotene, is a great neutralizer of singlet oxygen free radicals. So are selenium and vitamin E. As mentioned earlier, singlet oxygen free radicals are some of the commonly produced chemical species in the presence of salt, sodium, chlorine and water.

Vitamin C and the amino acids cysteine and methionine are good in removing many of the toxic metals that may exist in your drinking water.[10] Hence, if you don't trust the water you're drinking, you can at least aid yourself with the nutrients and supplements.

In summary, your overall health will greatly depend on both good nutrition and the quality of the water you drink. Since water occupies the largest volume in your body and since the multitude of biochemical processes that takes place in it happen in a water medium, the purity or integrity of this medium is very important for the efficiency and consistency of these processes.

Because polluted drinking water tends to depress your immune system, replacing your water supply with pure water will help you feel healthier and stronger. When your body fluids are "uncluttered" (as they are when you drink pure water), hormones can zip around the body quicker, oxygen and nutrients are transported faster and the enzymes and other chemicals work with higher efficiency. All these, in turn, can make you feel healthier and stronger. Pure water is truly a gift of nature. And you should give it to your body every day.

PART XIII
Exercise

Exercise Activities That Can Help Condition and Tone Your Body

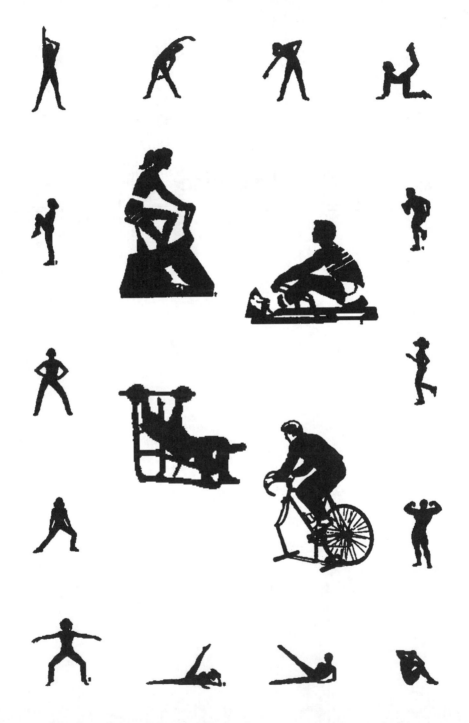

CHAPTER 35
Understanding Exercise

This book cannot be complete without including a chapter on exercise. Physical exercise is a spice of life. Just as food can be pretty bland, dull and boring, life without regular exercise can be equally dull and boring. It's not food, it's not water, and your body doesn't depend on it for its survival. Yet, for those who want to live longer and look and feel better and younger, exercise can make a world of difference in their health. It's the last piece in the puzzle that completes and optimizes one's picture of health.

Perhaps the first and immediate benefit of exercise is that it can help you release stress, depression and any other matters that may be clouding your mind at the time. Exercise heightens your awareness of your environment, how you think and feel about it and how you appreciate it. With exercise, you can also think more clearly, react more quickly and accomplish tasks more efficiently. Finally, exercise enables you to manifest fully the power of good nutrition in your health.

How It Works

There are a few different kinds of exercises, and each one affects your body and mind differently. The aerobic ones—like long-distance running, swimming, cycling, cross-country skiing, climbing stairs and rowing—help you by maximizing your cardiac output. With exercise, you use up more oxygen and force your heart to pump a higher volume of blood per minute to meet the fuel demands placed upon it by the various tissues. Aerobic activities such as the above therefore help strengthen your heart muscles. Aerobic exercise has many benefits:

1. Because the food gets completely burned into carbon dioxide and water, there is less buildup of toxic substances in the cells. This type of exercise which uses the Krebs cycle almost exclusively, was briefly discussed in Chapter 9. The Krebs cycle takes place in the mitochondria of the cells. During this type of exercise, you use up greater amounts of calories than you would in other forms of exercise (see below). Since aerobics enables you to burn fat at a higher rate, it can help you minimize the incidence of heart-related diseases. By increasing your HDL (the good cholesterol), aerobic exercises can protect you against heart attack and atherosclerosis (fat deposits in the arterial walls). For those who want

to lose weight, aerobic exercise is indeed very effective. The key is doing it regularly and in conjunction with other weight-reduction methods.

2. Aerobic exercise is perhaps the best for making you feel good overall and especially euphoric afterwards. During exercise, a variety of brain chemicals called endorphins and norepinephrine are produced. It is these chemicals that give you that heightened sense of well-being and keenness of mind and euphoria. As a neurotransmitter, epinephrine also enhances your memory and learning ability. When you are mentally sharp, you can accomplish a lot more in life.* That is what good, vigorous, regular exercise will do for you.

3. Because exercise in general, and aerobics in particular, pumps more blood through your circulatory system, more oxygen and nutrients are being delivered to the various tissues of your body. It's these nutrients and oxygen that enhance your looks and mental acuity. Notice how those who exercise regularly have something special about the way they look and relate to the world around them. Their skin may be clearer, smoother and more attractive than that of those who don't exercise regularly. These people also seem to be happier and have a higher energy level than their counterparts. As you can deduce from the above information, exercise indeed revitalizes your body and enhances the quality of your life. Since aerobic fitness enables you to burn more fat, it can also minimize the chance of death from diseases related to fat.

4. In another way, exercise rejuvenates your body by neutralizing free radicals—those molecular sharks that annihilate your body tissues at a cellular level. It's thought that since oxygen is used up in greater quantities when you exercise, it must also help neutralize the free radicals that form during metabolism. This seems contradictory at first, since we discussed in the section in Chapter 3 on free radicals that the most deadly of the free radicals (singlet oxygen and peroxides) are formed from oxygen. When the body is at rest, more of such radicals are formed than neutralized. With exercise, the numbers that are formed are equal to those that are neutralized. Since the oxygen molecule is a rich electron source, those generated from other metabolic sources get squelched by the oxygen molecules that bathe the tissue cells.

---

* In an experiment to show the benefit of exercise to human health, three groups of people were studied. Over a four-month period, one group did aerobics, another did strength exercises like weight lifting and the third (the control group) did nothing. It was found that all those who exercised had an improved reaction time, higher recall rate and improved analytical and reasoning abilities than those who did not exercise. Furthermore, the aerobics group performed even better than those who did strength exercises.[1] Incidentally, in a similar experiment, children who exercised performed better academically and in other tests that measured their mental and physical abilities.

5. Finally, exercise can induce the release of an important substance known as growth hormone (GH).* GH is your body's natural anabolic steroid that helps build muscle mass and strength. Unfortunately, like many other important substances that stop or slow down with age, the production of GH (by the pituitary gland in the brain) wanes after about age 30. In those over 30, however, the amino acids arginine and ornithine with vitamin B5 and choline cofactors were shown to increase the production and release of GH.[2]

Strength exercises like weight lifting, sprinting, shot putting and discus throwing, on the other hand, work by helping you build, strengthen and tone certain muscles. Although not as vigorously, the heart and lungs also work hard in this type of exercise to bring food and oxygen to meet the energy demands of those specific muscles.

This type of exercise tends to depend less on the Krebs cycle for extraction of energy from foods. Thus such exercises called *anaerobic* (without oxygen) exercise. The problem with this form of energy utilization is that food products are not completely burned, and as a result, lactic acid and other chemicals often collect in the muscle tissues. That is why weight lifters and sprinters commonly experience fatigue and cramps in their muscles when they engage in fast and highly intense exercises. If you want to lose weight or be in good shape, aerobic exercise is your best choice. Anaerobics are good for building strength and for increasing bone and muscle mass.

Another form of exercise that does not affect muscle endurance or the cardio vascular system is *isometrics*. This type of exercise strives to strengthen or firm muscles by pushing or pulling on a fixed object like a doorframe or parallel bars.

Isotonic is a similar form of exercise in which the body works against gravity (i.e., push-ups or free weights). Calisthenics and weight training are examples of isotonic exercise, and they can help you build endurance, muscle strength and muscle mass.

Although they began in Far Eastern countries, where the people practiced them as a way of purifying their minds and bodies through a series of mental and physical exercises, yoga and tai chi have found popularity in the West in the recent past. In these exercises, individuals attempt to attain maximum flexibility and coordination

---

* GH is also released during sleep time and when you have surgery, wounds or body damage. Because it is involved with growth and maintenance, these circumstances facilitate its secretion and availability in the body.

by stretching and breathing properly while simultaneously inducing the mind to free itself from unhealthy thoughts and desires. These exercises are unique in that they deal with the spiritual component of the body. To have a whole and totally integrated body and mind, it is important we work on our spiritual or subconscious mind. In most cases, our subconscious is more powerful in controlling our lives and destiny than any amount of muscles we are able to amass.

To build stamina and endurance and improve your cardiovascular efficiency, you need to do aerobics at least three times a week. Because this type of exercise strengthens capillaries and encourages the formation of new ones, many of the remote tissues (like the skin and scalp) will have more oxygen and nutrients delivered to them. As you must know, this is very important for the health and appearance of your skin and hair. This type of exercise can also increase the number and size of mitochondria, the cell's energy factories, which enable you to use more oxygen and burn more fuel.

When your heart is fit and strong, it pumps more blood (reportedly 25% and 50% per minute more blood while at rest and during exercise, respectively) and beats less frequently—60 to 70 times per minute as opposed to 80 to 100 times per minute when you are unfit. Besides making you feel good afterwards by relieving stress and depression, aerobics also minimizes the incidence of cardiovascular diseases such as stroke and heart attack.

To build strength and increase muscle mass, do weight lifting, sprinting and any number of other similar exercises that develop and tone specific muscle tissues. These exercises will enable you to lift, carry a load and push or pull on an object with power and strength. Simply speaking, these are your power exercises.

On the other hand, to improve flexibility and coordination, do isometric exercises like gymnastics and calisthenics. These improve your joints' and body's ability to do a whole range of motions—bending, stretching, rotating, etc. These exercises enhance the mechanical efficiency of the body. Unexercised muscles and joints become cranky and stiff—particularly as you get older. Thus, to maintain your youthful attributes and delay the process of aging, do these exercises regularly.

Finally, to achieve a fully integrated mind and body, include yoga, tai chi, meditation and visualization in your daily routine. These exercises will enable you to reach deep within yourself and release mental and spiritual toxins. No matter what you are able to do for your physical self (through various exercises discussed above), you're not completely fit unless you also do the same thing for your mental/spiritual self. Visualization is perhaps one of the most powerful techniques in achieving almost anything you want, including good health, power and strength, as well as in maintaining your youthful attributes.

In fact, true freedom (whatever that means to you) comes through the spiritual/ mental component of your self. The relief or freedom you experience after intense workouts lasts only through the duration of endorphins and epinephrine that your body produces during these physical exertions—and that is not very long. When you combine the mechanical/physical aspects of body fitness with your spiritual self, you enjoy and appreciate life, and you will look and feel your best.

Nutrition and Exercise

Exercise without a good nutrition program is like driving your car with very little oil and fuel in it. You may be able to drive it for a little while, but you're not going to get very far. Once all the oil or fuel is used up, the car will come to a grinding halt. This analogy is a good departure point for discussing your nutrition requirements while you pursue your exercise and fitness regimen. Let's follow the analogy a little further.

For your car to run properly, it needs fuel, oil and water. For fuel, you have regular, unleaded and supreme (a high-octane fuel). For oil you can get different grades: 40, 30, 10-40. Similarly, you can also use different water: tap water (which is bad because the minerals in the water can corrode your water tank and engine over time) or demineralized or distilled water (which is the best because it has no contaminants and does little damage to your car).

Your body has almost identical requirements. It needs fuel (food), oil (vitamins and minerals) and water. Just like your car, although it can run on regular (proteins) or unleaded (fats), its fuel of choice is supreme (carbohydrates—your body's high-octane fuel). Strictly as an energy source, proteins are not a good option. Just as regular gas releases lead and other pollutants into the atmosphere, protein burning can release ammonia* and other toxins. Ammonia can be very deadly if allowed to build up to a significant level. Fortunately, your body has a built-in safety mechanism by which it can quickly convert this dangerous substance into harmless urea and uric acid. These and other by-products are just as quickly filtered through your kidneys.

---

* The form that could temporarily build up is really not ammonia the gas but rather the water-soluble version (ammonium). It is this that the body quickly converts into uric acid. Bear in mind also that not all the amino acids from protein can be used as an energy source.

The other problem with excessive protein intake is the associated excessive loss of much water. This happens as the body naturally tries to purge itself of the protein-induced pollutants. Incidentally, this problem also burdens your kidneys with extra work—often a prelude to kidney-related diseases that may come later in life. So, when you plan to exercise, avoid eating protein-rich foods beforehand.

Fats would seem an ideal fuel source for individuals who exercise and do body training—because each molecule of fat has more than twice as much energy stored in it as a similar protein or carbohydrate molecule. (Each gram of fat contains 9 calories, while each gram of protein or carbohydrate contains only 4 calories.) Unfortunately, not only are fats metabolized differently in the body, but also they are very cumbersome substances that have many bad health consequences.*

Your best fuel supply is carbohydrates. These food groups are the cleanest (highest octane) and most readily available fuel. When athletes like sprinters, gymnasts or weight lifters or when you (in a fight-or-flight situation) need a burst of energy, you depend entirely on glucose—the smallest carbohydrate molecule, derived from foods like rice, pasta and potatoes and other food sources during digestion. This conversion is almost exclusively anaerobic (requiring no oxygen), and it happens in a flash. The problem with the anaerobic process is that glucose is not completely oxidized, which leads to potential buildup of lactic acid. These acids cause muscle cramps and fatigue when you engage in long and arduous weight lifting or repetitive sprints. They also waste energy because only 5% of the potential energy is extracted from food in this process.

As you may recall from the section "The Krebs Cycle," on page 91, this energy is transferred to ATP (adenosine triphosphate), which serves as a temporary storage medium. Bear in mind, though, that this is very temporary indeed. A sprinter's body, for instance, extracts energy from glucose, transfers it into ATP and uses this same ATP as his source of energy—all of which is done while he is still in motion.

The aerobic (oxygen-dependent) process, on the other hand, involves several steps and takes a little longer, comparatively speaking. This process uses the Krebs cycle exclusively and is the one in which 95% of the energy is extracted from each glucose molecule. In this reaction, all food molecules are completely oxidized into carbon dioxide and water. Long-distance runners, swimmers and cyclists who need

---

* Since it's not water soluble it does not get around the body very easily. It needs carrier mediums like HDL's (high density lipoproteins). So, eating large quantities of fat to get your concentrated energy can be a dangerous affair. Some of the fats are free radical generators, others clog the blood vessels leading to cardiovascular diseases.

steady sources of energy use the aerobic process almost exclusively.

The other benefit of the aerobic process is that your cells can burn other foods besides carbohydrates. Fats and proteins are equally "combustible" fuels that can be added to the furnace of the Krebs cycle. In endurance exercises like long-distance running, swimming and cycling, however, what becomes a limiting factor is the availability of enough oxygen.

Just as it takes a strong hand to fan and make a big fire for cooking or heating, it takes a strong heart that can beat steadily and pump large quantities of oxygen-carrying blood per stroke to the furnaces of the mitochondria. Your cardiovascular system has to be free of artery-clogging fats, not only to carry oxygen and nutrients but also to remove the "soot" (carbon dioxide and other waste matter) from the cells.

As you can see from the foregoing discussion, you need aerobic exercises not only to build stamina and endurance but also to lose weight and feel emotionally and physically good. As to shedding extra pounds, the problem most people have is how not to regain it once they lose it.

Traditionally, many weight-loss programs used the Krebs cycle theory to help people lose weight. Since carbohydrates are one of the three competing fuels in the aerobic reactions, it was believed that if you restricted your intake of pasta, rice and other starchy foods, your body would rely on its own fat for energy. By this method, it was thought that over a period of time you could literally melt your fat away.

Although those who endured the agony of this approach may have eventually dropped their extra baggage, they also found it difficult to maintain their new weight. The brain, in normal circumstances, is entirely dependent on glucose for its fuel supply. When you restrict your carbohydrates, you put the brain under a terrible stress. That is why most dieters have a tremendous craving for sweets and feel fatigued and exhausted when they are on a calorie-restrictive program.

Unfortunately, what happens 98% of the time is that these people either end up abandoning the program when they can no longer stand the ordeal or, once they have lost all they want and start eating normally again, regain all their dearly paid for poundage. Often, they may even gain more, because your body wants to store as many calories as possible in the event you starve it again. It might also possibly be interpreted as the body's punishment to you for putting it through this ordeal.

The best solution is to combine aerobic exercise with a high-carbohydrate diet. Carbohydrate-rich diets not only keep your mind sharp and full of energy but also will enable you to undertake your exercise regimen without feeling exhausted. Car-

Table 35.1 Suggested Weight For Adults

Height*	Weight in pounds**	
	19 to 34 years	35 years & above
5 0	97-128***	108-138
5'1"	101-132	111-143
5'2"	104-137	115-148
5'3"	107-141	119-152
5'4"	111-146	122-157
5'5"	114-150	126-162
5'6"	118-155	130-167
5'7"	121-160	134-172
5'8"	125-164	138-178
5'9"	129-169	142-183
5'10"	132-174	146-188
5'11"	136-179	151-194
6'0"	140-184	155-199
6'1"	144-189	159-205
6'2"	148-195	164-210
6'3"	152-200	168-216
6'4"	156-205	173-222
6'5"	160-211	177-228
6'6"	164-216	182-234

*Without shoes.

**Without clothes.

***The higher weights in the ranges generally apply to men, who tend to have more muscle and bones. The lower weights more often apply to women, who have less muscle and bone.

Source: Adopted from the National Research Council, 1989

bohydrate-based diets also encourage the burning of your body fat, as opposed to contributing to storing it. The key is, once you lose all the pounds you want to lose, keep exercising regularly. This will enable you to maintain your new weight and have overall good health.

Although there is no precise way of determining what a person's ideal weight should be, Table 35.1 can serve as a guideline to evaluate what your own healthy weight should be.

PART XIV
The Food Guide Pyramid

Food Guide Pyramid

A Guide to Daily Food Choices

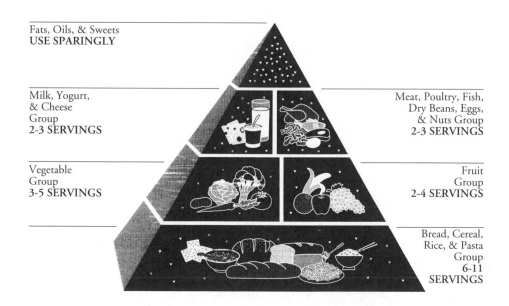

SOURCE: U.S. Department of Agriculture/U.S. Department of Health and Human Services

Figure 36.1 USDA Four Food Groups Pyramid Guide

CHAPTER 36
The Food Guide Pyramid

Thus far we have discussed many important health-related topics, including food components that may help you lead a healthy, happy and productive life. These topics range from certain nutritional conditions (such as subclinical and marginal malnutrition and obesity) to the various food components (such as vitamins, minerals, carbohydrates and proteins).

We have covered many key health-eroding factors, such as free radicals, the consumption of too many fat and cholesterol-containing foods, alcohol, processed foods and sweets. We have also covered those foods that are health enhancing, such as fibers and vitamins, minerals and amino acid supplements and herbs and phytochemicals. At various points in the book, we discussed the causes and nutritional remedies of many of the degenerative diseases we face today—e.g., cardiovascular diseases, cancer, osteoporosis and diabetes.

We have seen that good nutrition is also important to the reproductive system of both men and women. The fertility and sexual functioning of both sexes are strongly influenced by the quality and diversity of the nutrients they consume. Maladies such as impotence and frigidity may more often be caused by nutritional deficiencies than by other factors (such as psychological or physical disorders). Common female reproductive events or conditions, such as menopause and PMS, can be aided by good nutrition. During pregnancy and breast feeding, what the mother eats has a great influence on the health and proper development of the baby, both before and after birth.

Good health, happiness and well-being begin by how well the various foods are broken down, processed and absorbed by the digestive tract. To make you aware of the importance of these processes, we covered digestion at some length. Furthermore, since good health and well-being also depend on the quality of the water you drink and your level of physical fitness, we covered these two topics rather extensively.

From all these discussions, one thing must have been apparent to you. Your good health and longevity do not happen by accident. They can be achieved by your knowledge of the types of food you eat and by your actively and wisely configuring your daily meals.

It is often said that "living is an art." This may be so in the way you manage your personal or business affairs, but the art of living should really refer to how you manage your food intake and how you care for yourself. This means choosing and consuming health-providing nutrients and abstaining from many of the health-thwarting substances, such as drugs, cigarettes, too much alcohol and fats and too many sweets.

It is amazing how we seek pleasure or happiness from things that actually are detrimental to our health and yet take little care of our bodies or do not take the time to understand the foods we consume. It is also interesting that some of us find that cooking a decent meal for ourselves (in the absence of company) to be unimportant or irrelevant. In such circumstances, we often tend to grab anything from the refrigerator to kill our hunger or satisfy our craving.

Whether you live by yourself or with another person, have company or not, you need to be vigilant about the quality and diversity of foods you give your body, since food keeps you strong, healthy and productive. As was explained in the earlier chapters, many of the degenerative diseases that come later in life are largely a manifestation of cumulative nutritional inequities, as well as a result of consuming the wrong foods. So, what kinds of food do you need to nourish your body to achieve a long, productive, energetic and healthy life? A great portion of the answer to this question lies in the Food Guide Pyramid.

The Four Food Groups Pyramid Guide

The Food Guide Pyramid was configured in 1992 by the U.S. Department of Agriculture (USDA) in collaboration with the Department of Health and Human Services (HHS). It is based on the latest information about the connection between diet and human health, and hence, it is intended to enable us to make wise and healthy choices about our daily nourishment.

As was explained in earlier chapters, many of the current degenerative diseases are believed to be the result of the long-term consumption of the wrong foods as much as they may be from eating too few of the key nutrients. While cardiovascular disease and some cancers may be caused by excessive long-term consumption of fatty foods, our insufficient intake of certain key vitamins and minerals (particularly the antioxidants) can increase the problems we face with these degenerative diseases.

Similarly, osteoporosis is believed to stem from chronic consumption of insufficient calcium as well as from too much protein intake. Adult onset diabetes can come about from obesity and from long-term consumption of too many sweets.

On the other hand, foods such as grains, fruits and vegetables are found to be important contributors to good health. Not only are these foods some of the best sources of vitamins and minerals but also they are a great source of fiber, which, as explained in Chapter 6, has many healthful functions in the body.

Based on what you have learned so far, how would you go about configuring your daily meals to maximize the benefits of foods while minimizing their risks? Let's study Figure 36.1, "USDA Four Food Groups Pyramid Guide," on page 344.

Because carbohydrates are excellent fuels and are rich sources of vitamins, minerals and fiber (assuming you eat whole grains), we need to consume large amounts of these foods. For this reason, we allot the broad base of the pyramid to carbohydrates.

The next tier is for the vegetable and fruit group. These foods are rich in vitamins, minerals and fiber. Many vegetables and fruits contain substances that have not been fully studied but may have many healthful properties. The beauty of these foods is that they are also low in calories, and you can consume large amounts without having to worry about obesity.

The third tier contains the dairy and meat groups. Because of the health risks associated with these groups, we need to consume small amounts of them. This is indicated both by their location in the pyramid and by the serving sizes.

Fats, oils and sweets on the whole have very few vitamins and minerals, and thus, their nutritive importance is small. These foods are "pure calories," which only contribute to obesity. Since you also get calories from foods in the other tiers, the foods in this last tier may be superfluous. You need to consume these foods sparingly.

Serving Sizes

As you can see from the pyramid, the serving sizes given are shown as ranges. This is because when presented in this manner, people of different sexes and body sizes and those who are physically active can be adequately accommodated. Since different individuals have different caloric needs, body requirements vary accordingly

Thus, women, in general, and those who have sedentary types of employment, may need the smaller serving sizes. Men, teenagers and those women who are physically active may eat larger servings.

Since caloric demands determine serving size, let's first see what the suggested calories are for different groups of people. According to the USDA, if you are a

Table 36.1 Caloric needs for different groups of people

Caloric Level	Women and some older adults	Children, teenage girls, active women and most men	Teenage boys, most active men and some women
	Lower, about 1600	Moderate, about 2200	Higher, about 2800
Bread Group	6	9	11
Vegetable Group	3	4	5
Fruit Group	2	3	4
Milk Group*	2-3	2-3	2-3
Meat Group**	5	6	7

Source: Four Food Group Pyramid Guide, USDA, 1992

*Pregnant and breast-feeding women, teenagers and young adults up to age 24 need 3 servings.
**The amounts for the meat group are in total ounces per day.

sedentary woman or an older adult, your daily calories should be 1,600. If you are a teenage girl, an active woman or a sedentary man, your energy needs should be 2,200 calories daily.

Pregnant and breast-feeding women do not have a special category. Considering their higher nutrient needs (see Chapters 28 and 29), these women may need to consume more than 2,200 calories. Teenage boys, most active men and some very active women, on the other hand, can use up to 2,800 calories a day.

Table 36.1 summarizes the discussion above.

What Exactly Is a Serving?

A serving is an ounce, a cup or an "item equivalent" of a given food. For example:

- From the bread group, a serving is one slice of bread or one ounce of cereal or 1/2 cup of cooked rice, cereal or pasta.

- From the vegetable group, a serving is one cup of raw leafy vegetables, 1/2 cup of other vegetables (cooked or chopped raw) or 3/4 cup of vegetable juice.

- From the fruit group, a serving is one medium apple, a banana, an orange, half a cup of chopped, cooked or canned fruit or 3/4 cup of fruit juice.

- In the milk group, a serving is one cup of milk, 1-1/2 ounces of natural cheese or 2 ounces of processed cheese.

- From the meat group, a serving is 2-3 ounces of cooked lean meat, poultry or fish, 1/2 cup of cooked beans, 1 egg or two tablespoons of peanut butter.

How You May Use Serving Sizes in Your Daily Meals

Perhaps your first reaction when you look at the serving sizes outlined above is to wonder how someone can adhere to measuring or accounting for every component of the Food Guide Pyramid in an everyday meal! And, you may wonder, aren't some of the servings too large?

First, bear in mind that the servings are only meant as a guideline, a reference point, for you to keep track of your daily caloric intake. This is particularly so if you are trying to lose or maintain your weight. These serving sizes can also be useful for those who want to increase their caloric intake (for weight gain or for increased energy expenditure).

Second, serving sizes can help you better manage your food choice. For example, the consumption of many meats and dairy products may lead to a number of degenerative diseases. Thus, by limiting your intake to the suggested serving sizes, you may be able to minimize the health risks associated with these foods. On the other hand, grains, vegetables and fruits have been found to have many beneficial properties. Thus, the inclusion of the recommended serving sizes of these foods on a daily basis may enable you to lead a healthy life.

As for adhering to the serving sizes, you will find that after you have studied and followed the suggested amounts for each food category for a while, you should have no difficulty in estimating the equivalent amounts of the foods you consume in a meal.

Third, serving sizes will also enable you to know which foods to emphasize. As you can see from the pyramid, the bread group, with 6-11 servings, has the highest amounts (or portions). This food group is followed by the fruit (3-5 servings), and vegetable (2-4 servings) groups. The dairy and meat groups, in the third tier, have the least amounts (or portions) with 2-3 servings. Thus, aside from the food hierarchy shown in the pyramid, the appropriate suggested serving sizes should indicate to you what your order of preference should be.

In regard to the serving sizes (6-11 servings for the bread group, for example), they really are not very big. If you add up the various foods in this group (a slice of bread, one ounce of ready-to-eat cereal, etc.), you can reach the equivalent serving sizes quickly. From your three meals (breakfast, lunch and dinner), you should be able to attain the servings indicated.

Of course, these amounts should be adjusted according to your age, body size, sex or level of physical activity. Any extra calories, which are not used by the body, will be converted and stored as fat. This is particularly so for the bread, meat and milk groups. Since most vegetables and fruits consist largely of fiber, your concern about obesity gained from these foods should not be as great as for the others.

Finally, you notice that no serving size is allotted to the fats, oils and sweet group at the tip of the pyramid. Because these foods are pure calories and have very little nutritive value, large and prolonged intake of them can lead to a variety of degenerative diseases. You should consume these foods very sparingly.

Sodium and Salts

Although sodium and salts* are not mentioned in the food groups we discussed above, these substances are an important part of our dietary intake. Of all the inorganic minerals (salts) we consume every day (either as part of the foods we eat or in supplements), none has had such bad publicity as sodium. Like cholesterol, this important mineral has been maligned over the years.

Sodium has been associated with cardiovascular diseases (such as stroke, high blood pressure or hypertension) and other complications, such as edema (excessive fluid accumulation in the tissues), which is not good, as it can deprive the body of oxygen. Be that as it may, sodium is an important mineral in the body. All the cells in your body depend on sodium to function properly. This function includes nerve impulse transmission (as an electrolyte), as a regulator of fluids and nutrients in the cells (osmotic pressure) and as an antagonist partner to potassium, which bathes the inside of the cells. Like cholesterol, it becomes a problem when one consumes too much of the mineral. Because sodium has a great affinity for water, excessive amounts of the mineral (and, therefore, water) could lead to hypertension and edema.

The best solution to this problem is to maintain an intake of sodium at an acceptable level. According to some health professionals, our daily intake of sodium should be within 3,000 mgs. Some even suggest it should not be more than 2,400 mgs.

---

* Includes all the inorganic salts, such as magnesium chloride, calcium phosphate, copper sulfate, zinc oxide, that we obtain from our foods.

Unfortunately, not only is the salt shaker omnipresent in homes and restaurants, but there are also many hidden sources of sodium. Besides the fact that sodium is naturally found in grains, vegetables, fruits and others foods we consume every day, great amounts of the mineral are added to all types of foods by the manufacturers. These include cured meats, many cheeses, most canned soups and vegetables, luncheon meats, infant formulas and some of the flavor enhancers, such as soy sauce. To limit your consumption of sodium to an acceptable level, be aware of some the hidden sources, such as canned and packaged foods.

Just to give you a reference point for the above measurements, one teaspoon of salt contains 2,000 mgs of sodium. This is not very much. Sadly, the average American consumes many times more than that on a daily basis. No wonder we have over 50 million people who suffer from hypertension in this country.

Decision at the Table—What Food to Emphasize When

Referring back to the Food Guide Pyramid, for the food groups that appear at the top tier, eliminate or minimize your intake of sweets, saturated fats and certain oils. These include salad dressings, butter, cream, margarine, cooking oils, soy sauce, sugar, alcoholic beverages, candies, soft drinks and sweet desserts. These foods and drinks are pure calories, and thus you may want to watch out for them.

You may choose, instead, fat- and sugar-free sweets, drinks and condiments. For example, for your salad you might use light oil (preferably olive) and vinegar or salad dressings that are fat-free. With your sandwiches, you might use just catsup and mustard and exclude regular mayonnaise or use light mayonnaise. For drinks, you might want to have sugar-free drinks, water and natural (or unsweetened) juices.

From dairy products (in the second tier), you could emphasize cottage cheese, fat-free cheese, skim or lowfat milk and fat-free yogurt. From the meat group, you could choose water-packed tuna, fish, skinless chicken breasts or drumsticks or turkey. You could also boil some of these meats in water and throw away the liquid before you prepare your dish. This practice should help get rid of much of the saturated fat that some of these meats contain. When using eggs, you might do away with the yolk.

In the vegetable and fruit groups (the third tier), although you may not have to worry about fats, consuming fresh or unsalted or lightly salted canned or frozen ones will be healthful. Since these foods are also an important source of fiber, vitamins and minerals, as well as proteins (e.g., all beans, lentils and peas), you may want to have them as part of your regular meal.

From your bread group, go for the whole wheat or whole grain rolls or muffins, low-sugar cold cereals (such as Grape-Nuts, Life, Nutri-Grain, Bran Flakes, Shredded Wheat, Total, Wheaties) and oatmeal or Wheatena for hot cereals. Equally healthful are brown rice, air-popped popcorn, whole grain and unsalted pretzels, non-oil tortilla chips, pasta and others. Study the labels carefully.

On the opposite end of the spectrum, foods that you may want to avoid or minimize include whole milk, ice cream, cheeses (such as cheddar, American, Swiss), frozen yogurt, etc. from the dairy group; and pork, beefsteak, ham, hot dogs, bologna, eggs, chicken wings and thighs and others from the meat group. Aside from the fact that many of these foods contain a considerable amount of saturated fat, some of them are filled with salts, preservatives and coloring agents. You may want to be watchful about your intake of these foods.

From the vegetable and fruit group, you may want to avoid or minimize consumption of potato and corn chips, onion rings, French fries, avocado, coconut, cole slaw, some of the sweetened fruit drinks (read the label) and others. With these foods, you may be aware of the added salt, fat and sugar, which, as was discussed earlier, are not healthy when they are in excess in your system.

The bread group is perhaps the most diversified and the most omnipresent, and as a result, unless you are watchful of what you eat, you may bring upon yourself some unwanted health problems, such as obesity. The foods in this group are cakes, cookies, doughnuts, Danish pastries, crackers, pies, cakes, croissants, rice, cereals and all types of bread. The problems associated with many of these foods are the inclusion of sugar, salt and fat and the fact that many of them may be prepared from processed or refined flour. With these foods, you might have to worry not only about the added calories but also that you might not get all the vitamins and minerals your body needs. That is why, as explained in Chapter 2, the problems of subclinical and marginal malnutrition, as well as obesity, prevail in this country.

The Solution

First, let your conscience and wisdom, not your appetite, craving or whim, be your guide. The American food industry has long known that the best way to reach into your wallet is through your palate. It has for a long time enticed you into purchasing its fat-, oil- and sugar-filled foods or drinks. Massive consumption of these foods and drinks in the past few decades has resulted in unprecedented proportions of degenerative diseases and deaths in this country.

We now know the definite correlation between the high consumption of fatty foods and the incidence of obesity (which can lead to diabetes), cancer and cardio-vascular diseases, and between the high intake of salt and high blood pressure and between the frequent consumption of sugar and dental cavities, among other things. Our knowledge and these findings should lead us to be astute in our choice of foods and in our eating habits.

Second, for us to be aware of the beneficial aspect of foods and lead a healthy life, the U.S. Department of Agriculture recommends the following precautions:

- **Eat a variety of foods.** Since minerals, vitamins and other nutrients are found in different foods and in varying amounts, the best way of ensuring that you are getting these nutrients is by eating a variety of foods.

- **Maintain healthy weight.** When you become too fat, you predispose your body to a number of degenerative diseases. One way of minimizing this is by keeping your weight to an acceptable level. See Table 35.1 on page 342 as a guide for a healthy weight.

- **Chose a diet low in fat, saturated fat and cholesterol.** Since a high consumption of these foods can lead to heart diseases, certain cancers and diabetes, you may want to keep the intake of these foods to a minimum— particularly if you are an adult.

- **Choose a diet with plenty of vegetables, fruits and grain products.** These foods are generally rich in vitamins, minerals and fiber and low in fat. As was discussed earlier, fiber is an excellent lubricant of the gastrointestinal tract. Fiber can help minimize such chronic problems as diverticulosis, constipation and hemorrhoids.

- **Use sugar only in moderation.** Excessive consumption of pure sugar can lead to obesity and tooth decay. Sugar can also upset one's day-to-day living, creating wild mood swings, irritability and depression.

- **Use salt and sodium in moderation.** Salt (sodium chloride) and sodium are found in a variety of processed as well as whole foods. Since excessive intake of sodium can lead to high blood pressure, watch your consumption of this mineral.

- **If you drink alcoholic beverages, do so in moderation.** In addition to the fact that the excessive intake of alcohol can usurp your mental acuity and leave you vulnerable to hazards, it can lead to diseases such as cirrhosis of the liver and cancer of the esophagus. In pregnant women, alcohol can damage the health of the fetus.

Along with the proper choice of foods from the Food Guide Pyramid, you may want to include quality supplements. Vitamin, mineral and amino acid supplements can help to optimize your health and may even add years to your life. As was discussed in Chapter 20, there are many reasons why we can't depend on our regular food for all of our nutrient needs. Supplements may enable you to deal with these problems and help to optimize your health.

Conclusion

From everything we discussed in this book, living a long, healthy and happy life requires our personal commitment to nourishing our body properly and adequately. This means providing our body with all those nutrients that are known to be good and minimizing or abstaining from all those that are known to be bad or unhealthy for us. Thus, we need to cut out or limit our intake of fat- and cholesterol-rich foods and sweets, table salt and those foods that contain additives (preservatives, artificial coloring and flavoring agents).

Some of these may sound difficult at first, especially if you have been consuming such foods for a long time. Once you realize the deleterious effects of some of the foods, you should have no difficulty in developing an aversion to them; you should be able to let your mind master your gluttony whenever you are "confronted" with some of these bad foods. The key is knowing what they are and understanding the impact they have on your health.

For configuring your daily meals, the Food Guide Pyramid will certainly be a good starting point. Practice eating a well-balanced meal every day, and take quality supplements. Vitamins and minerals are crucial to your health. Considering the fact that those from regular foods are often poorly processed and absorbed, quality supplements may help minimize this problem.

As you must already know, without the presence of sufficient amounts of vitamins and minerals, none of the food groups from the pyramid will be properly and efficiently metabolized. As a result, your body may not get sufficient energy, build new tissues or synthesize millions of other substances (such as hormones, enzymes and neurochemicals), all of which contribute to your energy level and well-being.

Along with watching what you eat, you may also want to drink pure or distilled water. Since your body is nearly three-quarters water and since many of the metabolic processes that go on second by second happen in this medium, it is important that the water you consume be free of unnecessary foreign matter.

Exercise is an important component of good health. Besides giving you a sense of euphoria and well-being, exercise can make your muscles strong so that you can accomplish physical tasks easily. Exercise is also important for keeping your circulatory system free of artery-clogging fats, as well as for maintaining properly functioning bones and joints.

Do you have a weight problem? Regular exercise can help you lose weight or maintain a steady weight. According to the *Journal of the American Medical Association,* exercise can also help you live longer. It has been found that people who allow their weight to fluctuate often die younger than those who maintain a steady weight.

An integral part of good health is rest, meditation and relaxation. Considering that many of us lead a very stressful life, it is important that we have a quiet and peaceful time for ourselves at least for an hour every day. This practice will enable us to be in touch with our inner feelings and emotions as well as help our body and mind to relieve tension and stress. Excessive drinking, cigarette smoking and substance abuse are equally detrimental to your health. Thus, you may also want to distance yourself from these health hazards.

In summation, food is the foundation of who you are physically, emotionally and intellectually. Food is also the basis of your health, well-being and longevity. To take advantage of the many beneficial aspects of food, you may want to configure your daily meals according to your own specific needs or caloric demands. You may also want to choose your meals according to the known food values. For this, use the Food Guide Pyramid religiously and avail yourself of quality supplements regularly. These practices should enable you to live a long, happy and productive life.

PART XV
Appendices

(For the technically inclined and for those who want to know more.)

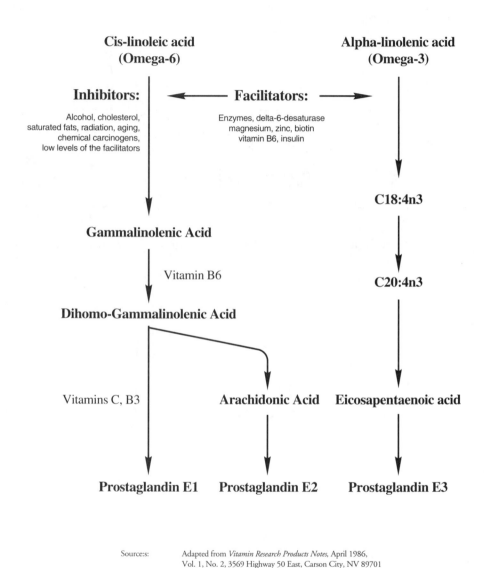

Figure A.1 Synthesis of Prostaglandins from omega-3 and omega-6 Fatty Acids

APPENDIX A
Prostaglandins

Prostaglandins are a rather intriguing group of molecules that have many benefits to you. Although they were first isolated from the prostate gland (thus their name) in the 1930s, their many roles in our health are still being discovered. Synthesized in the body from essential fatty acids, prostaglandins perform many critical functions in our bodies.

There are roughly 30 known prostaglandins, but of these, only about three have been extensively studied. Prostaglandin E1 is one of those on which we have an impressive amount of information. Formed from *cis*-linoleic acid (see Figure A.1 on page 358), this substance has many benefits to your health.

In the section Essential Fatty Acids (EFAs) on page 77, we briefly mentioned some of the important functions of prostaglandins in our bodies, but what makes them such intriguing substances are their peculiarities. They function like hormones in that they control the activities of enzymes, cells and organs. Yet unlike hormones, prostaglandins are more localized and shortlived—lasting, at most, a few seconds after being synthesized. The influence they have on our bodies during these fleeting moments, however, is pretty astounding.

By enabling the blood vessels to dilate and platelets to remain fully dispersed, E1 can help you minimize the incidence of cardiovascular diseases. When platelets stick together, they tend to form clots, which can obstruct blood vessels, causing heart attack or stroke. In the liver, E1 limits the production of cholesterol, which is equally important to the health of your circulatory system. Prostaglandin E1 similarly inhibits the production of potentially cancerous cells in the body.

Insulin, which helps us metabolize sugar, is empowered in the presence of prostaglandin E1. This is a bit of good news for diabetics. Those who suffer from arthritis can find relief with E1, because it has an ability to inhibit the production of inflammatory chemicals in the joints and elsewhere in the body. In the brain, E1 can increase the activities of the neurons that help elevate your mood and bring you a sense of well-being.

Your immune and reproductive systems are also greatly benefited by prostaglandin E1. Outwardly, this versatile molecule can also improve your skin and hair because it has an influence on the production of sebum and other chemicals that keep the skin healthy.

Unfortunately, as much as there are health-providing prostaglandins like E1, there are also others that have the opposite action on our bodies.[1,2] One particular culprit, called prostaglandin E2, can instigate many unwanted problems. These range from causing inflammation in the joints to causing the platelets to stick together and fluid to build up in the tissues, which are all not good.

Fortunately, the production of E2 is inhibited as long as you have more of E1.[3] It has been found that although both E1 and E2 have the same parent, the production of E1 is normally favored over E2. As it turns out, this is dependent on the amount of essential fatty acids you have in your body.[4] Flaxseed (discussed in Appendix B) and evening primrose oil are the best sources of these series of prostaglandins. The availability of the necessary vitamin and mineral cofactors shown in Figure A.1 is also very important for the conversion of the fatty acids into prostaglandins. The third, very well documented prostaglandins are the E3 series. These molecules can be derived from omega-3 fatty acids, but they also can come from eicosapentaenoic acid (EPA) found in fish oil. Considering E3's role in the proper functioning of the nervous system and its use in the synthesis of brain cells, the folklore about the importance of fish to the brain is not without basis.

In terms of their benefit to our health, E3s have many functions similar to E1s. Some of them were already covered in the section Essential Fatty Acids (EFAs), on page 83. These included their ability to reduce heart attack and stroke by lowering the production of cholesterol and triglycerides (fats) and their ability in helping to boost the immune system and in lowering the incidence of cancer. Prostaglandins, E3 as well as E1, are also involved in alleviating mental disorders such as depression and schizophrenia.

In another area, these prostaglandins also are essential for protection of the gastric mucosa (the mucous membrane) against the extreme acidity found in the stomach. The gastric side effects of drugs like Motrin happen because the levels of prostaglandins in the gastric mucosa are also reduced (not just those in the uterus), and hence one can get irritation of the gastric mucosa. Figure A.1 is assembled to help you see the paths the essential fatty acids take to give you the wonder workers of your health—prostaglandins. As you can see, the conversion of these important foods into those key end- products is not often an easy one. There are many factors that can impede, as well as aid, the processes.

The key is to distinguish those that aid your cells to manufacture the prostaglandins from those that block their synthesis.

APPENDIX B
Flaxseed—the Best Source of Essential Fatty Acids

This remarkable food once graced the meals of ancient Greeks, Romans, Egyptians and Babylonians with its rich nutrients and pleasant, nutty flavor. In many parts of the world, flaxseed is still used as food. In this country and in Europe, however, flaxseed has been relegated to serving mainly as a binder or protective material for the paint and printing industry.

Flaxseed is a rich source of essential fatty acids and a variety of key minerals, vitamins and amino acids. For instance, flaxseed oil can contain up to 60% of omega-3 and from 15% to 20% of omega-6 fatty acids. Both of these are precursors of prostaglandins, which we discussed in Chapter 7 and Appendix A. Prostaglandins are very important for good health.

Flaxseed itself contains important minerals such as potassium, magnesium, phosphorus, calcium, sulphur, sodium, zinc and chlorine. In addition, this important food product has a fair amount of copper, manganese, iron, aluminum, fluorine, nickel, cobalt, iodine, chromium and molybdenum.[1] Vitamins, such as A, C and D and thiamine and riboflavin, are also found in flaxseed. The protein content is equally impressive.

Flaxseed contains practically all the essential amino acids and another important substance called lecithin. Lecithin (a phospholipid) has many benefits to your health. One of its functions is to keep fat from settling or separating out in the blood. This function of lecithin is very important to the health of your heart and the rest of your circulatory system. In the presence of a sufficient amount of lecithin in the diet, fats and cholesterol can be made to remain suspended in the blood until they are metabolized or removed from the body. This avoids the possibility of clogging blood vessels. HDLs are rich in phospholipids. Lecithin is also an important source of choline, a key precursor of acetylcholine. Acetylcholine is a prominent neurotransmitter involved in memory and learning abilities. In addition, lecithin is found to be beneficial in improving muscle and nerve disorders. It also serves as a precursor to substances used in the manufacture of cell membranes.

Together with all of the above important nutrients, flaxseed also contains fiber. You know how important fibers are for your health and well-being. In the digestive tract, ground flaxseed can turn into mucilage, which has a laxative and purging effect. This can help you remove from the digestive tract many unhealthy substances, including cholesterol, fats, excess sugar and a number of toxins. In addition, flaxseed can help soothe irritations and ulcers in the stomach.

You probably wonder why such an important food is not commonly available in your neighborhood grocery stores. Well, despite its great importance to human health, flaxseed oil (also called linseed oil) has one weakness. Its molecules are pretty vulnerable and can oxidize quickly in the presence of light, heat and oxygen. This same property, which has made linseed oil unattractive to the food industry, has been made practicable in the paint and printing industry.

Because linseed oil has the ability to oxidize, harden and dry quickly, manufacturers of paint, varnish, printing ink and linoleum are the major commercial consumers of flaxseed. The protein and mineral rich refuse has also been used as an important feed for livestock in this country and in Europe. Before polyester, flax fibers were used to manufacture linen.

Needless to say, if you follow the simple preparative instructions below, you can greatly benefit from this important ancient food. Most health food stores carry flax, which they sell by the pound. You can buy as many pounds as you like, but depending on the frequency of use, one pound can last you up to two weeks.

Suggested Preparative Methods

The easiest way to prepare flaxseed is, first, to roast it. You can do it in a frying pan or in a pot, on low heat. Because it tends to splatter like popcorn, you need to cover it and frequently stir with a long wooden spoon. Once the seeds have become a shade darker than their original brown color, remove them from the fire, transfer them to a tray or plate and let them cool off. Next, pour them in a coffee grinder and mill them for about a minute or two. (Braun's top model is preferable. Other models tend to make the powder pastelike.) Nonetheless, you'll notice a pleasant redolence pervading your home while they're being ground.

Immediately after grinding, transfer the powder into a ziplock bag and store it in the freezer. Doing so minimizes oxidation.

How You Can Use Your Ground Flax

You can use flax powder with just about anything. As a dressing, you can sprinkle a spoonful of the powdered flax on your tossed salad, especially good if you use olive oil and vinegar as a base. Blue cheese and some of the other highly spiced dressings can dilute the delightful, nutty flavor and smell of the flax. You can also use it with your green vegetables such as green beans, cabbage, broccoli, collard greens and zucchini. Experiment with it in all your favorite dishes. Ground flaxseed can reward you with health, vitality and well-being.

You can also make a delicious drink with it. Just mix two heaping spoonfuls of the ground seeds with water in a tall glass containing a couple of ice cubes. You'll have a smooth, healthy and flavorful drink. Since it's rich in fiber and mucilages, it nicely lubricates your digestive tract, while its nutrients can nourish your body.

You can have this drink as part of your breakfast or dinner. You might want to have it as part of your dinner because many of the important nutrients (essential amino acids, minerals and vitamins) in this drink can be used for the repair and rejuvenation of your tissues at night. You don't want them wasted as fuel during the day.

APPENDIX C
State-of-the-Art Ingredients and Unique Technologies

Chelation

Chelation is a process of wrapping, cradling or encapsulating mineral particles (ions) with organic molecules such as amino acids, amino acid derivatives, proteins or other organic molecules. (An amino-acid chelate is illustrated in Figure C.1 on page 366.)

Chelation is derived from a Greek word, "chelate," which means "claw." It appears that the person who coined the term could visualize the similarity between a bird's claws trapping a rock or some other object and a metal ion wrapped in an organic molecule. This analogy is a very good one because chelation is similar to clawing or trapping a metal ion (a "rock") in an organic molecule.

Chelation in Nature

Nearly all the minerals in biological systems are found bound to organic molecules. The formations of some of these organometallic complexes (or chelates) are so important that life on earth as we know it now would not be possible without them. Let's take chlorophyll—the green substance found in most plants. Do you know that practically all forms of life (plant or animal) are dependent on chlorophyll for their existence?

In fact, it's believed that billions of years ago bacteria or other simple life forms evolved because a magnesium-chelated organic molecule (chlorophyll) was able to trap sunlight and produce sugar, oxygen and water. Now we take it for granted. Without oxygen, we can die in a few minutes. In this illustration, the magnesium that sits in the center of porphyrin (a square, planar organic molecule that makes up chlorophyll) serves as a catalyst for the absorption of the sun's energy and its utilization in the synthesis of sugars (our body's energy supply) and in the formation of water and oxygen.

How about the hemoglobin in our bodies? This globular (spherical or globlike) protein contains four chelated iron atoms at different sites of the molecule. It is the iron that enables the hemoglobin to pick up oxygen from the

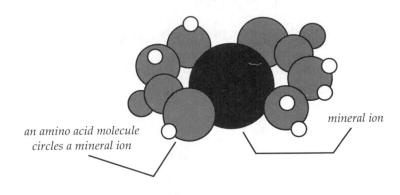

*an amino acid molecule
circles a mineral ion*

mineral ion

Figure C. 1 Amino Acid Chelate

lungs and deliver them to the cells. Similarly, myoglobin is an iron-containing protein that serves as a reservoir for storage of oxygen in the muscle tissues. In the mitochondria of the cells, another iron-chelated globular protein molecule, called cytochrome c, is responsible for the Krebs cycle's utilization of oxygen and the production of energy, carbon dioxide and water. Vitamin B12 is also chelated with cobalt (see the chemical structure for this vitamin on page 392.) This vitamin won't exist or function without cobalt.

There are thousands of other chelated organic molecules in both animals and plants. Each one of these molecules cannot be synthesized or function properly without its specific minerals. These include, in addition to those discussed above, thousands of enzymes, hormones and vitamins, and those molecules involved in the formation and configuration of DNA molecules. Let's look at each one separately.

As you must already know, enzymes are catalysts. From the breakdown of food in the digestive tract to its utilization in building and repairing tissues to the production of energy and many other metabolic processes, enzymes play an important part. Minerals are intimately involved in all these processes.

Hormones are chemical messengers that influence the function of various tissues and organs in our body. Hormones are usually produced by a gland (like the pituitary, adrenaline, the pancreas or thyroid gland) and are released into the bloodstream where they are carried to various parts of the body but only to influence a specific tissue or organ. From the metabolic processes to digestion to monitoring blood pressure and bodily fluids to growth and development and hundreds of other processes, hormones play vital functions in our daily lives. With these chemicals, too, minerals play an important role.

Vitamins are essential nutrients that we cannot live without. Although they don't become part of our tissues and organs (like proteins, fats and carbohydrates), vitamins are crucial to the proper function of many of the enzyme systems and practically all of the chemical processes that go on every second in our bodies. Interestingly, vitamins, too, cannot function efficiently and effectively without minerals.

From this brief discussion, you can see that minerals have a great influence on many of the fundamental body processes and functions, all of which should contribute to your health and well-being. According to one author, "minerals are involved in more body processes than any other basic nutrient—including protein, vitamins, fats, carbohydrates, and water."[1]

This is also to say that the true meaning and value of these nutrients can be captured only in the presence of diverse and adequate minerals in the body. Without minerals, the growth and repair of tissues, the production of energy and many of the other body processes may be severely compromised. According to one testament: "Even small departures from the normal mineral composition of the milieu interieur [the interior of the cell] may have profound physiological consequences, but may make no appreciable difference to composition of the body as a whole."[2]

Simply put, minerals give meaning and purpose to the food we eat and to life itself. Because these inert, tiny, earthly substances are so important to our health and yet are not easy to secure once they enter our system, nature has devised chelation as way of ensuring their stay and function in the body.

What Is the Importance of Chelating Mineral Supplements?

From the preceding discussion, you noticed that minerals are a crucial part of our daily nourishment. Unfortunately, as much as they are, they can also be some of the least available to our body. This is so not only because minerals have to be imported from outside through the foods we consume but also because there are many factors that limit their availability to our bodies. These may range from the natural variability in the soil's mineral content or its depletion (due to overused agricultural lands) to food processing, which removes a significant portion of the minerals naturally found in foods like wheat or sugar.

Table C.1 Minerals Lost through Food Processing

Wheat Milling		Refining Sugarcane	
Mineral	**Loss**	**Mineral**	**Loss**
Manganese	88%	Magnesium	99%
Chromium	87%	Zinc	98%
Magnesium	80%	Chromium	93%
Sodium	78%	Manganese	93%
Potassium	77%	Cobalt	88%
Iron	76%	Copper	83%
Zinc	72%	Phosphorus	71%
Copper	63%	Calcium	60%
Molybdenum	60%	Cobalt	50%

Source: Henry Schroeder, M.D. The *Trace Elements and Man.*[3]

Then there is the problem of absorption. This problem comes about largely from our body's inability to efficiently process and extract the minerals from the food we consume, as well as from the factors that interfere with the proper absorption of these nutrients. Some of these can be compounds such as oxalate, phytates or tannic acid (found in certain vegetables), which may combine with certain minerals in the digestive tract and make them unavailable. Similarly, fiber and the consumption of excessive alcohol and fat, as well as the presence of high amounts of competing minerals, may hinder the proper utilization of the minerals we get from food.

Whether you get minerals from conventional supplements or from foods, after they have been ionized* they first have to be chelated in the digestive tract by amino acids before they can be absorbed. The chelation process is random and requires the presence of a few synergistic factors; as a result, proper binding and absorption may be limited.

To minimize all the above possible problems and provide higher absorption, certain companies use amino-acid-chelated minerals. In addition, the molecular size and the special patented technique used to manufacture them are important.

In terms of their comparison to organic salts, Table C.2 illustrates the dramatic difference between iron amino acid chelate and the iron in organic salts you may find in your ordinary supplements.

In conclusion, chelation of minerals in bioavailable organic molecules is cer-

---

*The mineral-containing compound breaks apart leaving the mineral particle ion.

Table C.2 Mean Comparison of 59Fe (Iron) Retention and Distribution cc/m/gm)*

Body Part	[59] Iron Sulfate	[59] Iron Amino Acid Chelate	Change Chelated with Sulfate
Heart	63	151	+ 140%
Liver	136	243	+79%
Leg muscle	2	54	+2,600%
Jaw muscle	14	138	+886%
Brain	31	130	+319%
Kidney	2	327	+ 16,250%
Testes	20	109	+445%
Blood serum	700	1,797	+ 157%
Red blood cells	724	2,076	+180%
Whole blood	1,355	4,215	+211%
Feces	302,400	214,000	-29%

Source, Dr. H. DeWayne Ashmead. *Conversation on Chelation and Mineral Nutrition.*[4]

*Corrected counts per minute per gram of body portion being analyzed.

tainly nature's way of dealing with the potential scarcity or unavailability of minerals to the body. Considering the many problems we encounter involving soil mineral variability, food refining or poor absorption by the digestive tract, the best way to ensure we get adequate amounts of these vital substances is by chelating them with amino acids. There are companies that sell amino-acid chelated minerals. Look for supplements that contain chelated minerals in your health-food or drug store, or talk to your independent nutritional supplement distributor.

Chromium Picolinate

In the previous section, we talked about how minerals are a critical part of our bodies' processes and how our health, well-being and happiness are tied to diverse and sufficient amounts of these nutrients as well as others we consume every day. One mineral that has never been recognized as essential (although acknowledged as healthful) by the Food and Nutrition Board of the National Academy of Science, but become to be popular recently, is chromium.

From research findings that have been gathering in the past decade or so, chromium is shown to have many health-giving and life-enhancing properties. Its primary function is in enabling the body to process sugar at a higher rate in our tissues.

It has also been found to improve fat metabolism and increase muscle mass, and may help to tackle the problems associated with excess cholesterol in the blood.

How Chromium Picolinate Functions in the Body

First, bear in mind that chromium picolinate is made up of chromium and picolinic acid; the latter serves as a carrier to the former. What makes this particular compound of chromium (as opposed to chromium salts, like chromium chloride, for example) unique is that there is a higher absorption of the chromium into the bloodstream; and once it reaches the tissues, it easily converts to the biologically active form.

Second, chromium's position in our bodies is mainly as facilitator of processes involving sugar, fats, amino acids and other biochemicals. As you can see below, this job of chromium's is very crucial to your overall health as well as to your day-to-day living. Let's see how chromium does its job.

Insulin is the hormone responsible for the passage of nutrients and other substances across the cell membrane. Insulin can do this task efficiently only in the company of sufficient amounts of chromium. The metabolic and health significance of this is that in the presence of adequate insulin and chromium, your cells may have higher amounts of sugar, fats and amino acids delivered to them so that they can use these nutrients to produce energy as well as to build tissues. When you have higher amounts of energy, you will naturally feel energetic and become more productive.

As more fats are mobilized from circulating fluids into the cells, you may also have fewer problems involving cardiovascular diseases and hypertension—two of the most common degenerative diseases that come from an excess deposit of fats and cholesterol in the blood vessels.

How Chromium Picolinate May Help You in Losing Weight, Increasing Muscle Mass and Dealing with High Cholesterol

As was explained in Chapter 9, obesity comes about from the consumption of too many calories, lack of exercise and slowed metabolism. Each one of these problems will naturally lead to excessive accumulation of fat in our bodies. When supplied with larger quantities of high-calorie foods such as fat and sweets, and in the absence of regular exercise, the body has no way of shutting off its fat-making apparatus (the cells). In its propensity to save for the future, it simply converts those extra calories into and stores them as fat.

A corollary to the above statements is the fact that a low level of chromium in the body tends to lead to higher* amounts of insulin production by the pancreas, which concomitantly leads to a greater storage of body fat.[5] What a supplement like chromium picolinate may do for you is to deliver sufficient amounts of chromium to the body so that fat and cholesterol can have greater access to muscle and liver cells to be used as fuel and for other purposes. Chromium picolinate may also help you simultaneously reduce the LDL (bad) cholesterol and increase the HDL (good) cholesterol. All these events may contribute to weight loss.[6]

Another attribute of chromium regarding weight loss is its indirect role in curbing appetite by stabilizing the blood-sugar level. In conjunction with insulin, chromium is also believed to stimulate the thermogenesis[†] effect of carbohydrates as well as the production of the brain chemical serotonin, which among other things is believed to bring about a sense of satiation or fullness to the stomach. Both these effects of chromium may add to your weight-loss efforts.[7,8]

Regarding its role in increasing lean muscle mass, chromium (along with insulin) functions by enabling the muscle cells to absorb higher amounts of amino acids from the circulating fluid and by indirectly stimulating the synthesis of protein by the DNA. According to Dr. Fisher, when you combine these activities "with resistance exercise, it (may) result in more muscle development and fat loss."[9]

In summary, chromium picolinate is indeed a remarkable ingredient that may have many benefits to your health. To get all the beneficial results you need, make sure that you get this ingredient from your supplements.

As was discussed in Chapter 6 and in the section "Chelation" on page 365, the amount of minerals we obtain from our food sources may be inadequate. Besides the variation in the soil content, food processing and refining remove a great percentage of the minerals naturally found in foods. In addition, as we age, the body's ability to extract chromium from natural sources goes down dramatically. Again, the best way to enhance the availability of minerals is through quality supplements.

---

* In the absence of sufficient chromium in the body, there can be excessive amounts of sugar, fat and amino acids collecting in fluids and tissues and trying to gain entrance to the cells. To over compensate for the chromium shortage, the pancreas starts to release higher amounts of insulin, which leads to higher production of fat cells and fat storage.

† Increasing the body's metabolic rate, which may enable the body to lose weight.

L-Carnitine

This compound's primary function in the body is in enabling the cells to mobilize and utilize fat at a higher rate. L-carnitine does this by acting like a little pickup truck, which gathers fat molecules from within the cell and dumps them into the mitochondrial furnace, where they can be utilized as fuel.

L-carnitine is synthesized from the amino acids lysine and methionine. Although the body makes some of its own, the best way to maximize the beneficial effect of L-carnitine is obviously by including it as part of a daily supplement. Adequate amounts of L-carnitine may help reduce the health risks associated with excess fat in the circulating fluids and tissues. You can perhaps see the significance of L-carnitine when it is present in conjunction with chromium picolinate, as discussed above. Both of these ingredients may enable the body to utilize fat at a higher rate and optimize health. (See the section "Amino Acids for Your Heart" on page 285 for more information.)

Pycnogenol

Technically, this strange-sounding plant extract is very similar to the yellow, orange or green of fruits and vegetables you eat every day. A major portion of these different colors represents a group of organic substances known as bioflavonoids. There are over 20,000 bioflavonoids, but the pycnogenol you find in some supplements represents a special group of flavonoids, known as proanthocyanidins or, simply, procyanidins.

Jacques Masquelier, the French scientist who has done extensive work on bioflavonoids, is credited for naming these special flavonoids "pycnogenol" and for developing a patented extraction process from a bark of a certain type of pine tree, the richest known source of the extract. Let's see what pycnogenol may do for you.

Some of the traditional areas where pycnogenol has been found useful are in improving circulation, reducing stress, reducing joint inflammation (such as that caused by arthritis), enhancing mental clarity and visual acuity and in a number of other related areas, including making skin look better and healthier.[10]

The current area where pycnogenol has found popular use is in fighting free radicals, those molecular renegades we discussed in Chapter 4. This plant extract may help neutralize free radicals by itself or as a special helper of vitamin C. Pycnogenol helps vitamin C to do its job effectively. Ordinarily, once an antioxidant like vitamin C gives up its spare electron to a free radical, the vitamin self-

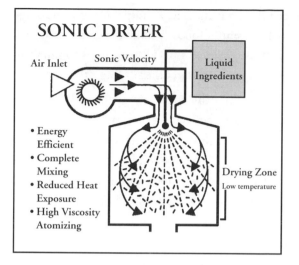

Figure C.2 Sonic Enhanced Drying

destructs. In the presence of sufficient amounts of pycnogenol, however, the vitamin can be regenerated and go on to neutralize more free radicals.

What all this means is that since free radicals are known to cause many unwanted health problems, keeping them in check with a group of weapons like pycnogenol, vitamin C and other phytoantioxidants becomes of paramount importance. All those traditional areas in which pycnogenol was found to be beneficial have something to do with this extract's role in fighting free radicals.

Ideally, you would want to obtain pycnogenol from a variety of fresh vegetables, fruits and nuts. These may include red peppers, grapes, lemons. cranberries, beans, kola nuts and other fruits and vegetables.[11] This is not practicable for *two* reasons, however: (a) to get enough pycnogenol from natural sources, you would have to consume large quantities of them and (b) eating a medley of vegetables and fruits is not something people do on a regular basis. Your best option, therefore, is to find a supplement that contains a concentrated amount of pycnogenol.

Sonic Enhanced Drying

Unless you consume foods that come fresh from the farm, chances are that you may not be getting all the nutrients that are naturally found in grains, vegetables and fruits. Refining, processing and canning foods may inactivate or partly remove many of the nutrients found in these natural foods.

Sonic enhanced drying is the new and upcoming technology designed to preserve the nutritional content of foods. Unlike the traditional method—which uses excessive heat (sometimes in excess of 300 degrees Fahrenheit)—sonic enhanced drying uses a lower temperature than other drying processes.

As shown in Figure C.2, this unique processor uses high-velocity air, which creates a partial vacuum around the wet, warm food particles that have been fed through a tiny opening in the top of the main chamber. These pressurized or atomized food particles are now able to dry at a low temperature. The vacuum created literally sucks the moisture out of the food and ultimately allows the dry, nutritionally intact powder to drop out of the bottom of the chamber.

Ester-C®*

In our discussion of antioxidants in both Chapter 4 and Chapter 12, we saw that vitamin C has many remarkable benefits to the human body. This versatile nutrient can minimize the symptoms of the common cold, serves as an antiviral and antibacterial agent, boosts the immune system, fights free radicals and lowers the cholesterol level in the blood. Vitamin C plays crucial roles in fighting certain cancers and is very important in the formation and development of connective tissues (collagen, elastin, tendons and ligaments). Both diabetics and hypoglycemics also benefit from this wonderful vitamin.

When you read about the great attributes of vitamin C, you may feel that you need to have this nutrient as part of your daily meals and in large quantities. Yes, you should have a regular intake of vitamin C and in amounts considerably larger than the 60 mg recommended by the RDA. The RDA amount may be enough to prevent scurvy (a vitamin C deficiency disease) or serve to meet some other basic needs. Much of the preventive, or even curative, benefits of this great nutrient come largely from one's consumption of higher doses.[12,13]

When we talk about "higher doses," perhaps you wonder, would there be health risks associated from taking too much of the vitamin? Vitamin C, in general, is a very benign nutrient, and you should have very little concern when taking it in larger doses. Some researchers have found, however, that ascorbic acid, the form you find in most multivitamin supplements, is not tolerated well by the gastrointestinal tract when consumed in considerably higher amounts, say 10,000 mgs/day. It turns out that this form of the vitamin is also poorly absorbed. For this reason, over

---

* Ester-C® is a trademark of Inter-Cal Corp.

the years, scientists have come up with vitamin C formulations that are much gentler and more absorbable by the digestive tract. (For more information about the safety of vitamins and minerals read Chapter 21).

The ascorbates, which are calcium or sodium salts of vitamin C, not only are gentler on the gastrointestinal tract but also are better absorbed. The recent addition to these forms of vitamin C is the one that goes by the trade name Ester-C®. Developed by Inter-Cal Corporation of Prescott, Arizona, Ester-C® has been hailed as the most absorbable (4 times better than ascorbic acid) and assimilable of vitamin C forms. Formulated by a patented process, this form of vitamin C is bonded or chelated with minerals such as calcium, potassium, sodium, magnesium and zinc, which make the nutrient more absorbable than ascorbic acid or the other ascorbates.[16]

Besides the fact that Ester-C® is the most absorbable and least irritating or discomforting to the gastrointestinal tract, it is also the most effective. Ester-C® also stays longer in the body than other forms of vitamin C. Considering the many great attributes of this nutrient and its tendency to be flushed out of the system easily (because it is water soluble), this feature of Ester-C® is a definite plus.

In summation, from the discussion above and elsewhere in the book, you have learned that vitamin C has many great benefits when taken in higher (than RDA) amounts. To take advantage of this nutrient's great benefits, make sure that you consume foods that are a good source of the vitamin and take supplements that contain Ester-C® in their ingredients.

APPENDIX D
The Krebs Cycle

The following diagrams illustrate how energy is extracted from the foods you eat.

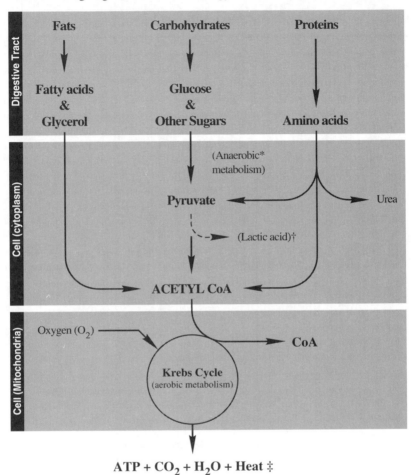

$$ATP + CO_2 + H_2O + Heat \ddagger$$

*   As in weight lifting, sprinting and other activities that require a quick burst of energy, this process does not require oxygen.

†   If such activities are continued repetitively for some time in the absence of sufficient oxygen, lactic acid can buildup causing cramps and a burning feeling in the muscles.

‡   When you engage in a long and continuous exercise like aerobics, running, swimming or bicycling, ATP is continually produced to provide energy for your muscles. The other byproducts of these types of exercise are a profuse amount of sweat and carbon dioxide. For these types of exercises you need good lungs and a strong heart, which effciently and continuously delivers oxygen-rich blood to the working muscles.

Net ATP Harvested:	1 glucose	2 ATP	(anaerobic)
	1 glucose	38 ATP	(aerobic)
	1 fatty acid (16:1)	129 ATP	(aerobic)

Figure D.1 The Krebs Cycle

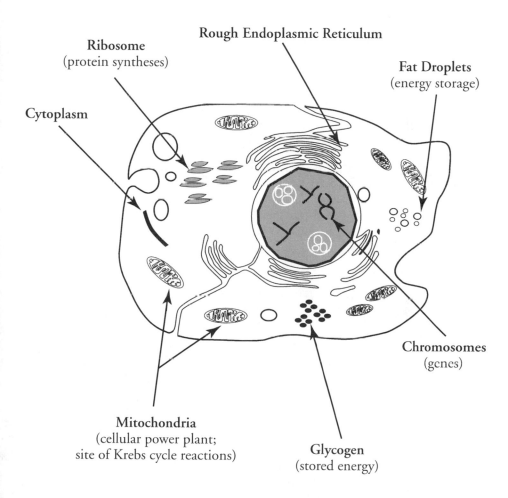

Figure D.2 A Cell with Its Life-Sustaining Apparatus

APPENDIX E
Molecular Structure of Fat Molecules

As we mentioned in Chapter 7, there are three general types of fats: saturated, monounsaturated and polyunsaturated. Although all these fats have the same backbone (glycerol); their difference is in the fatty acid portion of these molecules. Dangling like a set of strings attached to a stationary object, fatty acids can be saturated or unsaturated, be short or long or have *cis*- or *trans*- configuration around their double bonds.

The physical characteristics of fats (whether they're solid or liquid at room temperature), the effect they have on your health and how well they function as structural components of cell membranes are all determined to a large degree by the type of fatty acids they contain. Thus, if you are concerned about cancer and heart disease, as well as the proper functioning of your cells, you should be selective in your choice of fats or seek adequate protection from some of their harmful effects.

The molecular structures in Figure E.1 on page 382 show a glycerol molecule and representative examples of the different kinds of fatty acids found in our foods. In these illustrations, the C's stand for carbon, the H's for hydrogen and the O's for oxygen. The different fatty acids, shown in the same figure, can attach to the oxygen end of the glycerol molecule to give rise to different types of fats and oils.

As we said earlier, a given molecule of fat or oil can have monounsaturated, polyunsaturated, saturated, short or long chain fatty acids. Butter, for example, ordinarily contains roughly 35% oleic acid, 25% palmitic acid, 10% stearic acid and another 30%, which is a combination of butyric, capric, lauric, myristic, palmitoleic and linoleic acids. On the other hand, both sunflower and safflower oils contain largely linoleic and oleic acids.

With a few exceptions, unsaturated fatty acids predominate in plant oils, while saturated fatty acids are the major components of animal fat. These basic differences, together with the length of the carbon chains involved, determine the physical state of the triglyceride molecule. Animal and some vegetable fats, such as palm and coconut oils, contain relatively shorter chains of fatty acids—usually only up to 14 carbon atoms. At room temperature, coconut, palm and animal fats are solid,

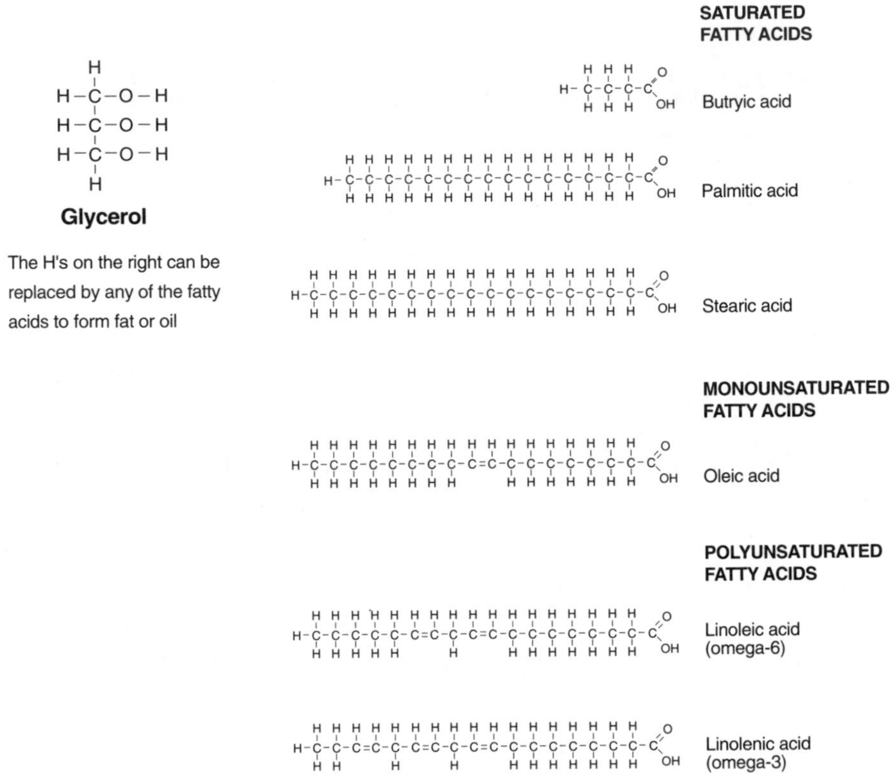

Figure E.1 Representative Structures of Various Fats

but because both these plant fats are liquid in the tropics where they are produced, they are classified as oils.

Most plant oils, on the other hand, contain longer carbon chains (often up to 18 and more carbon atoms) with double bonds interspersed throughout the chains. The most frequent number of double bonds encountered in these oils are 1, 2 and 3. Two essential fatty acids, called *eicosapentaenoic acid (EPA)* and *docosahexaenoic acid (DHA),* have 5 and 6 double bonds, respectively. These fats are found primarily in fish oils, as well as in the brain, testicles, eyes and adrenaline glands.

Fats, Oils and Your Health—a Mixed Blessing

One of the fundamental differences between saturated and unsaturated fats (i.e., between fats and oils) is the way the fatty acid chains pack or arrange themselves. This difference is illustrated in Figure E.2 on page 383. While the fatty acids

The space-filled model A represents a saturated fat. In this figure, the fatty-acid chains pack closely, thus making this class of fats solid at room temperature. Model B, on the other hand, illustrates an unsaturated fat. The kinked portion of the molecule represents a cis-configuration of hydrogens around the carbon atom. The same molecule is also shown in a different way of illustrating chemical structure in model C. Most of the unsaturated fats are liquid (oil) at room temperature.

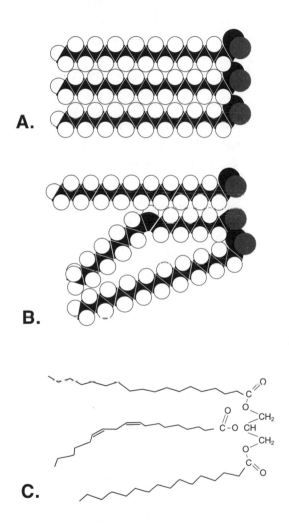

Figure E.2 Saturated and Unsaturated Fats

In the space-filled models A and B, above, the white spheres represent hydrogen atoms. The black skeletal frames show a chain of carbon atoms. Figure C is also a molecular model, but in this case, the hydrogen atoms on the fatty-acid chains (or tails) are not shown. Chemists find it timesaving to draw zigzagging (but sensible) chemical structures, as in C, rather than a string of carbon atoms. All the kinks in this structure represent carbon atoms.

in a saturated fat molecule pack neatly, as shown in molecular model A, the fatty acids in an unsaturated fat have a kink or bend in their chains.

This variation between the two acids leads to the difference in their chemical and physical properties, as well as to the difference in the way they function in your body. Because saturated fatty acids pack densely, they are solid or semisolid at room temperature. Unsaturated fats, on the other hand, are liquid (oil) at room temperature because the fatty acid portion of these molecules is rather loose. It makes sense, doesn't it?

Chemically, saturated fats are less interactive than unsaturated fats. Because of their highly reactive properties, unsaturated fats (particularly the polyunsaturates) in your body can make a number of useful substances out of them. Saturated fats function largely as insulators against cold and as cushions around the vital organs. Besides getting what its needs from fatty foods (such as milk and meats), your body can make its own saturated fats from proteins, carbohydrates and unsaturated fats.

Nutritionally, saturated fats may serve as precursors to cholesterol and for certain hormones. Some of the short-chained saturated fats can be used for energy. Overall though, saturated fats do more harm than good to your body, particularly if too many of them accumulate. A majority of the saturated fats that come from meats and dairy products are rather bulky molecules that clog up the highways and byways of your blood vessels.

When used as an integral part of the cell membrane, saturated fats can have a sealing effect, interfering with the free flow of nutrients, enzymes and other molecules. As a result, toxic and waste by-products can collect within the cell. Incidentally, trans-fatty acids, which we discussed in Chapter 7, have the same effect on cellular membranes. That is why fats like margarine and shortening are not good for you.

On the other hand, unsaturated fatty acids (UFAs), shown in the model B of Figure E.2, pack or arrange themselves loosely, which gives these molecules fluidity and flexibility. These are very important attributes, whether these fatty acids circulate in your blood or are used to make cell membranes, nerve fibers and sheaths. When the UFAs are part of cellular structures, for example, nutrients and other substances can move in and out of the cell readily—an important feature for the survival and proper functioning of the cell. As part of brain cells, muscle and nerve fibers, UFAs are involved in electrical impulse transmission—another important attribute for the health and proper functioning of your body.

Unfortunately, as much as UFAs have many benefits to your health, they also are vulnerable to destruction by free radicals, radiation, oxygen, light and other agents. Particularly vulnerable are those tissues such as those in the brain, which contain over 60% fat—most of which is polyunsaturated.

APPENDIX F
Molecular Structures of Fat-Soluble Vitamins

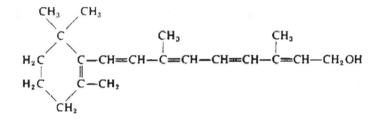

Retinol (Vitamin A)

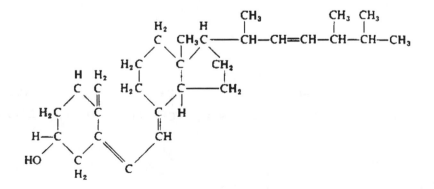

Cholecalciferol (Vitamin D)

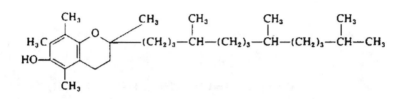

Tocopherol (Vitamin E)

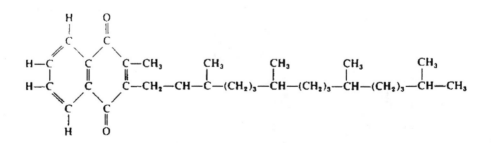

Phylloquinone (Vitamin K)

Molecular Structures of Water-Soluble Vitamins

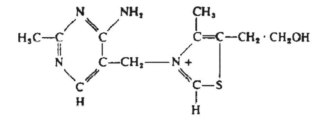

Thiamin (Vitamin B1)

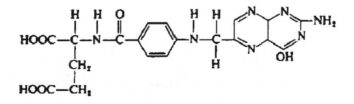

Folacin

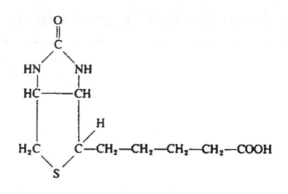

Biotin

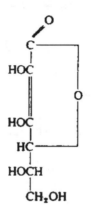

Ascorbic Acid (Vitamin C)

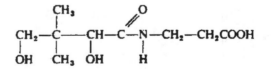

Pantothenic Acid

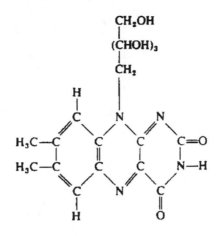

Riboflavin (Vitamin B2)

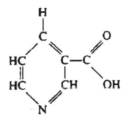

Niacin (Nicotinic Acid)

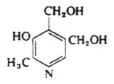

Pyrodoxine (Vitamin B6)

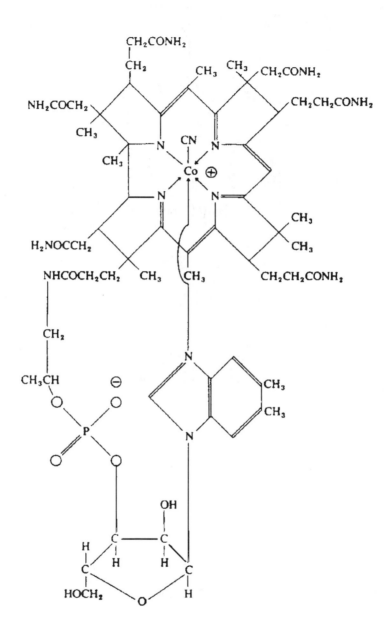

Vitamin B$_{12}$

APPENDIX H
Molecular Structures of Essential Amino Acids

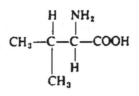

Valine

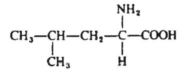

Leucine

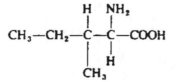

Isoleucine
(Branched-Chain Amino Acids)

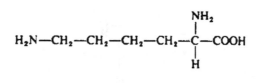

Lysine

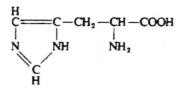

Histidine

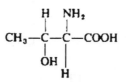

Threonine

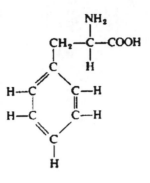

Phenylalanine

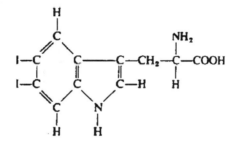

Tryptophan

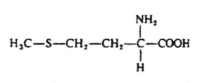

Methionine
(one of the sulfur-containing antioxidant amino acids)

APPENDIX I
Clinical Nutrient Analyses

In Chapter 2, we talked about how increasing and diversifying our nutrient intake can move us from where we are currently (normal or malnourished) to the optimal section of the nutrition continuum (shown in Figure 2.3 on page 23.) We also said that because of the many differences (biological, genetic, lifestyle, etc.) that exist among us, we cannot use some mythical RDA figures as our guideline to achieving optimal nutrition, good health and maximum life span.

Our approach to optimal health and optimal nutrition needs to be more stringent and systematic than what it has been, mere guesswork—mixing vegetables, fruits, grains, meat and dairy products in whatever way we choose.

Besides abstaining from some of the harmful substances, such as cigarettes, alcohol and other drugs, we need to understand the nutritional value of the foods we eat, as well as periodically assess our health and nutritional status. To do this, we have many tools available. For example, in Chapter 2 we discussed the various tests we can take to assess our health, nutritional levels and the existence of health-threatening substances within our bodies.

Samples of such test runs are shown in Appendix J. The Mineral Analysis Report on page 402 evaluates the various mineral levels, both nutritional and toxic, in a person's hair sample. In this test, when you compare the patient's mineral levels with the reference ranges for the first 16 elements, you'll see that 7 of them, or nearly 45%, are below the minimum reference values. Although the "toxic mineral" figures are within acceptable ranges, there are significant deviations in both the mineral ratios and the "additional mineral" levels.

The essential fatty acid report on page 406 is perhaps the most complete of its kind and can be useful in assessing the levels of essential fatty acids and their derivatives in a person's body. The relative concentration of the different fatty acids and their derivatives can indicate their potential benefits as well as their risks. This test compares diagnostic results with what is considered normal. Tests from SpectraCell Laboratories, however, are perhaps the most up-to-date in that the analysis is done on a cellular level. This test reportedly is also the most sensitive, as it can detect vitamin and other nutrient deficiencies that are not ordinarily picked up by other tests. Since vitamins have many key roles in the body, it's important that you know how well supplied you are with these nutrients.

The Sample CDSA Test Reporting Form on page 407 evaluates how well your digestive system processes and utilizes the food you eat. In addition, it assesses the levels of useful, as well as parasitic or harmful, bacteria that may exist in the digestive tract. Because it's in the digestive tract that food is broken down and made available for distribution to the rest of the body, the health and proper functioning of this system is very important. This test would be very useful for anyone who has chronic problems with digestion, constipation or any other gastrointestinal disorders.

The Amino Acid Analysis Report on page 405 is an equally useful indicator of how well your body processes and utilizes the amino acids in your diet. As you can see in Appendix J, this test can also be an important indicator of the level of certain key minerals and vitamins in your tissues. For instance, in the absence of sufficient amounts of vitamins B6 and B12 and biotin, a high level of G-amino-isobutyrate may be detected in a urine sample. Similarly, an unusually high level of phosphoserine may indicate the lack of adequate magnesium, phosphorus and zinc.

In addition to helping you determine your nutritional intake, tests such as those starting on page 402 can be used to trace any dysfunctional problems, such as metabolic imbalances, kidney malfunctions or problems associated with the endocrine system. Because nutrients are the basis of our existence, any major shortage or imbalance in any of them may cause many health-related problems.

Once, a young woman told me that her parents had gone to many doctors and had spent thousands of dollars trying to find a cure for her father's infertility. Her parents had already given up and had planned to divorce when someone suggested that they see a prominent nutrition doctor in Mexico City. As it turned out, there was nothing inherently wrong with the father other than inadequate levels of certain key nutrients. Much to their surprise and happiness, this couple had their first daughter (the woman who told me the story) within a year and three more children after her. So, if you have a problem with infertility or impotency, you might want to have a nutrition profile done before you spend thousands of dollars with psychologists or specialty doctors. Your problem may be as simple as the couple's above.

If you are recovering from alcoholism or other drug addiction, or are pregnant, elderly or a preoperative patient, it would be to your great benefit to take tests like those discussed here. If you smoke, work in a stressful environment or have a stressful job, you also might want to have your nutrient levels checked. As was mentioned earlier in this book, alcohol, other drugs, cigarettes and stress are some of the great robbers of your tissue's nutrients. They can lead to subclinical or marginal deficiencies in the mildest case and to outright malnutrition and deficiency in the worst case scenario.

To have a properly developed child and to avoid miscarriage, a pregnant woman would find nutritional tests equally beneficial. As we said earlier, about 50% of all preoperative patients are malnourished. Hence, assessing one's tissue levels of nutrients and correcting any deficiencies that may exist prior to the operation can make the surgery and the postoperative recovery much easier.

In summary, good nutrition is truly the basis of good health, happiness and maximum life potential.

APPENDIX J
Sample Nutrition Clinical Reports and Analyses

PHYSICIAN'S COPY

MINERAL ANALYSIS REPORT

D D DOCTOR'S DATA

P.O. Box 111   30W101 Roosevelt Rd.
West Chicago, IL 60185   U.S.A.   800/323-2784

LAB. NO.: 91277-9999		
PATIENT: B Patient		AGE: 42 SEX: M
DOCTOR: HMO-BOB SMITH		ACCT.: 15417
ACCT.:		

DATE SAMPLED: 10/01/91	DATE IN: 10/04/91		DATE OUT: 10/05/91 R
OFFICE CODE: 2-2	HAIR COLOR: gray	SAMPLE SIZE: 0.40 g	SAMPLE TYPE: head hair

James T. Hicks, MD, PhD, FCAP
Laboratory Director

Nutrient Mineral Levels

NUTRIENT MINERAL	PATIENT LEVEL (parts per million)	LOW ◆ REFERENCE RANGE ◆ HIGH	NUMERICAL VALUE OF REFERENCE ◆ RANGE ●
Calcium	112	★★★★★★★★★★★★★★★★★★★★	280- 600
Magnesium	9	★★★★★★★★★★★★★★★★★	30- 75
Sodium	109	★★★★★★★★★★★★★★★★	20- 90
Potassium	77	★★★★★★★★★★★★★★★★★★★	9- 40
Copper	8		11- 28
Zinc	97	★★★★★★★★★★★★★★★★★★★	115- 165
Iron	8	★★★★★★	5- 14
Manganese	0.16	★★★★★★★★★★★★★★★★★★	0.26- 0.75
Chromium	0.44	★★★★★★★★★★★★★★★★★	0.78- 1.00
Cobalt	0.19	★★★★★★★★★★★★★★★	0.26- 0.47
Iodine	n/a		not available
Molybdenum	0.56	★★★★★★★★★★★★★★★	0.21- 0.44
Phosphorus	134	★★★★★★★	120- 170
Selenium	0.29	★★★★	0.38- 0.70
Silicon	2.9	★★★	1.2- 5.0
Sulfur	43100	★★★★★★★★★★★★★★★★★★★	46500- 52000

ADDITIONAL MINERAL LEVELS

		LOW REFERENCE RANGE HIGH	NUMERICAL VALUE
Antimony	0.80	★★★★★	0.45- 1.35
Barium	0.21	★★★★★★★★★★★★★★	0.30- 2.10
Boron	1.8	★★★	1.1- 2.8
Germanium	0.48	★★★★★★★★★★★★★★	0.65- 1.00
Lithium	0.028	★★★★★★★★★★★★★★	0.038- 0.069
Platinum	0.70	★★★★★★	0.01- 1.00
Rubidium	n/a		not available
Silver	0.30	★★★★★	0.02- 0.70
Strontium	0.36	★★★★★★★★★★★★★★★	0.50- 4.80
Thorium	4.61	★★★★★★★★★★	1.50- 5.15
Tin	0.9	★★★	0.1- 1.6
Titanium	0.44	★★★★★	0.10- 1.00
Tungsten	0.52	★★★	0.05- 0.95
Vanadium	<dl .001	★★★★★★★★★★★★★★★★★★★★★	0.36- 0.80
Zirconium	0.70	★★★★	0.01- 1.20

dl = detection limit, n/a = currently not available

Additional Mineral Levels

TOXIC MINERAL	PATIENT LEVEL (parts per million)	➤ HIGH ONE STANDARD DEVIATION ABOVE MEAN / TWO STANDARD DEVIATIONS ABOVE MEAN / MORE THAN TWO STANDARD DEVIATIONS ABOVE MEAN
Lead	8.0	★★★★★★★★★★★★7.0★★
Arsenic	0.8	★★ 7.0
Mercury	0.90	★★★★ 2.5
Cadmium	0.30	★★★★ 1.0
Aluminum	<dl 1.00	
Nickel	<dl .300	
Beryllium	0.01	★★ .10
TOTAL TOXICS		★★★★★★★★★★★★★★★★★★★★★★★
RACE: caucasian	SAMPLE CONDITIONS:	
HAIR PREPARATIONS:		
SHAMPOO: glycerin soap		

Mineral Ratios

Ca/Mg	12.4	5-	15
Ca/Zn	1.2	2.5-	7.0
Ca/P	0.8	2.6-	6.1
Ca/Fe	14.0	40-	90
Mg/K	0.1	1.8-	5.0
Na/K	1.4	1.8-	4.0
Zn/K	1.3	3-	13
Zn/Cu	12.1	4-	12
Cu/Fe	1.0	1.2-	3.5
Cu/Cd	26.7	> 30	
Zn/Cd	323	>400	
Se/Hg	0.3	>0.4	
P/Al	149	> 10	

Lab Procedures According to ASETL Protocol
Laboratory Work Performed By Doctor's Data Laboratories, Inc.   CDC License No. 14L 041   IL License No. 13758   Copyright 1991 Doctor's Data Inc.

Figure J.1 Mineral Analysis Report

SpectraCell Laboratories, Inc.
Scatterplots of Patient Test Results

Interpretive Example

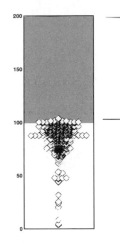

DEFICIENT RESULTS

The light blue area highlights the range of values that indicate deficient nutrient status.

REFERENCE RANGE

The diamond icons represent the distribution of test results for a reference population. Test values are the Percentage of Control Growth which is set to 100% for each patient.

PATIENT RESULTS

The patient's result as a percentage of control growth is depicted by

a GREEN square for an adequate value
a RED square for a deficient value

Patient Results

■ *Adequate*

■ *Deficient*

Values in this area represent a deficiency, and patient may require nutrient repletion or dietary changes.

Figure J.2 Essential Metaobolics Analysis (EMA™)

Requisition Number 79447
Sample Patient

SpectraCell Laboratories, Inc.

SPECTROX Total Antitoxidant Function

Status:

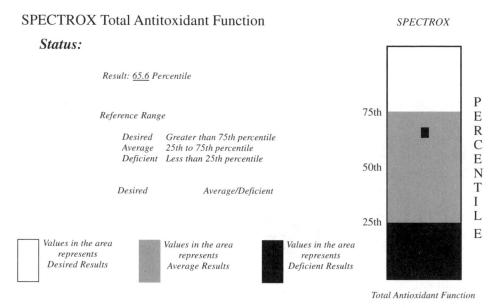

SPECTROX

Result: <u>65.6</u> *Percentile*

Reference Range

> *Desired   Greater than 75th percentile*
> *Average   25th to 75th percentile*
> *Deficient   Less than 25th percentile*

Desired   Average/Deficient

Values in the area represents Desired Results

Values in the area represents Average Results

Values in the area represents Deficient Results

75th

50th

25th

PERCENTILE

Total Antioxidant Function

Interpretation: Average

A SPECTROX value between the 25th and 75th percentiles indicates an average antioxidant function for apparently healthy persons. Since antioxidants are protective nutrients, an average status means an ability to resist an oxidative stress similar to the majority of persons. However, average status is not ideal, nor is it clearly deficient.

SPECTROX values below the 25th percentile indicate a deficient antioxidant function. A deficient antioxidant status may indicate decreased ability to resist oxidative stress or an increased oxidant load. A deficient antioxidant status may arise from lack of nutrient antioxidants, lack of uptake of dietary antioxidants, endogenous overproduction or exogenous exposure to free radicals and/or oxidative events, deficient synthesis of endogenous antioxidants, increased utilization of antioxidants, deficient cellular repair mechanisms, or any combination of these factors.

SPECTROX measures the lymphocytes' total antioxidant function by addition of a peroxide [oxidative stress] to complete medium. Lymphocyte growth response with peroxide is reported as a percentile of growth responses from a reference range of apparently healthy person. Since SPECTROX measures total antioxidant functions, clinical interpretation of results should consider physiological, pathological, environmental, lifestyle and dietary factors. Please consider that prior, current or additional supplementation with nutrient antioxidants [vitamin C, vitamin E, beta carotene, etc.] reflects only a part of the total antioxidant systems. Supplementation and lifestyle changes may or may not improve overall antioxidant functions, because of the many factors that affect antioxidant status.

Figure J.3 Spectrox: Functional Antioxidant Analysis of the Cell

Physician:	Acct Number:	410
Patient:	Lab Number:	89297-0016
Test: URINE AMINO ACID ANALYSIS	Page Number:	3

SECTION 4: Results related to renal dysfunction

Abnormal Condition	Abnormal Kidney Clearance	Acid/Base Imbalance	Mineral Imbalance	Toxicity or Nephritis
Abnormal Urine Volume				
Abnormal Creatinine				
Abnormal Urea				
Abnormal Ammonia	√	√		
Hyperglycinuria				
Hyperprolinuria				
Hypertaurinuria				
Elevated Phosphoserine			√	
Elevated Phosphoethanolamine				
Histidinuria				
Cystinuria				
Hartnup				
Dicarboxylic Hyperaminoaciduria				
Nonspecific Hyperaminoaciduria				
Hyperlysinuria				
Hyperdibasic Aminoaciduria				
Abnormalities Found	1	1	1	0

SECTION 5: Results related to mineral imbalance

Metabolite	Mg	P	Zn	Fe	Mn	Na	K
Serine							
Phosphoserine	√	√	√				
Ethanolamine							
Phosphoethanolamine							
Asparagine							
Met Sulfoxide							
Alanine							
Arginine							
Phenylalanine							
Taurine	√					√	√
Anserine							
Carnosine							
Abnormalities Found	2	1	1	0	0	1	1

SECTION 6: Results related to B-Vitamin dysfunction

Metabolite	B1	B2	B3	B6	B12	Folate	Biotin
A-Aminoadipate							
Alanine							
B-Alanine							
B-Aminoisobutyrate				√	√		√
A-Amino-N-Butyrate							
G-aminobutyrate				√			
Aspartic Acid							
Leucine							
Isoleucine							
Valine							
Tyrosine							
Ornithine				√			
Serine							
Glycine							
Met Sulfoxide							
Homocystine							
Cystathionine							
Sarcosine							
1-Methylhistidine							
3-Methylhistidine							
Abnormalities Found	0	0	0	4	1	0	1

Figure J.4 Amino Acid Analysis Report

Monroe Medical Research Laboratory
Route 17, P.O. Box I
Southfields, NY 10975
914-351-5134

RATIOS	VALUE	ANALYSIS NORMAL RANGE	INDICATION
Saturated Fatty Acids to Poly-Unsaturated Fatty Acids	2.69 H	1.42-2.43	
Arachidonic (20:4 w6) to Eicosapentaenoic (20:5 w3)	12.51 N	7.17-25.6	Low ratio indicates increased risk of bleeding. High ratio indicates increased risk of thrombosis.
Arachidonic (20:4 w6) ' to Linoleic (18:2 w6)	0.29 L	0.37-0.88	Low values indicate inefficient or inadequate conversion of Linoleic acid to Arachidonic acid
Linoleic (18:2 w6) to Gamma-Linolenic (18:3 w6)	57.95 L	89.70-177	high ratio indicates too much linoleate in diet or inadequate conversion to Gamma-Linolenic acid
Alpha-linolenic (18:3 w3) to Eicosapentaenoic (20:5 w3) & Docosahexaenoic (22:6 w3)	0.08 N	0.04-0.14	High ratio indicates inadequate or inefficient conversion of Alpha-linolenic acid to its metabolites.
Gamma-linolenic (18:3 w6) to Dihomogammalinolenic (DHGL) (20:3 w6) I	0.10 H	0.04-0.10	High ratio indicates inadequate or inefficient conversion of Gamma-linolenic acid to its metabolites.
Summation of: Myristoleic (14:1 w5) Palmitoleic (16:1 w7) Oleic (18:1 w9	11.43 N	7.69-13.44	Concentration increases in fatty acid deficiency liver swelling results.
Percent Concentration of trans fatty acids	0.16 N	0.00-1.00	

The Dietary levels of Linoleic (I8:2 w6) and Alpha-linolenic (18:3 w3) as well as their ratios affect the suppression of metabolism of each by the other. The optimum intake of each for a given patient is unique.

Wx = omega fatty acids, where x is the type of fatty acid that refers to the location of the first double bond from the methyl end of the fatty acid chain. (See molecular structure on page 382.)

The interpretation in the last column can give important clues about how the body utilizes and processes fatty acids. For example, low saturated fatty acids to polyunsaturated fatty acids ratio can indicate a high level of free radical generation in the body. In addition, excessive use of alcohol, high amounts of saturated fat consumption and low levels of certain nutrients can interfere with the efficient utilization of the essential fatty acids.

Figure J.5 Plasma Phospholipid Comprehensive Fatty Acid Profile

Comprehensive Digestive Stool Analysis®

Great Smokies Diagnostic Laboratory

SAMPLE (stamp overlay)

63 Zillicoa Street
Ashville, North Carolina 28801-1074
Phone: (704) 253-0621 Fax: (704) 253-1127

Patient Name:

Patient: ID# 23201   Age: 53_ Sex: M

Date Received: 2/8/97   Date Sent: 1/14/97

Digestion

	Normal	Abnormal	Reference
Triglycerides:	0.1		0.03%
Chymotrypsin:	24		6.2-41.0IU/gm
Valerate, Iso-butyrate:	6		0-10 umoles/gm
Meats Fibers		0cc	0
Veg. Fibers	3		0.4

Microbilogy

Beneficial Bacteria		IF	NF
Lactobacillus			4+
Bifidobacter			4+
E. Coli			4+ Additional
Bacteria NF	IF	PP	
gamma strep 4+			
mucoid E. Coli		3+	
beta Strep, not Group A or B		3+	
Mycology	NF		PP
No Yeast Isolated			

Yeast from parasite exam: N/A
NF= Normal Flora, IF= Imbalanced Flora, PP=Possible Pathogen

Please Note:

All negative and 1+ yeast cultures will be held for 7 days and reexamined. If additional growth occurs, you will receive a revised report.

Absorption

	Normal	Abnormal	Reference
LCFAs:	0.5		0-1.1%
Cholesterol:	0.1		0-0.3%
Total Fecal Fat:	0.6		0-1.6%
Total SCFA:	61		55-156 umoles/gm

Metabolic Markers

	Normal	Abnormal	Reference
n-Butyrate:	13		10-30 umoles/gm
beta Glucuronidase:	120		70-1000 IU/gm
pH		5.9	6.0-7.2
Acetate:	59		54 67%
Propionate	20		16-24%
Butyrate	21		14-23%

Immunology

	Normal	Abnormal	Reference
Fecal sIgA:	28		22-140 ug/gm

Macroscopic

	Normal	Abnormal	Reference
Color:	Brown		Brown
Mucus:	None		None
occult blood:	None		None

Dybiosis Index

Normal	Slight	Moderate	Severe
3			

DIGESTIVE MARKERS Meat and/or vegetable fibers are above the reference range. Elevated meat and vegetable fibers are indirect indicators of maldigestion due to hydrochloric acid/pepsin insufficiency, pancreatic enzyme insufficiency or rapid transit time.

ABSORPTION Markers for absorption are all within the reference range.

METABOLIC MARKERS while the short chain fatty acid distribution, butyrate and beta glucuronidase are within the reference range, stool pH is depressed (acidic). This may be due to bacterial flora producing greater than normal levels of short chain fatty acids, malabsorption of short chain fatty acids, or excessive protein metabolism. And acid fecal pH may also result from pancreatic insufficiency or rapid transit time.

IMMUNOLOGY Secretory IgA (S-IgA) is within the normal reference range. S-IgA is secreted by the intestinal mucosa and is the primary immunoglobulin in fluids. S-IgA acts as the first line of immunological defense in the gastrointestinal tract.

MICROBIOLOGY Sufficient amounts of E. coli, lactobacilli and bifidobacteria appear to be present in the stool. These "friendly bacteria" are important for gastrointestinal function, as they are involved in vitamin synthesis, natural antibiotic production, immune defense, detoxification of pro-carcinogens and a host of other activities. Maintaining these levels is important for supporting the health of the digestive system. A number of imbalanced bacteria are also present.

The presence of the organism(s) mucoid E. coli 3+, beta strep, not Group A or B3+, is best interpreted in the context of other CDSA markers. Imbalanced bacterial flora is a common finding. It can occur as a result of a parasite of bacterial infection, yeast overgrowth, or poor nutrition and maldigestion. The effects of imbalanced bacterial flora can be profound, and can lead to dermatologic, rheumatologic, and other systemic complaints, as well as GI disturbances.

DYSBIOSIS INDEX The Dysbiosis Index is within the normal range. This suggests that test results show little alteration in gut ecology, digestion and absorption. The Dysbiosis Risk Index is a calculated score based upon digestive, absorptive and metabolic markers, as well as gut microbiology.

Figure J.6 Sample CDSA Test Reporting Form

APPENDIX K
Clinical Conditions and Vitamin Assessments

According to research findings, the following clinical conditions are associated with vitamin deficiency and warrant vitamin assessments:

1. **Vitamin** B12
   Anemia (differential diagnosis)
   Malnutrition
   Stomach and small-intestinal
   surgery

2. **Folic Acid**
   Anemia (macrocytosis)
   Neurological damage
   Gastrointestinal disease and
   surgery
   Alcoholism
   Liver disease
   Food faddism
   Drug abuse
   Pregnancy

3. **Vitamin B6**
   Anemia (microcytosis)
   Neurological signs (e.g.,
   convulsive seizures)
   Peripheral neuropathy
   Malnutrition
   Alcoholism
   Liver disease
   Pregnancy
   Pre-menstrual tension

4. **Thiamine**
   Cardiomyopathy
   Neurological involvement
   (e.g., peripheral neuropathy)
   Alcoholism
   Malnutrition
   Liver disease
   Drug abuse

5. **Niacin**
   Malnutrition
   Dermatitis
   Diarrhea
   Dementia

6. **Biotin**
   Convulsive seizures
   Food faddism
   Alcoholism
   Skin lesions

7. **Riboflavin**
   Swollen lips and inflamed tongue
   Hypervascularity of conjunctiva
   Scrotal hypermia

8. **Pantothenic Acid**
   Neurological involvement
      (i.e., "burning-feet
      syndrome")
   Alcoholism
   Liver disease

9. **Vitamins A and B-Carotene**
   Xerosis
   Liver disease
   Malnutrition
   Dermatitis
   Gastrointestinal surgery
   Intestinal disease
   Alcoholism
   Kidney and liver disease
   Fat malabsorption

10. **Vitamin C (ascorbic acid)**
    Gum lesions
    Tissue bleeding
    Blood clots in the skin
    Scurvy (e.g., corkscrew hairs)
    Malnutrition
    Easy bruising
    Gastrointestinal disease

11. **Vitamin E**
    Liver disease
    Fragile red blood cells
    Gastrointestinal disease
    Cystic fibrosis
    Fat malabsorption

A complete vitamin profile should be ordered for the elderly, as well as for patients with signs of malnutrition, alcoholism, neurological disorders, blood disorders, neurological disease, hyperalimentation or pregnancy.

Source: Baker, Herman. *Jounzal of Medical Society of New Jersey,* 800:633-636 (1983).

APPENDIX L
Representative Test Laboratories

There are many laboratories that do different tests in various parts of the country. Only your doctor can order these tests. You can call or write them, however, to obtain literature and price information directly. The following labs are only representative of the many that exist in the U.S.

Bay Area Laboratory Cooperative (BALCO)
1520 Gilbreth Road
Burlingame, CA 94010
800-777-7122
—Analyzes hair, blood and urine samples for toxic and trace minerals.

Great Smokies Diagnostic Laboratory
18-A Regent Park Blvd.
Asheville, NC 28806
800-522-4762
—This lab can do extensive analysis of problems related to the digestive tract. See the list of tests it can do on page 407.

Immuno-Nutritional Clinical Lab (INCL)
6700 Valjean Ave.
Van Nuys, CA 91406
800-344-4646
—This lab specializes in food-allergy tests and other immunological disorders. It reportedly is one of the oldest and most advanced in this field.

Monroe Medical Research Laboratory
Route 17, P.O. Box I
Southfields, NY 10975
800-831-3133
—This lab specializes in evaluating essential nutrient status and function in the body, such as essential fatty acids and minerals.

Nichols Institute
26441 Via De Anza
San Juan Capistrano, CA 92675
800-553-5445
—With the use of liquid gas chromatography and elemental spectroscopy, this lab can do a variety of mineral and vitamin analyses, as well as evaluate hormonal and immunological conditions.

Doctor's Data, Inc.
170 West Roosevelt Rd.
West Chicago, IL 60185
800-323-2784
—This lab does extensive analysis of nutritional minerals as well as toxic ones. Hair, blood and urine samples can be sent to this lab, but your doctor and the lab will decide what they need, depending on your particular situation and what you wish to learn from the test results. If you have a problem with amino acid metabolism, you can also have this lab do an amino acids profile for you.

Pacific Toxicology Laboratories
1545 Pontius Ave.
Los Angeles, CA 90025
800-23-TOXIC or 213-479-4911
—Considering the amount of toxic chemicals we are constantly exposed to— from the air in our homes and in our workplaces or from the food we eat—it's important to have our level of exposure or tissue stores of harmful chemicals assessed. Pacific Laboratories does one chemical, such as PCB or chloroform, or multiple ones. The prices vary accordingly.

SpectraCell Laboratories, Inc.
515 Post Oak Boulevard, Suite 830
Houston, TX 77027
800-277-5227
—Specializes in analyzing the functional status of nutrients by measuring the growth of lymphocytes (white blood cells) in a process involving a patented technology. This laboratory also tests for antioxidant levels in cells. Currently it does only 20 tests, covering all of the B-complex vitamins, some amino acids and a few minerals.

Glossary

absorption The process of transferring food nutrients from the digestive tract into the bloodstream.

acetylcholine A brain chemical that facilitates the transfer of information from one nerve cell to another.

acid A substance that produces hydrogen ions (H+'s) when in solution.

adrenaline A hormone secreted by the adrenal gland. Also called epinephrine, adrenaline hormone is responsible for the arousal of the "fight or flight" response in the body.

aerobic metabolism The oxygen-dependent, final breakdown of food molecules occurring in the mitochondria to release energy, carbon dioxide, water and heat.

age spots A light to dark brown patch of skin that appears on the body as a person ages. This coloration is usually a result of incomplete oxidation of fats (known as lipofuscin deposits).

alkaloids A group of nitrogen-containing compounds that are of plant or animal origin and that have medicinal or pharmacological activity. Examples of alkaloids are morphine, nicotine and quinine.

alpha-tocopherol The most biologically active and widely distributed natural form of vitamin E.

alterarive A substance that has a restorative or balancing effect on the body.

amino acid A group of nitrogen containing compounds that serve as building block for protein molecules.

amino acid chelation The cradling or trapping of inorganic minerals to increase their absorption from the digestive track.

anabolism The building or synthesis of bigger molecules, such as proteins, fats and carbohydrates, from their respective simple precursor molecules by living tissues. Anabolism is an energy-requiring process, and it is provided by the adenosine triphosphate (ATP).

anaerobic metabolism The breakdown of glucose molecules without oxygen which occurs in the cytoplasm (of the cell). Through this process, only 5% of the potential energy is extracted from glucose; the other 95% is extracted when the partially processed glucose molecules enter the Krebs cycle in the mitochondria. Anaerobic metabolism takes place usually during intense short-duration physical exertion such as sprinting, weight lifting and downhill skiing.

antibiotic A substance that inhibits the production or growth of bacteria. Most medicinal antibiotics are undiscriminating in their destruction of bacteria. Herbal antibiotics such as garlic, on the other hand, do not harm helpful bacteria such as those found in the GI tract.

antibody A specialized group of protein molecules produced by the body to deactivate, destroy or neutralize foreign or invading substances (antigens).

antioxidants Electron-rich chemicals or nutrients used to minimize or eliminate oxidation. A number of nonfood-and food-based chemicals are used for this purpose. For example, vitamins A, C and E and the amino acids cysteine, methionine and taurine are well-documented antioxidants used to neutralize the damaging effect of free radicals. Nonfood chemicals, such as butylated hydroxytoluene (BHT) and butylated hydroxyanisole (BHA), are common antioxidants added to food to slow down the aging or spoiling of foods.

ascorbic acid An alternate name for vitamin C. Vitamin C helps the absorption of iron and is an excellent antioxidant. It is also important for the health, growth and normal functioning of teeth, bones, gums and muscles.

ascorbyl palmitate The fat-soluble form of vitamin C. This form of the vitamin stays longer in the body.

astringent An agent or substance that causes contraction of tissue.

ATP (adenosine triphosphate) Serves as temporary storage of food energy extracted during aerobic and anaerobic metabolism.

B

basal metabolic rate The metabolic rate of the body at rest.

basal metabolism The minimum amount of energy needed by the body to maintain vital processes, i.e., circulation, respiration and digestion.

base A molecule that produces hydroxyl ions (-OH) when dissolved in solution.

beriberi A disease arising from vitamin B1 deficiency.

beta carotene also called provitamin is usually a plant carotene that can be converted into two vitamin A molecules.

beta-carotene Precursor of vitamin A found mostly in yellow vegetables.

Beta carotene is an excellent antioxidant, particularly against the singlet oxygen free radicals. This water-soluble vitamin also has many other healthful properties.

beta cells The cells in the pancreas that manufacture insulin.

bile A pigmented fluid secreted by the liver and stored in the gallbladder that helps with the digestion of fats upon entry into the duodenum (upper portion of the small intestine). Bile can be yellow, green or brown, depending on the relative concentration of salts, acids, cholesterol, lecithin (a fat-emulsifying agent) and a number of other colored compounds. When these pigmented chemicals mix with digestion by-products in the intestine, they give feces its brown color.

bilirubin A bile component that is a breakdown of hemoglobin of the red blood cells. Bilirubin is responsible for the brown appearance of stool

bioavailability The amount of nutrient (or chemical) that is available to the body in relation to the total ingested amount.

biochemistry The study of the chemical processes that takes place in living things.

bioflavonoids A group of related compounds that act as special helpers of vitamin C. These pigmented substances team up with vitamin C to help us maintain a healthy immune system as well as properly working muscular and other tissues.

biological aging The physical condition of a person compared to his/her chronological age.

biotin One of the B-complex vitamins that is involved in the metabolism of fat. Biotin is also vital for the health and growth of tissues.

blood-brain barrier A membranous tissue that prevents the passage of material from the blood into the brain.

Bromelain A protein-digesting enzyme obtained from pineapple.

C

caffeine A chemical substance obtained from coffee, tea and chocolate that serves as a stimulant to the nervous system.

calcium A major component of bones and teeth is also involved in muscle contraction, nerve impulse transmission and blood clotting.

calcium ascorbate A less acidic form of vitamin C that is also a highly absorbable form of calcium.

calmative A substance that has calming or sedative action.

calorie A measurement of energy that is equivalent to the amount of heat required to raise the temperature of one gram of water by one degree Celsius. In nutrition, "calorie" is used to indicate the energy value of foods. One calorie (also referred to as a kilocalorie) is equal to 1,000 calories.

capillary The smallest blood vessels that bring nutrients to the cells. In the capillaries, each blood cell passes through one at a time.

carbohydrates One of the three classes of food substances that provide the body with energy. There are generally three classes of carbohydrates: monosaccharides (*i.e.,* glucose, galactose and fructose), disaccharides (*i.e.,* table sugar, lactose and honey) and polysaccharides (wheat, corn, potatoes, etc.). Chemically, carbohydrates are made up of carbon, hydrogen and oxygen atoms.

carcinogen A substance that causes cancer in living tissues.

(See also **anabolism** and **metabolism**)

carminative An agent used to expels gas from the intestine.

carotene A fat-soluble plant pigment some of which can be converted into vitamin A in the body.

casein A protein found in milk.

catabolism The breakdown of nutrients (carbohydrates, proteins and fats) or body tissues to provide energy and other necessary metabolic functions. (See also **anabolism and metabolism**)

catalyst A substance that speeds up the rate of chemical reaction without being consumed itself.

catecholamines A group of substances generated by the brain and the adrenal glands that have important physiological functions. They include epinephrine, norepinephrine and dopamine, each of which has different functions, but mainly work as neurotransmitters and stimulators of the sympathetic and central nervous systems.

cell The basic building block of body tissues.

cell membrane The outer covering of a cell.

cellulose fiber A form of carbohydrate made up of thousands glucose molecules and is a major constituent of plants. Cellulose fiber is important for the healthy functioning of the digestive tract.

ceruloplasmins The combination of copper with plasma protein believed to protect the red blood cells from free radicals.

chelated minerals Amino acid (or other organic molecule) complexed (or bound) minerals to enhance their absorption across the digestive tract.

cholecalciferol A form of vitamin D-3 important for calcium absorption and in the calcification of bones.

cholesterol A fatlike substance found in the blood and in most animal tissues. Cholesterol is one of the important constituents of cell membranes and it serves as precursor to many hormones and bile salts. Cholesterol is not found in plants.

chronological age The age of an individual as measured by the passage of time.

coenzyme A nonprotein organic substance that assists enzymes in doing their job well. Coenzymes often contain B vitamins in their molecular structures.

cofactor Another nonprotein substance that is involved during an enzyme catalyzed reaction. Certain minerals often function as cofactors.

cold pressed A process of extracting oils, without heat or chemicals, to preserve all the nutrients found naturally in vegetable oils.

cold processed A process of using chemicals (as opposed to heat) to extract vegetable oils. This process is also used to minimize damage to the nutrients found in vegetable oils. The chemicals are later removed.

colic Severe, spasmodic pain the abdomen -that comes in waves.

colitis Inflammation of the colon.

collagen A form of protein found throughout the body but which is highly concentrated in the skin, bone and cartilage tissues.

colostrum The first batch of a mother's breast milk, which is secreted shortly after, or sometimes before, birth. Colostrum is rich in antibodies and white blood cells, which serve as protection to the brand-new digestive tract of the baby.

compress Also known as fomentation, a compress is the application of herbal containing linen or gauze pad to increase circulation and relieve pain or swelling. The pad or gauze is usually socked in the tea of the herb and applied on the affected surface.

constipation An abnormally difficult or infrequent passage of stool. An increased consumption of dietary fiber, the use of laxatives or an enema can often be an effective solution to constipation.

cyanocobalamin A form of vitamin B12 that is important for the development of red blood cells, as well as for the proper function of the nervous system.

D

decoction A liquid extraction of a root, bark or leaves of a plant obtained by simmering either one of these plant materials in a closed container for 15-30 minutes

degenerative disease The gradual atrophying of organs or tissues in a biological system, which arises from the dysfunction or damage done to those organs or tissues.

demulcent A substance that soothes and softens inflamed tissues such as those found in the digestive tract.

dendrite The branch or rootlike extensions of a nerve cell that receive messages from neighboring neurons and transfer them toward the body of the cell.

dextrose see glucose

diabetes A degenerative disease characterized by abnormally high blood sugar as a result of a malfunctioning pancreas and thus an insufficient production of insulin.

diarrhea A frequent and rapid passage of abnormally soft or watery feces. Diarrhea may be caused by a number of things, including intestinal inflammation, anxiety, malabsorption or infection.

diet The variety of foods that a person consumes habitually.

dietary fiber The indigestible part of food (i.e., of fruits, vegetables and carbohydrates) that is not processed and absorbed for energy or other bodily purposes. Dietary fiber is divided into four groups: cellulose, hemicellulose, legnins and pectins. Dietary fiber is believed to be important in minimizing the incidence of colon cancer, diverticulosis, diabetes, obesity, constipation and a number of intestinal disorders.

digestion The breakdown of foods in the digestive tract into their simpler components for absorption and processing by the body.

digestive tract All the organs (mouth, esophagus, stomach, small intestine and colon) involved in the digestion and absorption of food.

disaccharide A form of carbohydrate consisting of only two sugar molecules.

diverticulosis An often painful ballooning or outpouching of the intestine or colon wall. It is believed to arise from eating foods low in fiber.

DL-alpha tocopherol Synthetic vitamin E. This form of vitamin is less biologically active than d-alpha tocopherol.

DNA The genetic material found in the cells of nearly all living things, which controls the transmission of heredity or hereditary traits. DNA stands for deoxyribonucleic acid.

duodenum The first 12-inch portion of the small intestine that receives bile and pancreatic juice from the gallbladder and pancreas, respectively.

E

edema The accumulation of excess water in body tissues. This problem is often observed in protein deficiency conditions.

Eicosapentaenoic acid (EPA) A fatty acid found primarily in cold-water fish, flax seeds and primrose oil.

elastin The yellowish, elastic protein fiber found in the connective tissues.

electrolyte A substance that has dissociated into positively and negatively charged ions, which are capable of conducting electricity. For example, when table salt dissolves or melts, it gives rise to sodium (positively) and chloride (negatively) charged ions. These are capable of conducting electricity.

electron A negatively charged particle that revolves around the nucleus of an atom.

emetic A substance that causes vomiting.

emulsifier A fat- or oil-dispersing agent when added to water.

emulsify The breakdown of large fat globules into smaller uniform droplets .

enrichment The process of adding four nutrients (thiamine, riboflavin, niacin and iron) back to food that has been processed or refined. When you see a food label that says "enriched," it may sound to you like that food has more than it naturally had. In actuality, the processed food may have lost as many as 22 different nutrients during the refining process.

enzyme A biological substance (usually a protein) that initiates and speeds up a biochemical reaction.

essential amino acids A group of (8 to 9) amino acids that are not synthesized by the body and that must be obtained from dietary sources.

essential fatty acids One group of unsaturated fatty acids that are not synthesized in the body and that are involved in many bodily functions and processes.

essential oils Also called volatile oils or essences, essential oils are a complex mixture of organic compounds containing phenols, alcohols, ketones, acids, ethers, esters, oxides and aldehydes that evaporate when exposed to air.

Ester-C® A highly bioavailable form of vitamin C.

estrogen A female hormone that is responsible for the sexual development, growth and function of the female sexual organs and secondary sexual characteristics.

extract A concentrated form of a natural product obtained by treating an herbal with a solvent and then completely or partially removing the solvent. In this manner a variety of extracts called liquid extracts, solid extracts, powder extracts, tinctures and native extracts can be obtained.

F

fats One of the three classes of nutrients that provide your body with energy. Fats can supply 9 calories per gram. There are three different types of fats: saturated (found mostly in animal products), monounsaturated and polyunsaturated (obtained from plants).

fat-soluble vitamin A vitamin molecule that is transported by fats in the body. Vitamins A, E, D and K are the only known fat-soluble vitamins.

fatty acid An organic molecule consisting of a chain of hydrogen-containing carbon atoms with a few oxygen atoms.

fiber See dietary fiber

flavonoid A term used to refer to a group of flavon-containing compounds or plant pigments such as anthocyanins, anthoxanthins, bigflavonols, flavonols, flavons and apeginens. It is now know that the flavonoids have a tremendous effect on the human body.

fortification The addition of one or more nutrients to foods to improve their nutritional quality. The nutrient added may already exist in the food to which it is added. Fortification is intended to increase the food's quality. (For example, vitamin D is added to milk and vitamin E is added to margarine.)

free radical A very unstable and highly reactive molecular fragment, which is known to cause a number of problems in the body, including aging.

frigidity Typically applied to a woman who lacks interest in sexual intercourse or has an inability to reach orgasm.

fructose One of the simple sugars found mostly in fruits and as part of honey and table sugar (sucrose).

G

galactose A monosaccharide that results from the breakdown of lactose (milk sugar).

gastric juice The colorless secretions of the gastric glands of the stomach. The major constituents of gastric juices are hydrochloric acid (which makes it very acidic, pH 2), pepsin, mucin and renin (in infants). The gastric juice is a very powerful neutralizer and deactivator of bacteria, viruses and a number of unwanted substances. It also is important for the absorption of minerals and vitamin B12.

glucose The most common monosaccharide found in fruits, sugars and starch. Glucose (sometimes called dextrose) is an important source of energy for the body and a primary source of fuel for the brain. In the blood, the optimal level of glucose is 5 millimole/liter. In a healthy person, the constancy of glucose is monitored by two hormones: insulin and glucagon. When there is an abnormally high level of glucose, insulin helps bring it down to normal by facilitating the cells' uptake of the sugar. Glucagon does the opposite: it helps break down glycogen (the body's stored sugar) when there is an abnormally low level of glucose in the blood.

glucose tolerance test (GTT) A test administered to determine how well a person's body utilizes sugar. GTT is usually given to someone who is suspected of having diabetes or hypoglycemia.

glutathione peroxidase A powerful free-radical quenching enzyme produced in the body from the sulfur-containing amino acid glutamine and the mineral selenium.

glycogen Often referred to as animal starch, glycogen is a polysaccharide made by the body from excess glucose. The conversion of glucose into glycogen and the storing of this energy source are nature's ways of dealing with excesses or shortages.

goiter An appendage or enlargement around the neck arising from an abnormal functioning of the thyroid gland due to a deficiency of iodine.

goitrogens Substances or agents that cause the onset of goiter when ingested. These substances or agents often interfere with the normal production or function of the hormone thyroxine (produced by the thyroid gland), thus creating goiters.

H

hair follicle A bed of cells in the epidermis and connective tissues that anchor the root of the hair.

hair papilla The core of the hair bulb (root) and part of the dermis that is supplied with capillaries, which bring nutrients to the growing hair.

HDL (high-density lipoprotein) cholesterol A tightly "packaged" cholesterol that can easily and efficiently move through the blood vessels.

helper T cell A type of white blood cells that fight in the army of the immune forces.

hemoglobin The iron-containing protein made by the bone marrow that helps transport oxygen to the various tissues throughout the body.

homeostasis The process by which the body maintains many of its physiological components (body temperature, electrolytes, acid-base balance and blood pressure) within constant or near constant states.

hormone A chemical that is produced in one part of the body and transported by the bloodstream to another part of the body, where it can influence the function of a specific organ or tissue. Examples of such hormones are the epinephrine or glucagon secreted by the adrenal and pancreas glands, respectively, which influence the liver to convert glycogen into glucose whenever there is a low level of this sugar in the blood. Similarly, the pituitary gland at the base of the brain secretes (among many others) growth hormones, which help with development of muscle tissues and in the healing of wounds.

hydrogenation The addition of hydrogen to vegetable oils (i.e., unsaturated fats) to make them solid at room temperature. Examples are margarine and vegetable shortening.

hypoglycemia An abnormally low level of blood sugar resulting from the excessive production of insulin.

I

immunity The body's ability to fend off infections due to the production of specialized cells such as the white blood cells and antibodies.

immunoglobulin (Ig) A group of related proteins (so-called gamma globulins) that serve as antibodies in the body.

immunology The study of the immune system.

impulse In neurology, it refers to the transmission of electrical signals (i.e., information) from the cell body down the axon and on to the next neuron.

infertility In a woman, infertility means the inability to conceive a child; in a man, infertility means the inability to induce conception.

inflammation A localized defensive reaction by the body due to an infection, chemicals or abrasion. Inflammation is characterized by swelling, heat, redness, pain and a temporary loss of function by the affected tissue.

infusion The removal or extraction of the active ingredients of a plant material by steeping or immersing it in a liquid such as water.

inositol A quasi B vitamin and a six carbon alcohol found mostly in grain, brans and certain vegetables. When an inositol molecule combines with a phosphate molecule, it forms phytic acid, a substance believed to have anticolorectal-cancer properties. Some intestinal, carcinogenic bacteria thrive in the presence of high amounts of iron. Phytic acid, by combining with iron suppresses the proliferation of the offending microorganisms in the digestive tract.

insulin A sugar-metabolizing hormone that is secreted by the pancreas gland.

intercellular Something, such as fluid, that exists between cells.

interferon A group of proteins produced by the cells infected by a virus to coat and protect the neighboring, healthy cells. Interferons work only within the species that produces them.

intestinal flora Microorganisms found in the intestinal tract that are believed to have many useful functions, including the production of vitamin K, the blood-clotting nutrient.

intracellular Situated, or existing, inside a cell.

intrinsic factor A protein-based substance produced in the stomach that helps with the absorption of vitamin B12. Failure of its secretion by the gastric cells leads to pernicious anemia, a usually fatal disease.

in vitro Something that occurs outside a living organism and in an artificial environment.

in vivo Something that occurs in the living body of an animal or a plant.

K

keratin A fibrous protein found in hair, nails and the topmost layer of the skin.

ketone Any organic compound containing a ketone group (CO).

ketosis An abnormally high formation of "ketone bodies" in the body tissues. Ketones are produced from an incomplete burning (oxidation) of fats. During starvation or in diabetic conditions, however, ketone bodies can be the last energy source.

Krebs cycle An energy-producing process that occurs in the mitochondria of the cell. It's in the Krebs cycle that the maximum amount of energy is extracted from the food you eat. The other by-products of this process are carbon dioxide, water and heat.

L

lactic acid A by-product of glucose metabolism formed due to inadequate levels of oxygen in the cell. Lactic acid is generally formed during strenuous physical activities such as weightlifting, sprinting and other continuous, repetitive physical exertions.

lactose A sugar found in milk. Lactose consists of two disaccharide molecules, glucose and galactose.

lactose intolerance An inability to metabolize lactose because of the absence of the enzyme lactase, which is responsible for the breakdown of lactose. The expressed symptoms are diarrhea and gas.

L-carnitine-L-tartrate The salt form of L-carnitine which helps transport long chain fatty acids across the mitochondrial membrane to be used for energy production.

LDL (low-density lipoprotein) cholesterol One of the forms in which cholesterol is transported in the blood vessels. LDLs are often regarded as "bad guys" because they are sluggish and tend to increase the risk of heart diseases.

lecithin A type of fat (containing phosphates) found in the cell membranes that serves as a fat-metabolizing agent in the liver. In commercial food products, lecithin is used as an emulsifying agent.

leukocytosis An abnormally high production of white blood cells, which often happens in the presence of antigens (foreign elements) in the blood.

liniment A thin medicinal liquid rubbed on the affected area of the body to relieve pain or a bruise.

lipid A group of organic substances consisting of fats, cholesterol, phospholipids, steroids and prostaglandins.

lipoprotein A complex of fats (lipids) and protein molecules found in the blood serum. Lipoprotein serves to transport cholesterol and fats to the cells for metabolism or to the liver for excretion.

liver spots See age spots

M

macronutrient Refers to foods that the body utilizes in large quantities.

malignant A condition in the body (such as cancer) that gets worse in time and eventually cause death.

malnutrition A nutritional condition in which the body is under- or overnourished. Malnutrition can be subclinical, which means it cannot be detected through normal medical examination. It can be marginal, in which case there may be overt symptoms, such as unexplainable irritability, depression or fatigue. Obesity is often the result of excessive intake of the wrong foods and is a form of malnutrition as well.

MAO see monoamine oxidase

MAO inhibitor A drug that interferes with the activity of the enzyme monoamine oxidase in the brain and that as a result affects a person's mood.

mast cells A group of cells found throughout the body that cause the allergic response of sneezing or inflammation by secreting histamine and other related substances.

medicinal A substance used to cure or treat a disease.

megaloblast An immature red blood cell with an enlarged nuclei. This occurs usually from a vitamin B12 deficiency.

melanin A dark or brown pigment usually found in the skin, hair and the iris of the eyes.

menopause That time in a woman's later reproductive cycle when the ovaries cease to produce an egg cell at regular intervals. With the cessation of menstruation, a woman's childbearing capacity ceases. Menopause normally occurs anywhere between the ages of 35 and 55.

menstruation The discharge of blood from the uterus of a woman of childbearing age once every month.

metabolism All the chemical and physical processes that take place within the body to ensure survival and proper development of the body.

minerals All the inorganic nutrients that are used during metabolism, as well as those that serve as structural components.

mitochondria A cellular power plant. In a process called the Krebs cycle, all oxygen-dependent reactions take place in the mitochondria.

monoamine oxidase (MAO) An enzyme that catalyzes the breakdown of monoamines such as epinephrine, serotonin and norepinephrine. MAO is found in all tissues, but in particularly rich quantities in the liver and the nervous system. Drugs that inhibit the activity of this enzyme are effective in the treatment of depression.

monosaccharide A simple one molecule sugar such as fructose or glucose.

monounsaturated fatty acid A fatty acid that contains one double bond in its carbon chain. Because of its heat stability, monounsaturated fat is excellent for cooking: for example, olive oil, peanut oil and canola oil.

mucilage A substance that gels when placed in water to give rise to a soft and slimy product.

mucopolysaccharide One of a group of complex carbohydrates containing amino sugar. Mucopolysaccharides function mainly as structural components in connective tissues such as tendons and cartilages.

mucus The slimy fluid secreted by the mucous membrane to lubricate and protect it.

myelin A fatty tissue that covers the axon of a nerve fiber.

N

nerve impulse See impulse

neuron A single nerve cell containing a body, dendrites and an axon.

neurotransmitter A chemical messenger in the nervous system that transfers electrical activity (or information) from one neuron to the next.

niacinamide One of the B-complex vitamins that is essential for energy production. Also known as vitamin B3, this nutrient is important for healthy skin and proper functioning of the nervous and digestive systems.

nonessential amino acids Amino acids that are synthesized in the body. Although these amino acids are important for the growth and repair of tissues, because they are made within the body, it is not essential that we get them from food sources. (See also **essential amino acids**)

nutrient A food substance that is essential for the growth, repair and maintenance of body tissues.

nutrient density The ratio of nutrients to calories obtained from a food source. If a food contains a small amount of calories in relation to its nutrient content, that food is thought to be nutrient dense.

O

obesity The accumulation of excess fat in a person's body. A person is said to be obese if he/she is 20% above the recommended weight for his/her height and build.

oil A fat that is liquid at room temperature.

organic foods Foods grown without the use of artificial fertilizers or pesticides.

osmosis The passage of particles or solvents through a semipermeable membrane from a high to low concentration. This will eventually bring the two solutions to an equilibrium.

osteomalacia The softening of the bones in adults arising from vitamin D deficiency or a loss of calcium from the body.

osteoporosis The depletion of calcium from the bones that causes them to become thin and porous. This leads to easy fracture or breakage of the bones. Osteoporosis is most frequency observed in postmenopausal women.

oxidation A chemical reaction in which oxygen is added to a substance or a hydrogen atom is removed from it.

P

papilla Any tiny nipple-like protrusion, or a clump of cells, that gives rise to hair.

pectin A dietary fiber that absorbs cholesterol and fats from the digestive tract. This helps lessen fat buildup in the blood vessels.

pepsin An enzyme in the stomach that breaks down protein into smaller chunks or peptones.

peptide A molecule consisting of two or more amino acids linked by bonds between an amino group (-NH) and a carboxy group (-CO). This bond is referred to as a peptide bond.

peristalsis A wavelike muscular motion of the intestines which causes food to move through them.

pica A craving or desire for nonfood items such as clay, grass, chalk or clothes. This abnormal desire is normally experienced by pregnant women or by women who may have an iron deficiency.

placebo An inert substance used to test the efficacy of another substance.

platelets Tiny disc-shaped particles found in the blood. Their main function is to help stop bleeding when you have a cut.

polysaccharide A carbohydrate containing three or more glucose molecules.

polyunsaturated fatty acids Fatty acids containing two or more double bonds.

poultice A warm and soft herbal material spread over a thin clothe and applied on the skin to impart heat and relieve pain or serve as antiseptic.

powdered extract A solid extract that has been dried as powder.

prostaglandins Hormonelike substances synthesized in the body from omega-3 and omega-6 fatty acids. Prostaglandins have many healthful benefits, which include dilating blood vessels, lowering cholesterol and limiting the development of cancerous cells.

protein One of the three classes of foods that are used for structural and functional purposes. Proteins are built from a chain of amino acids. Proteins differ from carbohydrates or fats by the nitrogen atom in their chain.

purgative A substance that causes vigorous bowl movement.

pyruvate A partially metabolized glucose molecule occurring during anaerobic metabolism.

R

Recommended Dietary Allowance (RDA) Officially recommended amounts of various nutrients.

S

sacchride A sugar molecule.

salve A healing or relieving ointment.

saturated fat A fat molecule containing the maximum number of hydrogen atoms in its fatty acid portions.

sedative A substance the calms or tranquilizes the body.

serotonin A neurotransmitter made from the amino acid tryptophan, which induces sleep. Serotonin is also important for weight reduction.

solid extract Extracts that have all their residual solvent removed.

stimulant An agent that temporarily hyperactivates a tissue or an organ.

subcutaneous Occurring or existing below the skin.

sucrose A sugar made of glucose and fructose, also known as table sugar.

suppressor T cells A group of white blood cell controlled by the thymus gland and that suppress the overproduction of other immune cells or antibodies.

synapse A contact point between two neurons where nerve impulses are transmitted.

T

tea An infusion made by adding hot water to an herb for use as medicine or as a beverage. Herbal tea is usually made by steeping one teaspoon of the herb in eight ounces of water.

T cell A group of white blood cells that mature in and populate the thymus gland.

thiamine mononitrate A vitamin B complex (also known as vitamin B1) that is crucial for the extraction of energy from the food you eat. It acts like a spark plug that ignites carbohydrates and other foods in the body.

tincture An alcoholic solution of herbal active ingredients prepared by percolation or dilution of their corresponding fluid or native extracts. Although the alcohol amount may vary, the tincture strength is usually 1:10 or 1:5.

thyroxine A hormone produced by the thyroid gland, which is important for energy production.

tonic A substance that nourishes, restores and strengthens the entire body.

toxic A poisonous substance that can be of a plant or animal origin

Trans-fatty acid A type of fat such as margarine or shortening produced by applying hydrogen gas under a high pressure and temperature to vegetable oils.

triglyceride A fat molecule assembled from three fatty acids and an oily alcohol called glycerol. Nearly all the fats in foods and body tissues are made up of triglycerides.

U

unsaturated fatty acids A fatty acid containing at least one double bond.

urea A waste product of protein metabolism that is eliminated from the body through urine.

V

vegetarian A person who consumes vegetables and grains exclusively—anything but animal products.

vein A blood vessel that brings blood to the heart (arteries take blood from the heart).

vitamin Essential nutrient that must be obtained from food sources for the proper growth and function of the body.

vitamin A palmitate One of the antioxidant vitamins that is also important for growth and the proper functioning of the eyes, healthy skin, hair and the lining of the digestive tract.

W

western diet A diet in Western societies that consists of high fat, low fiber and refined and processed foods.

water-soluble vitamin A vitamin that dissolves in water. All of the eight B vitamins and vitamin C are water soluble.

References

Introduction

1. Lavenstein, F.W., *Bibleotecha Nutrio et Dieta*, vol. 30, 1981
   Hamilton, E., et al., *Nutrition: Concepts and Controversies*, St. Paul: West Publishing, 1985, p. 53.
2. Quillin, Patrick, p. 28.
   Ginter, E., *World Review of Nutrition and Dietetics*, vol. 33, 1979, p. 104.
3. Berger, Stuart M., *How to Be Your Own Nutritionist*, New York: Avon Books, 1987, p. 34.
4. McDougall, John, *The McDougall Plan*, New Century Publishers, 1983, p. 97.
5. Quillin, Patrick, pp. 15, 16.

Chapter 1: Nutrition Allowances

1. National Research Council, *Recommended Dietary Allowances*, National Academy Press, Washington, D.C., 1989, p. 1.
2. Quillin, Patrick, Ph.D., *Healing Nutrients*, Chicago, New York: Contemporary Books Inc., 1987, pp. 26, 27.
   Wurtman, R.J., et al., *Nutrition and the Brain*, vol. 7, 1986, p. 23.
   Cathcart, R.F. *Medical Hypothesis*, vol. 14, 1984, p. 423.
   Styslinger, L., et al., *American Journal of Clinical Nutrition*, vol. 41, Jan., 1985, p. 21.
   Pauling, L., *American Journal of Psychiatry*, vol. 131, no. 11, Nov. 1974, p. 1251.
   Reed, P., *Nutrition: An Applied Science*, St. Paul, Minn.: West Publishing, 1980, p. 14.
3. Kanofsky, JO, et al, *New England Journal of Medicine*. July p. 173, July 6, 1981
4. Lee, p. 25-29.
   Schneider, H.A., et al., (eds.), *Nutritional Support of Medical Practice*, Hargerstown, Md.: Harper & Row, 1977, p. 26.
   Journal of American Medical Association, vol. 231, no. 4, Jan. 27, 1975, p. 360.
   Habibzadeh, N., et al., *British Journal of Nutrition*, vol. 55, 1986, p. 23.
5. Enstrom, et al., *Epidemiology*, vol. 3, no. 3., 1992, p. 194.
6. *Time*, May 31, 1993, p. 57.
7-13. The information for references 7-13 is based on an FDA publication called *Backgrounder: Current and Useful Information from the Food and Drug Administration.*

Chapter 2: Optimal Nutrition

1. Dychtwald, Ken, *The Age Wave*, New York: Bantam Books, 1990, p. 6.
2. Schloss B: Possibilities for prologing life in the near future. *Rejuvenation* 1981; 9 (20:30-32.

3. Kinsella K: Changes in life expectancy 1900-1990. *Am J Clin N* 1992;55:1196S-1202S.

4. Lipschitz D, McClellan J: Impact of nutrition on the age-related decline in immune and hematologic function. *Cont Nutr* 1990;15(2):1-2.

5. Sacher, George A. " Life Table Modification and Life Prolongation." *Handbook of Biology of Aging.*

6. Quillin, Patrick, p. 16

7. Masoro E: Nutrition and aging: A current assessment. *J Nutr* 1985;115 (7):842-848.

8. Kushi, M., and Cottrell, M.C., M.D., *AIDS, Macrobiotics and Natural Immunity.* Tokyo, New York: Japan Publication, Inc., 1990, p. 21.

9. Niedorf A, Rath, M. et al. Morphological detection and quantification of lipoprotein (a) deposition in atheromatous lesion of human aorta and coronary arteries. *Virchow's Archives of Pathological Anatomy,* 417:105-111, 1990. See also Quillin p.83.

10. Houston, MC. *Archives of internal medicine,* vol.146, p.179, Jan.1986.

11. Wilson, TW. *lancent,* p.784, April 5, 1986

12. Altura, BM. *Medicinal hypotheses,* vol.5, p.843, 1979.

13. Schleettwein-Gsell D: Nutrition and the quality of life: A measure for the outcome of nutritional intervention? *Am J clin N* 1992;55:1263s-1266s.

14. Quillin, Patrick. *Healing Nutrients,* Chicago, New York: Contemporary Books, Inc., 1987

15. Block G, Dresser C. Hartman A, et al:Nutrient sources in American Diet: Quantitative Data from the NHANES II survey. 2. Macronutrients and fats. *Am J Epidem* 1985;122(1):27-40.

16. Haines, P, Hungerford D, et al: Eating patterns and energy nutrient intakes of U.S. women. *J Am Diet A,* 1992;92:168-174.

17. Quillin, Patrick, p. 127.

18. Pietrzik K: Concept of borderline vitamin deficiencies in Hanck A, Horning D (eds.): Vitamins: Nutrients and therapeutic agents. *Int J vit.N* 1985; Suppl 27:61-73.

19. Baker, H., and Frank, O., "Sub-Clinical Vitamin Deficits in Various Age Groups," *International Journal of Vitamin and Nutrition Research,* 27:47-59, 1985.

20. Mindell, Earl, *The Vitamin Bible,* New York: Warner Books, 1985, p. 6.

21. *Recommended Dietary Allowances 10th Edition,* Washington D.C .: National Academy Press, 1989., pages 101, 117, 150, and 189.

22. Kovda, V.A. Loss of productive land due salinization of , *Ambio* 12 (1983)

23. Colgan M. We have poisoned the land. *Nutrition and Fitness,* 1990;9:170-171

24. *Recommended Dietary Allowance 10th Edition,* Washington D.C.: National Academy Press, 1989. (This fact was illustrated by the decline of magnesium in human diet over a period of 80 years.)

25. Kushi, M., and Cottrell, M.C., M.D., *AIDS, Macro Biotics and Natural Immunity,* Tokyo, New York: Japan Publication, Inc., 1990, pp. 153, 155.

26. Malone, Wilfred F, Studies evaluating antioxidants and beta carotene as chemoprentivees, *Am J Clin Nutr* 1991;53:305S-13S

27. London R, Sundoram, G. Murphy L. et al. The effect of alpha-tocopherol during on premenustral symptomologoy: a double-blind study. *J. Am Col Nutr,* 1983, 2:115. See also Quillin p.35.

28. Somer, Elizabeth, *Nutrition for Women.* New York: Henry Holt and company, 1993, p. 304

29. Grey, Fred, Pushka, Pekka et al. Inverse correlation between plasma vitamin E and mortality from ischemic heart disease in cross-cultural epidemiology, *Am J Clin Nut,* 53:326, Supplement

30. Esterbauer, Herman, et al. Role of vitamin E in preventing the oxidation of low density lipoprotein, *Am J clin Nutr* 1991, 53:314s-21S.

31. Mitchell, H. et al. *Nutrition in Health and Disease,* 16th ed.18: Philadelphia, PA: JB Lippin Cott co, 1976.

32. Welsh, SO, et al. *Food Technology,* p.70, Jan., 1982.

Leaf, A., *New England Journal of Medicine,* vol. 310, March 15, 1984, p. 718.

C.F. Finch and L. Hayflick, 582, 1st ed., New York: Van Nostrand Reinbold, 1977

Kushi, L.H., et al., *New England Journal of Medicine,* vol. 312, March 28, 1985, p. 811.

Fortmann, S.P., *American Journal of Clinical Nutrition,* vol. 34, Oct. 1981, p. 2030.

Hubbard, J.D., et al., *New England Journal of Medicine,* vol. 313, July 4, 1985, p. 52.

Spector, L., et al., *Proceedings of the Society of Experimental Biology and Medicine,* vol. 100, 1959, p. 405.

Willett, W.C., et al., *New England Journal of Medicine,* vol. 330, March 8-15, 1984, p. 633

Michell, H., et al., *Nutrition in Health and Disease,* 16th ed.,Philadelphia: J.P. Lippincott, 1976, p. 18.

Pearson, J.M., et al., *Journal of the American Dietetics Association,* vol. 86, March 1986, p. 339.

Schroeder, H., *American Journal of Clinical Nutrition,* vol. 24, May 1971, p. 562.

Cathcart, R.F., *Medical Hypotheses,* vol. 14, 1984, p. 21.

Enstrom, et al., *Epidemiology,* vol. 3, no. 3, 1992, p. 194.

Time, May 31, 1993, p. 57.

Chapter 3: Aging

1. Pelton, Ross, *Mind Foods and Smart Pills,* New York: Doubleday, 1989, p. 186.
   Dean, Ward, *Biological Aging Measurement, Clinical Applications.* Los Angeles: The Center for Bio-Gerontology, October 1988.

2. Gerber, Jerry, et al., *Life Trends,* New York: Avon Books, 1991, p. 168.

3. Walford, Roy L. *The 120 Year Diet,* New York: Pocket Books, 1986, p. 56.

McCay, C. M. *Cowdry's Problem of Aging, Biological and Medical Aspects* (A.I. Lansing, ed.). Baltimore: Williams and Wilkins, 1992, p. 130.

Merry, B.J., and Holehan, A. M. *13th International Congress on Gerontology,* New York, July 12-17, 1985.

4.   Kushi, M., and Cottrell, M.C., M.D., *AIDS Macro Biotics and Natural Immunity,* Tokyo, New York: Japan Publication, Inc., 1990, p. 134.

Watson, Ronald, et al. Effect of beta carotene on lymphocte subpopulations in elderly humans: evidence for a dose-response relationship, *Am J Clin Nutr,* 1991;53:60-4.

Cutler, Richard G. Antioxidants and Aging, *Am J Clin Nutr,* 1991; 53:373S-9S

Mazes, Richard B and Barden, Howard S. Bone density in premenopausal women: effects of aging, dietary intake, physical activity, smoking and birth-control pills, *Am J Clin Nutr,* 1991: 53:132-42.

Masoro, Edward. Nutrition and Aging —A current Assessment, *J Nutr* 1985; 115(7):42-848

Norton, Lee and Wozny, Mark C. Residential location and nutritional adequacy, *J Geron,* 1984;39(5):592-595.

Garry, Philip, et al. Nutritional status in a healthy elederly population: dietary and supplemental intakes, *Am J Clin Nutr,* 1982;36:319-331.

Schlettwein-Gsell, Daniela, Nutrition and the quality of life: a measure for the outcome of nutritional intervention?, *Am J Clin Nutr,* 1992;55:126S-6S.

Chapter 4: Free Radicals and Antioxidants

1.   Halliwell, B. and Gutteridge John M.C. *Free Radicals in Biology and Medicine,* Oxford: Clarendon Press, 1989, pp. 454-458.

2.   Pelton, Ross. *Mind foods and Smart Pills,* N.Y.: Double Day 1989, pp. 49-50.

3.   Aust. S.D. et al. The role of metals in oxygen radical reactions. *J. Free Radicals Bio. Med.* 1,3, 1985. Rice-Evans and Halliwell, B. (eds.) Free Radicals and concepts. London:Richeliev Press, 1988.

4.   Demopoulos, H.B. The basis of radical pathology, *Federation Proceedings,* 1973, vol.32, pp. 1859-61.

5.   Halliwell & Gutteridge, p. 317.

6.   Ibid 142-43.

7.   Pelton, 53-54.

8.   Mediacal Tribune, vol. 17, N26, Aug. 18, 1976. P.7.

9.   Passwater, Richard. *Selenium as Food and Medicine,* New Canaan, Ct.: Keats Publishing 1980, pp. 22,53.

10. Bosco, Dominick. *The people's Guide to Vitamins and Minerals,* Chicago: Contemporary Books, 1980, p.2 48.

11. Berger Stuart M. *How to be Your Own Nutritionist,* New York: Avon Books, 1987, p.229.

12. Pelton, 218.

13. Ibid

14. Quillin, Patrick. *Healing Nutrients,* Chicago: Contemporary Books, pp. 341, 347, 349.

15. Zang, Y. et al. *Proceedings of the National Academy of Sciences of the United States of America.* 1972, March 16, 89 (6):2399-403.
16. Prigen, K. and Hager, M. *Newsweek,* March 25, 1994, p.46.
17. Murray, Michael T., Powerful herbal antioxidants, *Health Counselor,* vol. 5, no.2, p. 40.
18. Karcher, L. Zagerman, P. and Kreglstein, J. Effect of an extract of Gingko biloba on the rat brain energy metabolism in hyproxia. *Naunyn-Schmiedeberg's Arch Pharmacol.* 327:31-5, 1984.
19. Chatterjee, SS and Gabard B, Studies on the mechanism of action of an extract of Gingko biloba, a drug for the treatment of ischemic vascular diseases, *Naunyn- Schmiedeberg's Arch on Pharmacol.* 320-R52, 1982
20. Halliwell and Gutteridge p. 256. See Also, Mindell, Earl, *The Vitamin Bible,* N.Y.: Warner Brooks, 1985, p.78.

    Alfthan, Gerg, et al. Selenium metabolism and platelet glutathione peroxi dase activity in healthy Finish men: Effects of selenium yeast, selenite, and selenate *Am L Clin Nutr* 1991;53:120-5.

    Block, Gladys. Vitamin C and cancer prevention: the epidemiologic evidence *Am L Clin Nutr* 1991;53:270S-82S.

    Comstock, George W. et al. Prediagnostic serum levels of carotenoids and vitamin E as related to sugsequent cancer in Washington County, Maryland *Am L Clin Nutr* 1991;53:260S-4S.

    Diplock, Anthony. Antioxidant nutrients and disease prvention: an overview, *Am L Clin Nutr* 1991;53:189S-93S.

    Di Mascio, Paolo, Murphy, Michael E. and Sies, Helmut. Antioxidant defense systems: the role of carotenoids, tocopherols, and thiols, *Am L Clin Nutr* 1991;53:194S-200S

    Esterbauer, Hermann, et al. Role of vitamin E in preventing the oxidation of low density lipoprotein *Am L Clin Nutr* 1991;53:314S-21S. *Am L Clin Nutr* 1991;53:326S-34S.

    Ferrari, R. et al. Role of oxygen free radicals in ischemic and reperfused myocardium, *Am L Clin Nutr* 1991;53:215S-22S.

    Hhorwitt, Max, et al. Serum concentration of alpha tocopherol after

Chapter 5: Macronutrients, Micronutrients, and Fibers

1. Quillin, Patrick, Ph.D., *Healing Nutrients,* Chicago, New York: Contempo-rary Books Inc., 1987, pp. 351.

    Chasnof, I.J., et al., (eds.) *Family Medicine and Health Guide,* Skokie, Ill.: Publications International, 1984, p. 240.

    Painter, J., *British Medical Journal,* vol. 2, 1971, p. 156.

    Eastwood, M.A., et al., *American Journal of Clinical Nutrition,* vol. 43, March 1986, p. 343.

2. Berger, Stuart M., *How to Be Your Own Nutritionist,* New York: Avon Books, 1987, p. 80.
3. Quillin, Patrick, pp. 335, 336.

    Ershoff, B.H., *American Journal of Clinical Nutrition,* vol. 27, 1974, pp. 94-95.

    Ershoff, B.H., *American Journal of Clinical Nutrition,* vol. 41, 1976, p. 949.

4. Quillin, Patrick, pp. 133, 134, 335, 336.
5. Berger, Stuart M., p. 81.
6. Quillin, Patrick, pp. 300-331.

Chapter 7: Fats And Oils, Including Cholesterol

1. *Nutrition Action Healthletter,* September 1990, cover story.
2. Cleeman, James, M.D. "The National Cholesterol Education Program,"
   Journal of Reproductive Medicine, September 1989, 34(9 suppl):675-90.
   "Highlights of the Report of the Expert Panel on Blood Cholesterol."
   American Family Physician, May 1992, 45(5) 2127-26.
3. Dept. of R & D, *Meal Replacement Diet Program,* TwinLab, 1990, p. 18.
   "Study Suggests We Are What—Not How Much—We Eat," *Explore,*
   September/October 1988, [citing Stanford Center for Research in
   Disease Prevention].
   "Nutrition News," *Prevention,* May 1988, [citing Mark Hegsted, Ph.D.,
   Harvard Medical School].
4. Debra Lynn Dadd, "Is Your Diet Killing *You?," Men's Fitness,* September
   1990, p. 22.
5. Quillin, Patrick, Ph.D., *Healing Nutrients,* Chicago, New York:
   Contemporary Books Inc., 1987, p. 312.
   Documenta Geigy Scientific Tables, 1970.
   Recker, R.R., et al. *American Journal of Clinical Nutrition,* vol. 41., Feb.
   1985, p. 254.

Chapter 8: Energy

1. Airola, Paavo, *Hypoglycemia: A Better Approach,* Sherwood, Ore.: Health
   Plus, 1977, p. 28.
2. Dobersen, M.J., et al., *New England Journal of Medicine,* vol. 303, 1980,
   p. 1493. See also Quillin, Patrick, Ph.D., *Healing Nutrients,* Chicago,
   New York: Contemporary Books Inc., 1987, p. 297.
   Dobner, G., et al., *Experimental Clinical Endocrinology,* vol. 84, no. 2, March
   1985, p. 1558.
3. Quillin, Patrick., p. 295.
4. O'Dea, K., *Diabetes,* vol. 33, June 1984, p. 596. See also Quillin, Patrick.,
   p. 296.
   Henry, R. R., et al., *Diabetes,* vol. 35, Feb. 1986, p. 155.
5. Haas, Robert, *Eat to Win,* New York: Signet, 1983, p. 216.

Chapter 9: Causes of Obesity and Possible Solutions

1. Flatt, J.P., "The Biochemistry of Energy Expenditure," in Bray, G.A., ed.
   Recent Advances in Obesity Research II, London: Newman Publishing Ltd.,
   1978:211-28.
2. "Study Suggests That We Are What—Not How Much—We Eat," *Explore,*
   September/October 1988.
3. "Nutrition News," *Prevention,* May 1988.
4. Nutrition Committee, American Heart Association. "Dietary Guidelines for
   Healthy American Adults," *Circulation,* 77:3, March 1988.

5. U.S. Department of Agriculture, Economic Research Service. *Food Consumption, Prices, and Expenditures,* Washington, D.C.: Annual.
6. de Vries, H., and Gray, D., "After-effects of Exercise Upon Resting Metabolic Rate," *Res. Q. American Association of Health and Physical Education,* 34:314-321, 1963.
7. Dohm, G.L., Barakat, H.A., Tapsott, E.B., and Beecher, G.R., "Changes in Body Fat and Lypogenic Enzyme Activities in Rats after Termination of Exercise Training," *Proceedings of the Society for Experimental Biology and Medicine,* 155:157-59, 1977.
8. Evans, G.W., "The Effect of Chromium Picolinate on Insulin Controlled Parameters in Humans," *International Journal of Biosocial Medical Research,* 11:2, 1989, pp. 163-180.
9. Evans, G.W.,
10. Story, J. "Dietary Fiber and Lipid Metabolism" in *Medical Aspects of Dietary Fiber,* eds. G. Spiller and R. Kay, New York: Plenum Publishing Co., 1980, pp. 137-152.
11. Despres, J.P., et al., "Level of Physical Fitness and Adipocyte Lipolysis in Humans," *Applied Physiology: Respiratory, Environmental and Exercise Physiology,* 56:1157-1161, 1984.
12. Department of Research and Development, Twin Laboratories, Inc., 1990, p. 30.
13. Ibid.

Chapter 11: Fat-soluble Vitamins

Vitamin D

1. Garrison, R.H., and Somer, E., *The Nutrition Desk Reference,* New Canaan, Conn.: Keats Publishing, Inc., 1990, p. 215.
2. Ibid, pp. 126-127.
3. Berger, Stuart M., *How to Be Your Own Nutritionist,* New York: Avon Books, 1987, p. 188.
4. Garrison and Somer, pp. 98, 226.
5. Ibid, p. 40.

Vitamin E

1. Bosco, Dominick, *The People's Guide to Vitamins and Minerals,* Chicago: Contemporary Books, 1980, p. 176.
2. Lieberman, S., and Bruning, N. *The Real Vitamin & Mineral Book,* Publishers Group West, Garden City Park, N.Y.: 1990, p. 69.

Vitamin K

1. Garrison, R.H. and Somer, E., *The Nutrition Desk Reference,* New Canaan, Conn.: Keats Publishing, Inc., 1990, p. 43.

Chapter 12: Water-soluble Vitamins

Vitamin C

1. Bosco, Dominick, *The People's Guide to Vitamins and Minerals,* Chicago:

Contemporary Books, 1980, p. 133.
2.   Ibid., p. 148.

Riboflavin

1.   Bosco, Dominick, *The People's Guide to Vitamins and Minerals,* Chicago:
     Contemporary Books, 1980, p. 48.

Niacin

1.   **Lieberman, S., & Bruning, N., *The Real Vitamin & Mineral Book,***
     Publishers Group West,Garden City Park, N.Y.: 1990, p. 87.
2.   Bosco, Dominick, *The People's Guide to Vitamins and Minerals,* Chicago:
     Contemporary Books, 1980, p. 55.
3.   Ibid., p. 57.

Pantothenic Acid (Vitamin B5)

1.   Bosco, Dominick, *The People's Guide to Vitamins and Minerals,* Chicago:
     Contemporary Books, 1980, p. 109.
2.   Ibid., p. 108.

Pyridoxine (Vitamin B6)

1.   Bosco, Dominick, *The People's Guide to Vitamins and Minerals,* Chicago:
     Contemporary Books, 1980, p. 63.
2.   Ibid., p. 64.

Biotin (Vitamin H)

1.   Bosco, Dominick, *The People's Guide to Vitamins and Minerals,* Chicago:
     Contemporary Books, 1980, p. 103.

Choline

1.   Bosco, Dominick, *The People's Guide to Vitamins and Minerals,* Chicago:
     Contemporary Books, 1980, pp. 116, 117.

Chapter 13: Bulk Minerals
Calcium

1.   Quillin, Patrick, Ph.D., *Healing Nutrients,* Chicago, New York:
     Contemporary Books Inc., 1987, pp. 307-314.
     Fisher, S., et al., *American Journal of Clinical Nutrition,* vol. 31, 1978,
        p. 667.
     Lee. C.J., et al., *American Journal of Clinical Nutrition,* vol. 34, May 1981,
        p. 819.
     Haspels, A.A., et al., *Maturitas,* vol. 1, June 1978, p. 15.
     Journal of the American Medical Association, vol. 252, Aug. 1984, p. 799.
     Schnitzler, C., et al., *South African Medical Journal,* vol. 66, no. 19, Nov.
        1984, p. 730.
     Schwartz, R., et al., *American Journal of Clinical Nutrition,* vol. 26, May
        1973, p. 519.

2. Ibid.

    Documenta Geigy Scientific Tables, 1970, p. 312.

    Recker, R. R., et al., *American Journal of Clinical Nutrition,* vol. 41, Feb. 1985, p. 254.

    Smith, T.M., et al., *American Journal of Clinical Nutrition,* vol. 42, Dec. 1985, p. 1197.

    Jacobs. D.H., *New England Journal of Medicine,* vol. 314, May 1986, p. 1389.

Magnesium

1. Quillin, Patrick, Ph.D., *Healing Nutrients,* Chicago, New York: Contemporary Books Inc., 1987, p. 101.

    Lee, C.M., et al., *Annals of Clinical and Laboratory Science,* vol. 14, 1984, p. 151.

    Anderson, R.A., et al., *American Journal of Clinical Nutrition,* vol. 36, Dec. 1982, p. 1184.

Potassium

1. Quillin, Patrick, Ph.D., *Healing Nutrients,* Chicago, New York: Contemporary Books Inc., 1987, p. 96.

    Houston, M.C., et al., *Archives of Internal Medicine,* vol. 146, Jan. 1986, p. 179.

    Weaver, C.M., et al., *Food Technology,* vol. 40, Dec. 1986, p. 99.

2. Ibid., p. 99.

    Krombout. D., et al., *American Journal of Clinical Nutrition,* vol. 41, June 1985, p. 1299.

    Henningsen, N.C., et al., *Lancet,* January 15, 1983, p. 133.

    Smith, S.J., et al., *Lancet,* Feb. 12, 1983, p. 362.

    Materson, B.J., *Archives of International Medicine,* vol. 313, Aug. 12, 1985, p. 582.

Chapter 14: Trace Elements

Copper

1. Quillin, Patrick, Ph.D., *Healing Nutrients,* Chicago, New York: Contemporary Books Inc., 1987, p. 318.

    Walker, B.C., et al., *Agents and Actions,* vol. 6, 1976, p. 454.

    Huber, W., et al., *Clinics in Rheumatic Diseases,* vol. 6, 1980, p. 465.

    American Journal of Medicine, vol. 74, 1983, p. 124.

    Frank, B., *Nucleic Acid and Antioxidant Therapy of Aging and Degeneration,* New York: Rainstone Publishing, 1977.

Iron

1. Quillin, Patrick, Ph.D., *Healing Nutrients,* Chicago, New York: Contemporary Books Inc., 1987, p. 222.

    Leibel, *R.L., Journal of the American Dietetic Association,* vol. 71, 1977, p. 398.

Oski, F.A., et al., *Journal of Pediatrics,* vol. 92, Jan. 1978, p. 21.

Oski, F.A., *Pediatrics Clinics of North America,* vol. 32, April 1985, p. 493.

Oski, F.A., et al., *Pediatrics,* vol. 71, January 1983, p. 877.

Voors, A,W., et al., *Public Health Reports,* vol. 54, Jan. 1981, p. 45.

Pastides, H., *Yale Journal of Biology and Medicine,* vol. 54, 1981, p. 265.

Seoane, N.A., et al., *Journal of the Canadian Dietetic Association,* vol. 46, Nov. 1985, p.298.

Nickerson, H.J., et al., *American Journal of Diseases of Children,* vol. 139, Nov.1985, p.1115.

Brune, M., et al., *American Journal of Clinical Nutrition,* vol. 43, March 1986, p. 438.

2. Lieberman, S., and Bruning, N., *The Real Vitamin and Mineral Book,* Publishers Group West, Garden City Park, N.Y.: 1990, p. 153.

3. Quillin, Patrick, Ph.D., *Healing Nutrients,* Chicago, New York: Contemporary Books Inc., 1987, p. 257.

Villar, J., et al., *International Journal of Gynecology and Obstetrics,* vol. 21, 1983, p. 271.

Belizan, J., et al., *American Journal of Clinical Nutrition,* vol. 33, 1980, p. 202.

Belizan J., et al., *American Journal of Obstetrics and Gynecology,* vol. 146, 1983, p. 277.

Altura, B.M., et al., *Science,* vol. 221, July 1983, p. 376.

Elliot, J., *American Journal of Obstetrics and Gynecology,* vol. 147, Oct. 1983, p. 277.

Oski, F.A., *Pediatric Clinics of North America,* vol. 32, April 1985, p. 493.

Molybdenum

1. Quillin, Patrick, Ph.D., *Healing Nutrients,* Chicago, New York: Contemporary Books Inc., 1987, p. 335.

Ershoff, B.H., *American Journal of Clinical Nutrition,* vol. 27,1974, p. 1395.

Ershoff, B.H., *American Journal of Clinical Nutrition,* vol. 41, 1976, p. 949.

Selenium

1. Bosco, Dominick, *The People's Guide to Vitamins and Minerals,* Chicago: Contemporary Books, 1980, p. 249.

Chapter 15: The Significance of Supplements to Your Health

1. Ashmead, Dewayne, Ph.D., *Conversation on Chelation and Mineral Nutrition,* New Canaan, Conn.: Keats Publishing, Inc., 1989, p. 134.

2. Dadd, Deborah Lynn, "Is Your Diet Killing You?," *Men's Fitness,* September 1990, p. 27.

3. Quillin, Pattrick, Ph.D., *Healing Nutrients,* Chicago, New York: Contemporary Books, Inc., 1987, p. 48.

4. Ibid, p. 46.

5. Simon, Barry, M.D., Meschino, James, D.C., *The Winning Weight,* Ontario, Canada: Elite Publications, Inc. 1993, pp. 128-29.

6. Ashmead, Dewayne.

Chapter 15: Phytochemicals

1. *Proceedings of the National Academy of Sciences of the United States of America*, 1992 March 15, 89(6): 2399-403.
2. *Proceedings of the National Academy of Sciences of the United States of America*, 1994 April 12, 91(8): 3147-50.
3. *Newsweek*, April 25, 1994, society section.
4. Mendil, Earl. *Earl Mindel's Anti-Aging Bible*, New York: Simon & Schuster, 1996 pp.150-151.
5. *Cancer Research*, 1994 April1, 54(7 Suppl):1976s-1981s.
6. R.W. and Castonguay. Antimutagenic effects of polyphenolic compounds, *Cancer Letter* 66, no.2 (Spetember 1992), 107-113
7. *Proceedings of the National Academy of Sciences of the United States of America*, 1994 April 12, 91(8):3147-50.
8. Hocaman, Gabriel. *Prevention of cancer: vegetables and plants Comparative Biochemistry and Physiology* 93B, no.2 (1989):210-212.
9. *Annals of the New York Academy of Sciences*, 1992 Sept. 30, 669:7-20.
10. *Men's Health*, November, 1995, nutrition section.
11. *Consumers' Research Magazine*, August, 1992.

Chapter 16: The World of Herbs

1. Lust, J.B. *The Herb Book*, New York, Toronto, London, Sydney, Aukland: Bantam Books, 1974, P.4
2. Tierra, Michael. *The way of Herbs*, New York, London, Toronto, Sydney, Tokyo, Singapore: Pocket Books, 1990, xxiv - xxvii,
3. See ref. 2, p.13.

Chapter 17 Herbal Samplers

1. Hendler, S.S., *The Doctors Vitamin and Mineral Encyclopedia*, New York: Simon and Schuster, 1991, p.279.
2. Murray, M.T., *The Healing Power of Herbs*, Roklin: Prima Publishing, 1992, p.121.
3. Clostre, F., From the Body to Cellular Membranes: The different Level of Pharmacological Action of Ginkgo Biloba Extract. In Rokan (Ginkgo Biloba) - *Recent Results in Pharmacology and Clinic*. Funfgeld, E.W., ed., New York: Springer-Verlag, 1988, pp.180-98.
4. Schaffler, V.K., and Reeh, P.W.: Double-blind Study of the Hypoxia-protective Effect of Standarized Ginkgo Bilobae Preparation After Repeated Administration in Healthy Volunteers. *Arzneim-Forsch* 35:1283-6, 1985.
5. Foster, S. Making wise choices in herbal energy boosters, in *Better Nutrition for Better Living*, Jan, 1995, 121.
6. Ibid.
7. Shibata, S., Tanaka, O., Shoji, J., and Saito, H., Chemistry and Pharmacology of Panax, *Economic and Medicinal Plant Research* 1:217-84, 1985.
9. Brekham II and Dardymov IV: New Substances of Plant Origin which Increase Non-specific Resistance. *Ann. Rev. Pharmacol.* 9:419-30, 1969.

10. Brekham II and Dardymov IV: Pharmacological Investigation of glycosides from Ginseng and Eleutherococcus, *Lloydia* 32:46-5, 1969.

11. Saito, H., Yoshida, Y. and Takagi, K: Effect of Panax Ginseng Root on Exhaustive Exercise in Mice. *Jap. J. Pharmacol.* 24:119-27, 1974.

12. Avakia E.V. and Evonuk, E., Effects of Panax Ginseng Extract on Tissue Glycogen and Adrenal Cholesterol Depletion During Prolonged Exercise. *Planta Medica* 36:43-8, 1979.

13. Petkov, W. The Mechanism of Action of P. Ginseng. *Arzniem-Forsch*, 11:288-95, 418-22, 1961.

14. Kaku, T., Miyata, T., Uruno, T., et al, Chemicopharmacological Studies on Saponins of Panax Ginseng, C.A. Meyer. *Arzniem-Forsch* 25:539-47, 1975.

15. Mowrey, Daneil B. *The Scientific Validation of Herbal Medicine*, Keats Publishing: New Cannan, CT, 1986, p. 102.

16. Heinerman, John, Herman's *Encyclopedia of Fruits, Vegetables and Herbs*, Parker Publishing Company: West Nyak, N.Y., 1988, p. 157.

17. Fulder, S.J.: The Growth of Cultured Fibroblasts Treated with Hydrocortisone and Extracts of Medicinal Plant Panax Ginseng. *Exp Geronol* 12:125-31, 1977.

18. Foster, S.: Making Wise Choices in Herbal Energy Boosters, in *Better Nutrition for Better Living*, Jan.1995, P.66.

19. Ritchason, Jack, *The Little Herb Encyclopedia*, Woodland Health books: Pleasant Grove, UT, 1994, p.214, 215.

Chapter 20: Supplements: What You Should Know About Them

1. Mareschi J., Magliola, C. Couzy F., et al. The well balanced diet and the at-risk micronutrients: A forcasting nutritional index. *Int J Vit N.* 1987:57:79-85.

2. *Am J Clin Nutr*, Jan 1991.

3. Lowenstein, FW. *Bibliotheca Nutritio et Dieta.* vol. 30, p.1 1981.

4. Block G, Dresser C., Herman A, et al. Nutrient sources in the American diet:Quantitative Data from the NHANES II Survey. 2. Macronutrients and Fats. *Am J Epidem*, 1985; 122(1):27-40.

5. Pennington, J and Young, D. Total diet study nutritional elements 1982-1989. *J Am Diet A*, 1991;91:179-183.

6. Mareschi J, Magliola C, et al. The well balanced diet and the at-risk micronutrients: A forcasting nutritional index. *Int J Vit N* 1987;57:79-85.

7. Hulme AC., Ed. *The Biochemistry of Fruits and Their Products*, Vol. 1: NY: Academic Press, 1970.

8. Harris R, Karmas E. Eds. *Nutritional Evaluation of Food Processing*, Westport, Ct: Avi Publishing, 1975.

9. *Recommended Dietary Allowances 10th Edition.* Washington DC: The National Academy Press, 1989.

10. Ge K, Yang G. The epidemology of selenium deficiency in the etiological of endemic diseases in China. *Am J Clin Nutr*,1993:57:259S-263S.

11. Matkovic, V. Kostial K. et al. Bone status and fracture rates in two regions of Yugoslavia. *Am J Clin Nutr* 32:540-549.
12. Colgan, M. *Science.* 1981; 214:744.

Chapter 21: Do You Have To Worry About A Vitamin and Mineral Overdose?
1. San Francisco Bay Area Regional Poison Control Center, *Community Newswire,* Poison Prevention and Hazardous Materials Information, Vol. 9, No.1, Winter 1993.
2. From the American Association of Poison Control Centers, National Center for Health Statistics, *Journal of the American Medical Association,* Centers for Disease Control, March of Dimes Consumer Product Safety Commission, FDA Reports.
3. Rosenbaum, M.E, M.D, Bosco, D. *Super Supplements,* New York: New American Library, 1989, p. 181.
4. Ibid p.182.
5. See ref. 1.
6. Colgan, Michael. *Optimum Sports Nutrition,* New York: Advanced Research Press, 1993, p. 223.
7. Schmidt, K.H, et al. Urinary Oxalate Secretion After Large Intakes of Ascorbic Acid in Man. *American Journal of Clinical Nutrition* 1981, 34:305-311.
8. Wardlaw, Gordon M. and Insel, Paul M. *Perspective in Nutrition.* 2d ed. St. Louis: Mosby 1993, p. 363..
9. McCord, Holly. Vitamins and Beyond, *Prevention* November 1994
10. See refs. 1 and 3.
11. Arcus, Amy, and Kim, Allegra N., Pediatric Iron Poisoning: A Killer Returns, California.Epidemiologic Investigation Service Emergency Preparedness and Injury Control Branch, March 1995, p. 7.
12. See ref. 9.
13. Hathcock, John N. Quantitative Evaluation of Vitamin Safety, from *The Nutritional Debate: Sorting out Some Answers* by Gussow, Joan Dye, Thomas, Paul R. Palo Alto, CA: Bull Publishing Company 1986, p. 303.

Chapter 23: The Essential Amino Acids
1. Vitamin Research Products, July 1989, p. 1.
2. Leibovitz, Brian, "Amino Acids and Performance," *Muscular Development,* August 1989, p. 19.

Chapter 25: Amino Acids and the Immune System
1. Walker, Morton, M.D., *The Chelation Way,* Garden City, N. Y.: Avery Publishing Group Inc., 1990, p. 183.
2. Erdmann, Robert, *The Amino Acid Revolution,* New York: Simon & Schuster, Inc., 1987, p. 160.
3. Ibid., p. 162.

Chapter 26: Amino Acids for the Heart and Digestive System
1. Stryer, Lubert. *Biochemistry,* San Francisco: W. H. Freeman and Company, 1975, pp. 410, 411.

Chapter 27: Amino Acids and Your Sex Life

1. Erdmann, Robert, *The Amino Acid Revolution,* New York: Simon & Schuster, Inc., 1987, pp. 164, 165.
2. Ibid., pp. 167, 168.
3. Quillin, Patrick, Ph.D., *Healing Nutrients,* Chicago, New York Contemporary Books Inc., 1987, p. 274.
4. Erdmann, Robert, p. 169.
    Hartoma, P. A., et al., *Lancet* vol. 2., 1977, p. 1125.
    Medical News, vol. 249, no. 20, May 27, 1983, p. 2747.
    Kohengkull, S., et al., *Fertility and Sterility,* vol. 23, 1977, p. 1333.

Chapter 28: The Importance of Amino Acids and
Other Nutrients During Pregnancy

1. Quillin, Patrick, Ph.D., *Healing Nutrients,* Chicago, New York: Contemporary Books Inc., 1987, p. 244.
2. Malhotra A, Fairweather-Tail, S. Whantron, P. et al. Placental Zinc in normal and intra uterine growth-retarded pregnancies, *Br. J. Nutr* 1990; 63: 613-621. see also Somer, Elizabeth, *Nutrition for Women,* N.Y.: Henry Holt and Company, 1993, p.167.
3. McGarney S, Zinner, S. Willett W, et al. Material prenatal dietary potassium, calcium, magnesium and infant blood pressure. Hypertensio 1991;17:218-224.   See also Quillin, pp. 249-250.
4. Oski, FA et al. Pediatrics, vol. 7, p. 877, Jan. 1983.
    Meadows, N.J., et al., *Lancet,* Nov. 21, 1981, p. 1135.
    Mutch, P. B., et al., *Journal of Nutrition,* vol. 104, 1974, p. 828.
    Collipp, P. J., et al., *Annals of Nutrition and Metabolism,* vol. 26, 1982, p. 287.
    Hambridge, K.M., et al., *American Journal of Clinical Nutrition,* vol. 29, 1976, p. 734.
    Butrimovitz, G.P., et al., *American Journal of Clinical Nutrition,* vol. 31., 1978, p. 1409.
    Gipoulox, J.D., et al., *Roux's Archives of Developmental Biology,* vol. 195, 1986, p. 193.
    Breskin, M., et al., *American Journal of Clinical Nutrition,* vol. 38, Dec. 1983, p. 943.
    Sandstead, H.H., *Nutrition Reviews,* vol. 43, May 1985, p. 129.

Chapter 29: Nutrition and Breast Feeding

1. Dana, N., Price, A., *Successful Breast Feeding,* Deepheaven, Minn.: Meadowbrook, 1985, p.
2. Quillin, Patrick, Ph.D., *Healing Nutrients,* Chicago, New York: Contemporary Books Inc., 1987, p. 266.

Chapter 33: Enzymes

1. Santillo, H. *Food Enzymes,* Prescott, Ariz.: Hohm Press, 1993, p.14.
2. Howell, Edward. *Enzyme Nutrition,* Wayne, NJer: Avery Publishing Group, Inc, 1985, p. 27.

3. Ibid.
4. Ibid., pp. 81- 83.
5. Ibid., p. 6.

Chapter 34: The Importance of Good, Clean Water to Your Health and Happiness

1. Quillin, Patrick, Ph.D., *Healing Nutrients,* Chicago, New York: Contemporary Books Inc., 1987, 325.
2. Banik, Allen E., Dr., *The Choice Is Clear, P. O.* Box 9547, Kansas City, Mo.: Acres, U.S.A, 1975, pp. 1-23. Phone: (816) 737-0064.
3. Quillin, Patrick, p. 327.
4. Ibid., p. 327.
5. Ibid., p. 326.
6. Pearson, Durk, and Shaw, Sandy, *Life Extension,* New York: Warner Books, 1981, pp. 259, 260.
7. Banik, Allen E., *The Choice Is Clear,* P.O. Box 9547, Kansas City, Mo.: Acres, U.S.A, 1975, pp. 9-14.
8. Ibid., p. 12.
9. Ibid.
10. Wade, Carlson, *Amino Acids Book,* New Canaan, Conn.: Keats Publishing, Inc., 1985, p. 72.Chapter 35: Understanding Exercise
1. Pelton, Ross, *Mind Foods and Smart Pills,* New York: Doubleday, 1989, pp. 250-251.
2. Erdman, Robert, Ph.D., *The Amino Acid Revolution,* New York: Simon & Schuster, Inc., 1987, p. 79.

Chapter 35: Understanding Exercise

1. Pelton, Ross, *Mind Foods and Smart Pills,* New York: Doubleday, 1989, pp. 250-251.
2. Erdman, Robert, Ph.D., *The Amino Acid Revolution,* New York: Simon & Schuster, Inc., 1987, p. 79. ingestion of various vitamin E prepartions. *Am L Clin Nutr* 1984;40:240-245.
   Krinsky, Norman. Effects of carotenoids in cellular and animal systems, *Am L Clin Nutr* 1991;53:238S-46S.
   Luc, Gerald and Fruchart, Jean-charles. Oxidation fo lipoproteins and atheriosclerosis, *Am L Clin Nutr* 1991;53:206S-9S.
   Malone, Winfred, Studies evaluating antioxidants and beta carotene as chemopreventives *Am L Clin Nutr* 1991;53:305S-13S.
   Niki, Estuo et al. Membrane damage due to lipid oxidation, *Am L Clin Nutr* 1991;53:201S-5S.
   Pryor, William. The antioxidant nutrients and disease prevention what do we know and what do we need to find out, *Am L Clin Nutr* 1991;53:391S-3S.
   Schmidt, Karlheinz. Antioxidant vitamins and beta carotene: effects on immunocompetence, *Am L Clin Nutr* 1991;53:383S-5S.
   Singh, Visha and Gaby, Suzanne. Premalignant lesions: role of antioxidant vitamins and beta carotene in risk reduction and prevention of

malignant transformation, *Am L Clin Nutr* 1991;53:386S-90S.

Stahelin, Hannes et al. Beta carotene and cancer prevention: The Basel Study, *Am L Clin Nutr* 1991;53:265S-9S.

Stich, Hans F. et al. Remission of precancerous lesions in the oral cavity of tobacco chewers and maintenance of the protective effects of beta carotene or vitamin A *Am L Clin Nutr* 1991;53:298S-304S.

Weisburger, John H. Nutritional approach to cancer prevention with emphasis on vitamins, antioxidants, and carotenoids, *Am L Clin Nutr* 1991;53:226S-37S.

Trout, David L. Vitamin C and cardivascular risk factors. *Am L Clin Nutr* 1991;53:322S-5S.

Appendix A: Prostaglandins

1. Erasmus, Udo, *Fats And Oils,* Vancouver, Calif.: Alive Books, 1986, p. 258.
2. Graham, Judy, *Evening Primrose Oil,* Rochester, Vt.: Healing Arts Press, 1984, p. 33.
3. Erasmus, Udo, p. 258.
4. Ibid.

Appendix C: State-of-the-Art Ingredients and Unique Technologies

1. Ashmead, Dr. H. Dewayne, *Conversation on Chelation and Mineral Nutrition,* New Canaan, Conn.: Keats Publishing, 1989, p. 11.
2. Widdowson and Dickerson, in C. Comar and F. Bronner, eds., *Mineral Metabolism,* vol. 2 (New York: Academic Press, 1964), p. 57 (cited in Ashmead, p. 13).
3. Schroeder, Henry, M.D., *The Trace Elements and Man.* Devon-Adair Co., 1973.
4. Ashmead, H. Dewayne, p. 28.
5. Fisher, Jeffrey A., M.D., *The Chromium Program,* New York: Harper and Row, 1990, p. 23.
6. Passwater, Richard, Ph.D., *Chromium Picolinate,* New Canaan, Conn.: Keats Publishing, 1992, p. 16.
7. Ibid., p. 15.
8. Fisher, Jeffrey, p. 34.
9. Ibid, p. 22.
10. Passwater, Richard, Ph.D., *The New Superantioxidant-Plus: The Amazing Story of Pycnogenol, Free-Radical Antagonist and Vitamin C Potentiator,* New Canaan, Conn.: Keats Publishing, 1992, pp. 8, 9.
11. Ibid.
12. Goodman, Sandra, Ph.D., *Vitamin C, The Master Nutrient,* New Canaan, Conn: Keats Publishing, 1991, p. vii.
13. Quillin, Patrick, Ph.D., *Healing Nutrient,* Chicago, New York: Contemporary Books Inc., 1987, p. 105.
14. Bland, Jeffrey, Ph. D., *The Key to the Power of Vitamin C and Its Metabolites,* New Canann, Conn.: Keats Publishing, 1989, p. 25.

Bibliography

Airola, Paavo, Ph.D., *Hypoglycemia: A Better Approach,* Sherwood, Oregon: Health Plus, 1977.

Ashmead, Dewayne, Ph.D., *Conversation on Chelation and Mineral Nutrition,* New Canaan, Ct: Keats Publishing, Inc., 1989.

Bailey, Covert, *Fit or Fat,* Boston: Houghton Mifflin Company, 1991.

Balch, James F., M.D., and Balch, Phyllis A., *The Prescription for Nutritional Healing,* Garden City Park, N. Y.: Avery Publishing Group Inc., 1990.

Banik, Allen E., M.D., *The Choice Is Clear,* P.O. Box 9547, Kansas City, Mo.: Acres, U.S.A., 1975. (Talks about water.)

Berger, M. Stuart, M.D., *Dr. Berger's Immune Power Diet,* New York: Signet, 1986.

Berger, M. Stuart, M.D., *How to Be Your Own Nutritionist,* New York: Avon Books, 1987.

Berger, M. Stuart, M.D., *Forever Young,* New York: Avon Books, 1989.

Bland, Jeffrey, Ph.D., *The Key to the Power of Vitamin C and Its Metabolites,* New Canaan, Conn: Keats Publishing, Inc., 1989. (a 30-page booklet)

Bliznakov, Emile G., and Hunt, Gerald L., *The Miracle Nutrient: Coenzyme Q10,* New York: Bantam Books, 1989.

Bosco, Dominick, *The People's Guide to Vitamins and Minerals,* Chicago: Contemporary Books, 1980.

Bruce Miller Enterprices, Inc. Medicinal Herbs - A Quick Reference Guide. Dallas Texas: Bruce Miller Enterprices, Inc. 1995

Carper, Jean. The Food Pharmacy. New York: Bantam Books, 1989.Bosco, Dominick. The People's Guide to Vitamins and Minerals. Chicago: Contemporary Books, 1980.

Chase, Deborah, *The New Medically Based No-Nonsense Beauty Book,* New York: Henry Holt and Company, 1989.

Colgan, Michael, Ph.D. The New Nutrition. Sandiago, California: C.I. Publication, 1994.

Cooper, J.T., M.D., *Dr. Coopers Fabulous Fructose Diet,* New York: Fawcett Crest, 1979.

Colgan, Michael, Ph.D. Optimum Sports Nutrition. New York: Advanced Research Press, 1993.

Dana, N., and Price, A., *Successful Breast Feeding*, Deepheaven, Minn: Meadowbrook, 1985.

deVries, Herbert A. and Housh Terry J. Physiology of Exercise. Madison, Wisconson: Brown & Benchmark, 19940

Epstein, Emanuel, *Mineral Nutrition of Plants: Principles and Perspectives*, New York: John Wiley and Sons, Inc., 1972.

Erasmus, Udo, *Fats and Oils*, Vancouver, Canada: Alive Books, 1986.

Erdmann, Robert, Ph.D., *The Amino Acid Revolution*, New York: Simon & Schuster, 1989.

Evelyn, Nancy. The Herbal Medicine Chest. Freedom, California: The Crossing Press, 1986.

Fisher, Jeffrey, M.D., *The Chromium Program*, New York: Harper & Row, 1990.

Fisher, Patty, and Bender, Arnold, *The Value of Food*, Oxford University Press, 1979.

Fleck, Henrietta, Ph.D., *Introduction to Nutrition*, Macmillan Publishing Co., Inc., 1981.

Garrison, Robert, and Somer, Elizabeth, *The Nutrition Desk Reference*, New Canaan, Conn.: Keats Publishing, 1990.

Gerber, Jerry, Wolfe, Janet, Klores, Walter, and Brown, Gene, *Life Trends*, New York: Avon Books, 1991.

Gittleman, Ann Louise, *Beyond Pritikin*, New York: Bantam, 1988.

Goodman, Sandra, Ph.D., *Vitamin C—The Master Nutrient*, New Canaan, Conn.: Keats Publishing, 1991.

Goodwin, T.W., Mercer, E.I., *Introduction to Plant Biochemistry*, New York: Pergamon Press, 1972.

Graham, Judy, *Evening Primrose Oil*, Rochester, Vt.: Healing Arts Press, 1984.

Guthrie, Helen, Ph.D., *Introductory Nutrition*, St. Louis: The C.V. Mosby Company, 1979.

Haas, Elson, M., *Staying Healthy with Nutrition*, Berkeley, Calif. Celestial Arts, 1992.

Haas, Robert, Ph.D., *Eat to Win*, New York: Signet, 1985.

Halstead, Bruce W., M.D., *The Scientific Basis of EDTA Chelation Therapy*, Colton, Calif.: Golden Quill Publishers, Inc., 1979.

Halliwell and Gutteridge, John M.C. Free Radicals in Biology and Medicine. Oxford, England: Clarndon Press.

Hayflick, Leonard, Ph.D. How and Why We Age. New York: Balantine Books, 1994.

Hendler, Sheldon, S. M.D., Ph. D. The Doctors' Vitamin and Mieral Encylopedia. New York: Simon and Shuster, 1991.Hendrickson, James B., Ph.D., *The Molecules of Nature,* New York: W. A. Benjamin, Inc., 1965.

Horton, E.S., M.D. and Terjung, R.L., Ph.D., Exercise, Nutrition & Energy Metabolism. New York: Macmillan Publishing Company, 1988.

Howell, Edward, Ph.D. Enzyme Nutrition; Wayne Newjersey: Avery Publishing Group, Inc., 1985.Kronhausen, Eberhard, Ed.D., and Phyllis, Ed.D., *Formula for Life,* New York: William Morrow and Company, Inc., 1989.

Kamen, Betty, Ph.D. The Chromium Diet, Supplement & Exercise Strategy. Notato, California: Nutrition Encounter, Inc. 1992.

Kushi, M., and Cotrell, M.C., M.D., *AIDS Macrobiotics and Natural Immunity,* Tokyo, New York: Japan Publication, Inc., 1990.

Lamb, D.R., Knuttgen, H.G. and Murray, R. Physiology and Nutrition For Competitve Sport. Carmel, Indiana: Cooper Publishing Group, 1994.

Lehninger, Albert, L., Ph.D., *Biochemistry,* New York: Worth Publishers, Inc., 1970.

Litt, Jerome Z., M.D. *Your Skin,* New York: Dembner Books, 1989.

Lust, John, N.D., D.B.M., The Herb Book. New York: Bantam Books, 19974

Marshall Editions Limited, *The Human Body,* New York: Arch Cape Press, 1989

McArdle, William D. Katch, Frank I. and Katch Victor, L. Exercise Physiology. Philadelphia, Pennsylvania: Lea & Febiger, 1991.

Mindell, Earl, *The Vitamin Bible,* New York: Warner Books, 1985.

Moffett, D.F., Moffett, S.B. and Schauf, C.L. Human Physiology Foundations and Frontiers. St. Lous, Missouri : Mosby, 1990.

Morrill, Judi, S., *Science, Physiology, and Nutrition,* San Jose, Calif.: San Jose State University, 1991.

Mowrey, Daniel, B. Ph.D. The Scientific Validation of Herbal Medicine. New Canaan, Connecticut: Keats Publishing, 1986.

Murray, Michael, Ph. D. The Healing Power of Herbs.Rocklin, California: Prima Publication, 1992.Noller, Carl R., Ph.D., *Chemistry of Organic Compounds,* Philadelphia: W.B. Saunders Company, 1966.

Null, Gary and Howard Robins, DR. Ultimate Training. New York: St. Martin's Press, 1993.

Parsed, Keran N., Ph. D. Vitamins in Cancer Prevention & Treatment. Rochter, Vermont: Healing Arts Press.

Passwater, Richard, Ph.D., *Chromium Picolinate,* New Canaan, Conn.: Keats Publishing, Inc., 1992. (a 48-page booklet)

Passwater, Richard, Ph.D., *The New Superantioxidant—Plus,* New Canaan, Conn.: Keats Publishing, Inc., 1992. (a 48-page booklet, Pycnogenol)

Passwater, Richard, Ph.D., *Selenium as Food and Medicine,* New Canaan, Conn.: Keats Publishing, 1980.

Pauling, Linus, *How to Live Longer and Feel Better,* San Francisco: W.H. Freeman, 1986.

Pearson, Durk, and Shaw, Sandy, *Life Extension,* New York: Warner Books, 1980.

Pelton, Ross, Ph.D., *Mind Food and Smart Pills,* New York: Doubleday, 1989.

Reader's Digest Family Guide to Natural Medicine. Pleasanton, New York: The Reader's Digest Association, Inc.

Richason, Jack, N.D. The Little Herb Encyclopedia. Peasant Grove, Utah: WoodLand Health Books, 1994.

Rosenbaum, Michael E., M.D. and Bosco, Dominick, *Super Supplements,* New York: Signet, 1987.

Quillin, Patrick, Ph.D., *Healing Nutrients,* Chicago: Contemporary Books, 1987.

Santillo, Hurbert. Food Enzymes - the Missing Link to Radiant Health. Prescott, Arizona: Hohm Press, 1987.

Schechter, Steven R., *Fighting Radiation and Chemical Pollutants with Foods,* Herbs, & Vitamins, Encinitas, Calif.: Vitality, Inc., 1990.

Simons, Barry, M.D., Meschino, James, D.C., *The Winning Weight,* Downsview, Ontario: Elite Publications Inc., 1993.

Stryer, Lubert, Ph.D., *Biochemistry,* San Francisco: W.H. Freeman and Company, 1975.

Tierra, Michael, C.A. N.D., The Way of Herbs. New York: Pocket books, 1990.

Vogel, H.C. A. The Nature Doctor. New Canaan, Connecticut: Keats Publishing, 1991.

Wade, Carlson, *Amino Acids Book,* New Canaan, Conn.: Keats Publishing, Inc., 1985.

Walford, Roy L., M.D., *The 120 Year Diet,* New York: Pocket Books, 1988.

Walker, Morton, *The Chelation Way,* Garden City, N. Y.: Avery Publishing Group Inc., 1990.

Weiner, Michael, Ph.D. Weiner's Herbal. Mill Vally, California: Quantum Books, 1990.

Whitney, Eleanor Noss and Rolfe, Sharon Randy, Understanding Nutrition, Minneapolis/St. Paul, In: West Publishing Company, 1993

Wolinsky, Iraa and Hickson, J.F., Jr., Nutrition in Exercise and Sport. Boca Raton, Florida: CRC Press, 1993.

Index